T0207133

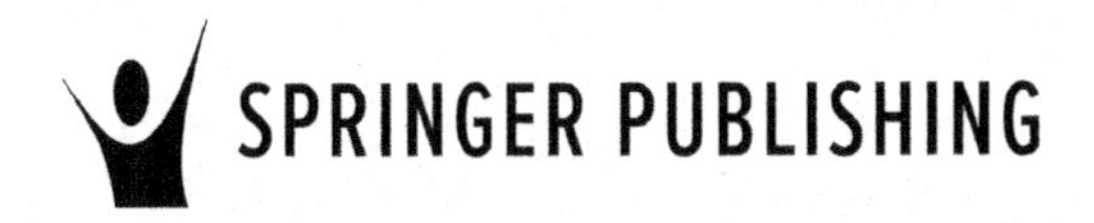

GET THE MOST FROM YOUR BOOK

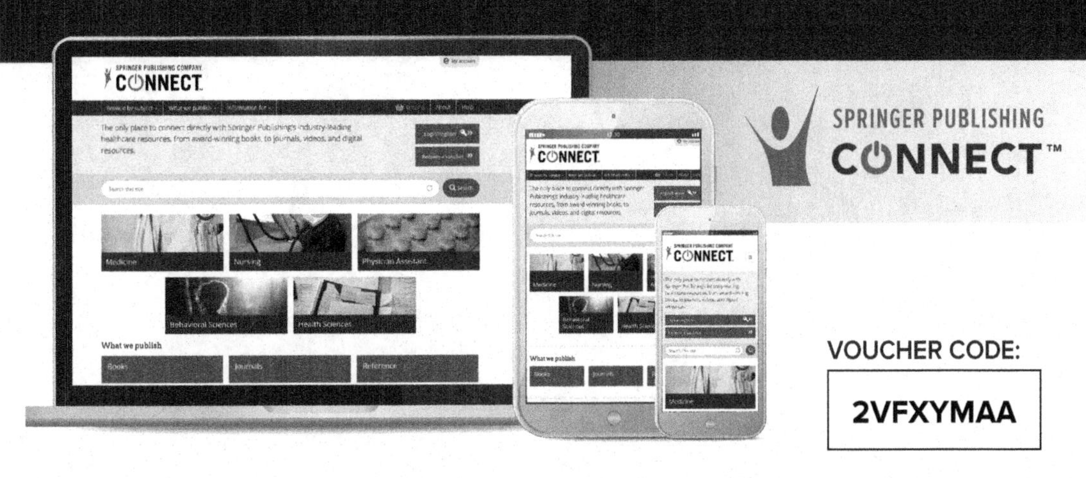

VOUCHER CODE:

2VFXYMAA

Online Access

Your print purchase of *Practical Implementation Science* includes **online access via Springer Publishing Connect**™ to increase accessibility, portability, and searchability.

Insert the code at http://connect.springerpub.com/content/book/978-0-8261-8693-5 today!

Having trouble? Contact our customer service department at cs@springerpub.com

Instructor Resource Access for Adopters

Let us do some of the heavy lifting to create an engaging classroom experience with a variety of instructor resources included in most textbooks SUCH AS:

INSTRUCTOR'S MANUAL

POWERPOINTS

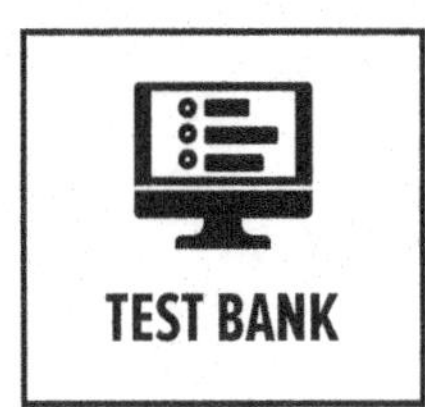

TEST BANK

Visit **https://connect.springerpub.com/** and look for the **"Show Supplementary"** button on your **book homepage** to see what is available to instructors! First time using Springer Publishing Connect?

Email **textbook@springerpub.com** to create an account and start unlocking valuable resources.

PRACTICAL IMPLEMENTATION SCIENCE

Bryan J. Weiner, PhD, is a professor in the Department of Global Health and the Department of Health Systems and Population Health at the University of Washington. He serves as the Strategic Hire in Implementation Science for the School of Public Health at the University of Washington and Director of the Implementation Science Program for the Department of Global Health. His research focuses on the implementation of innovations and evidence-based practices in healthcare. Over the past 25 years, he has examined a wide range of innovations including quality improvement practices, care management practices, and patient safety practices, as well evidence-based clinical practices in cancer, cardiovascular disease, infectious disease, mental health, maternal and child health, and traumatic brain injury. His research has advanced implementation science by creating knowledge about the organizational determinants of effective implementation, developing new theories of implementation, and improving the state of measurement in the field.

Cara C. Lewis, PhD, is a clinical psychologist, senior investigator at Kaiser Permanente Washington Health Research Institute, and affiliate faculty in the Department of Psychiatry and Behavioral Sciences, as well as the Department of Health Systems and Population Health at the University of Washington. She is a Beck Scholar with expertise in cognitive behavioral therapy. She is past president of the Society for Implementation Research Collaboration (SIRC) and co-founding editor-in-chief of *Implementation Research and Practice*, a journal published in partnership with SIRC. Her research focuses on advancing pragmatic and rigorous measures and methods for implementation science and practice and informing tailored implementation of evidence-based practices across diverse settings, populations, and problem areas. She is also co-director of the Social Needs Network for Evaluation and Translation (SONNET), which is a national coordinating center for bringing research, evaluation, and implementation support to bear across Kaiser Permanente in the service of addressing social risk among its members.

Kenneth Sherr, PhD, is a professor in the Department of Global Health at the University of Washington. Dr. Sherr's research focuses on developing and testing implementation strategies to support data-driven decision-making and service integration into the primary healthcare framework as a means of increasing the coverage and quality of evidence-based interventions. Dr. Sherr has led the development of implementation science training curricula at the University of Washington Department of Global Health, including the development of the PhD program in implementation science in 2012, and directs the Implementation Science Core of the NIH-supported UW/FH Center for AIDS Research. Dr. Sherr received his PhD in Epidemiology and MPH in International Health/Health Services from the University of Washington, and a BA in Anthropology/Sociology from Kenyon College.

PRACTICAL IMPLEMENTATION SCIENCE

MOVING EVIDENCE INTO ACTION

Bryan J. Weiner, PhD

Cara C. Lewis, PhD

Kenneth Sherr, PhD

EDITORS

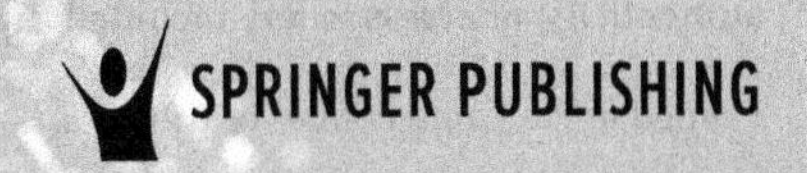

Springer Publishing Company, LLC
11 West 42nd Street, New York, NY 10036
www.springerpub.com
connect.springerpub.com/

Acquisitions Editor: David D'Addona
Compositor: S4Carlisle Publishing Services

ISBN: 978-0-8261-8692-8
ebook ISBN: 978-0-8261-8693-5
DOI: 10.1891/9780826186935

SUPPLEMENTS:
Instructor Materials:

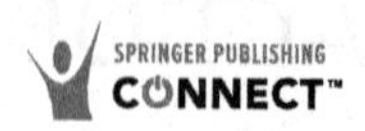

A robust set of instructor resources designed to supplement this text is located at http://connect.springerpub.com/content/book/978-0-8261-8693-5. Qualifying instructors may request access by emailing textbook@springerpub.com.

Instructor's Manual ISBN: 978-0-8261-8695-9
Instructor's PowerPoints ISBN: 978-0-8261-8694-2
Instructor's Syllabus ISBN: 978-0-8261-8696-6

Printed by BnT

Library of Congress Cataloging-in-Publication Data

Names: Weiner, Bryan J. editor. | Lewis, Cara C., editor. | Sherr, Kenneth H., editor.
Title: Practical implementation science : moving evidence into action / Bryan J. Weiner, Cara C. Lewis, Kenneth Sherr, editors.
Identifiers: LCCN 2021061995 (print) | LCCN 2021061996 (ebook) | ISBN 9780826186928 (cloth) | ISBN 9780826186935 (ebook)
Subjects: LCSH: Evidence-based medicine—Textbooks. | Medical care—Textbooks.
Classification: LCC R723.7 .P73 2023 (print) | LCC R723.7 (ebook) | DDC 610–dc23/eng/20220211
LC record available at https://lccn.loc.gov/2021061995
LC ebook record available at https://lccn.loc.gov/2021061996

Printed in the United States of America.

To Megan Lewis, for encouraging and supporting me to make this textbook a reality.

~ BJW

To Shannon Dorsey, for championing the idea that implementation science **should** *be made practical.*

~ CCL

To Steve Gloyd, for his mentorship and leadership in defining implementation science in global health.

~ KS

CONTENTS

CONTRIBUTORS

Kimberly T. Arnold, PhD Postdoctoral Fellow, Center for Mental Health, Department of Psychiatry, Perelman School of Medicine, University of Pennsylvania, Philadelphia, Pennsylvania

Bijal Balasubramanian, PhD, MBBS Professor, Department of Epidemiology; Regional Dean, School of Public Health, University of Texas Health Science Center at Houston (UTHealth), Dallas, Texas

Rinad S. Beidas, PhD Associate Professor, Departments of Psychiatry, Medical Ethics and Health Policy, and Medicine; Director, Penn Implementation Science Center; Associate Director, Leonard Davis Institute of Health Economics (PISCE@LDI), Center for Health Incentives and Behavioral Economics (CHIBE), Perelman School of Medicine, University of Pennsylvania, Philadelphia, Pennsylvania

Ross C. Brownson, PhD Steven H. and Susan U. Lipstein Distinguished Professor, Prevention Research Center, Brown School and School of Medicine, Washington University in St. Louis, St. Louis, Missouri

Heather L. Bullock, PhD Waypoint Centre for Mental Health Care, Penetanguishene, Ontario, Canada; Department of Health Research Methods, Evidence, and Impact, McMaster University, Hamilton, Ontario, Canada

Margaret E. Crane, MA PhD Student, Department of Psychology, Temple University, Philadelphia, Pennsylvania

Laura Damschroder, MS, MPH Veterans Affairs (VA) Ann Arbor Center for Clinical Management Research, VA Ann Arbor Healthcare System, Ann Arbor, Michigan

Cam Escoffery, PhD Professor, Rollins School of Public Health, Emory University, Atlanta, Georgia

Christine Fahim, PhD Knowledge Translation Program, Li Ka Shing Knowledge Institute, Unity Health Toronto, Toronto, Ontario, Canada

Peter Fajans, MD, MPH Secretariat Member, ExpandNet, Gex, France

Maria E. Fernandez, PhD Professor, Department of Health Promotion and Behavioral Sciences; Director, Center for Health Promotion and Prevention Research, School of Public Health, University of Texas Health Science Center at Houston (UTHealth), Houston, Texas

Kevin Fiori, MD, MPH, MSc Assistant Professor, Departments of Pediatrics and Family and Social Medicine, Albert Einstein College of Medicine, Montefiore Health System, Bronx, New York

Laura Ghiron, MPH Secretariat Member, ExpandNet; President, Partners in Expanding Health Quality and Access, Davis, California

Christian D. Helfrich, PhD, MPH Research Investigator, Seattle–Denver Center of Innovation for Veteran-Centered & Value-Driven Care, VA Puget Sound Healthcare System, Seattle, Washington

Lisa R. Hirschhorn, MD, MPH Professor, Department of Medical Social Sciences; Associate Director, Center for Global Cardiovascular Health, Northwestern University Feinberg School of Medicine, Chicago, Illinois

Heidi La Bash, PhD Clinical Psychologist and Research Psychologist, National Center for PTSD, VA Palo Alto Healthcare System, Menlo Park, California

John N. Lavis, PhD, MD Department of Health Research Methods, Evidence, and Impact, McMaster Health Forum, McMaster University, Hamilton, Ontario, Canada

Jennifer Leeman, DrPH Professor, School of Nursing, University of North Carolina at Chapel Hill, Chapel Hill, North Carolina

Cara C. Lewis, PhD Senior Investigator, Kaiser Permanente Washington Health Research Institute, Seattle, Washington

Hueiming Liu, PhD, MD, MIPH Senior Research Fellow, Process Evaluation (Lead), The George Institute for Global Health, University of New South Wales, Sydney, New South Wales, Australia

Sarah J. Masyuko, PhD, MBChb, MPH Ministry of Health, Nairobi, Kenya; Postdoctoral Scholar, Department of Global Health, University of Washington, Seattle, Washington

Barbara R. Majerczyk, MPH, BA Research Health Science Specialist, Seattle–Denver Center of Innovation for Veteran-Centered & Value-Driven Care, VA Puget Sound Healthcare System, Seattle, Washington

Arianna Rubin Means, PhD, MPH Assistant Professor, Department of Global Health, University of Washington, Seattle, Washington

Nicole Nathan, PhD Clinical Research Fellow, Hunter New England Population Health; Investigator Fellow, Department of Medicine and Wellbeing, College of Health, The University of Newcastle, Newcastle, Australia

Katherine L. Nelson, MPH PhD Student, Department of Health Management and Policy, Dornsife School of Public Health, Drexel University, Philadelphia, Pennsylvania

Elspeth Nolen, MSc Program Manager, Implementation Science, Department of Global Health, University of Washington, Seattle, Washington

Melanie Pellecchia, PhD Assistant Professor, Center for Mental Health, Department of Psychiatry, Perelman School of Medicine, University of Pennsylvania, Philadelphia, Pennsylvania

Jonathan Purtle, DrPH Associate Professor, Department of Health Management and Policy, Dornsife School of Public Health, Drexel University, Philadelphia, Pennsylvania

Lisa Saldana, PhD Senior Scientist, Oregon Social Learning Center, Eugene, Oregon

Rachel C. Shelton, ScD, MPH Associate Professor, Department of Sociomedical Sciences, Mailman School of Public Health, Columbia University, New York, New York

Kenneth Sherr, PhD Professor, Department of Global Health, University of Washington, Seattle, Washington

Ruth Simmons, PhD Professor Emerita, Department of Health Behavior and Health Education, University of Michigan School of Public Health, Ann Arbor, Michigan; Secretariat Member, ExpandNet, Inverness, California

Ryan R. Singh, PhD, MPH Early Career Scientist, Oregon Social Learning Center, Eugene, Oregon

Shannon Wiltsey Stirman, PhD Implementation Scientist, National Center for PTSD, VA Palo Alto Healthcare System, Menlo Park, California; Associate Professor, Department of Psychiatry and Behavioral Sciences, Stanford University School of Medicine, Stanford, California

Sharon E. Straus, MD, MSc, FRCPC Knowledge Translation Program, Li Ka Shing Knowledge Institute, Unity Health Toronto, Toronto, Ontario, Canada

Fiona C. Thomas, PhD Postdoctoral Research Fellow, Department of Psychology, Ryerson University, Toronto, Ontario, Canada

Liza Tomczuk Clinical Research Coordinator, Center for Mental Health, Department of Psychiatry, Perelman School of Medicine, University of Pennsylvania, Philadelphia, Pennsylvania

Bradley H. Wagenaar, PhD, MPH Assistant Professor, Department of Global Health; Adjunct Assistant Professor, Department of Epidemiology, University of Washington, Seattle, Washington

Anjuli D. Wagner, PhD, MPH Assistant Professor, Department of Global Health, University of Washington, Seattle, Washington

Mary Wangen, MPH Research Associate, Center for Health Promotion and Disease Prevention, University of North Carolina at Chapel Hill, Chapel Hill, North Carolina

Bryan J. Weiner, PhD Professor, Department of Global Health, Department of Health Systems and Population Health, University of Washington, Seattle, Washington

Michael G. Wilson, PhD Department of Health Research Methods, Evidence, and Impact, McMaster Health Forum, Hamilton, Ontario, Canada

PREFACE

This book addresses a growing concern. Implementation science seeks to close the research-to-practice gap by identifying the barriers that impede the adoption, implementation, sustainability, and scale-up of evidence-based health interventions, and by identifying the best methods for overcoming those barriers. As implementation scientists, our aspiration for the field is to generate useful and usable scientific knowledge to improve the *practice* of implementation. Put differently, we envision the field of implementation science producing the knowledge and tools to support the evidence-based implementation of evidence-based health interventions. The rapid growth of implementation science as a research enterprise, however, has given rise to concerns that we and other implementation scientists share: that implementation science itself will replicate the research-to-practice gap that the field was intended to address. This book represents the first systematic attempt by leading implementation researchers to "translate" implementation science for implementation practitioners by making accessible and *practical* the wealth of scientific knowledge and associated tools that implementation science has produced.

This book also addresses an unmet need. Although a growing number of colleges and universities offer courses in implementation science, there are no textbooks in implementation science geared specifically for graduate health professional students or advanced undergraduate students. Instead, instructors teaching such courses must rely on peer-reviewed articles published by implementation researchers for implementation researchers. These articles focus on developing and reporting scientific knowledge about implementation; they do not focus on how such knowledge could be used to support implementation *in practice*. Although suitable for educating doctoral students who want to become researchers, they are not well suited for educating graduate health professional students or advanced undergraduate students who want to learn *how to* implement evidence-based practices effectively using the knowledge and tools of implementation science. Several colleagues have written excellent books for researchers interested in learning about the field's historical development, research methods, conceptual frameworks, study designs, measurement challenges, scientific status, and future directions. However, these books are not intended for use as textbooks for classroom teaching of practice-oriented audiences like graduate health professional students or advanced undergraduates in public health.

Practical Implementation Science: Moving Evidence Into Action is organized into 14 chapters, suitable for a semester-long course but also useful for a quarter-long course. The core of the book consists of eight chapters organized by common tasks or steps involved in planning, executing, and evaluating implementation efforts. These tasks or steps include assessing the knowledge-practice gap (also known as the know-do gap); selecting an evidence-based practice (EBP) to reduce the gap; assessing EBP fit and adapting the

EBP; assessing barriers and facilitators of implementation; engaging stakeholders; creating an implementation structure; implementing the EBP; and evaluating the implementation effort. The focus of each chapter is on "how to" conduct the task or step using implementation science theory, frameworks, models, research findings, and tools. The textbook also includes four chapters on topics of practical importance: disseminating EBPs, scaling up EBPs, sustaining EBPs, and de-implementing practices that are no longer effective or never were. Again, the emphasis in these chapters is practical: The aim is to present and "translate" implementation science into practical guidance and tools that graduate health professional students and advanced undergraduate students could use to effectively implement EBPs in practice. For instructors who adopt this text, we have also designed several ancillary materials, including an instructor's guide and accompanying lecture slides.

Producing a textbook amid a global pandemic is no small feat. We are deeply indebted to the leading scholars in implementation science who contributed chapters to this book despite the sickness and death, social and economic disruption, parenting and caregiving challenges, and personal and collective trauma wrought by the COVID-19 pandemic. The chapter authors wholeheartedly embraced our call to make useful and usable the scientific knowledge and associated tools of implementation science, to write for a practice audience rather than the more familiar research audience, and to attend to health equity concerns and global health applications of implementation science. The chapter authors themselves would like to thank the following:

- Chapter 3 – Our colleagues in the Cancer Prevention and Control Research Network, who contributed their expertise in implementation practice, as well as the U.S. Centers for Disease Control and Prevention for its support of the network.
- Chapter 4 – Kera Swanson for her help putting together the slides that accompany this chapter, the textbook editors for their helpful feedback that strengthened our chapter, and all of the research participants, who allow us to advance our understanding of implementation science to best serve the greater good in promoting EBPs.
- Chapter 5 – Dr. Lara S. Savas, Ms. Preena Loomba, and Ms. Crystal Costa for their assistance, especially with the SEMM DIA case example. Aaron Rome for editing and for his persistent nudge for clarity.
- Chapter 6 – Our community stakeholders who partner with us on implementation efforts to improve the quality of care for individuals with health and mental health needs across Philadelphia, including the Philadelphia Infant and Toddler Early Intervention System, the Department of Behavioral Health and Intellectual disAbility Services, Community Behavioral Health, and the School District of Philadelphia, as well as the many agencies, providers, and families who provide and receive care through these systems.
- Chapter 8 – Caroline Dennis for editing, formatting, and providing feedback throughout the preparation of this chapter, as well as the many contributors of data to the SIC website that allowed us to learn more about the implementation process.
- Chapter 11 – The Bill and Melinda Gates Foundation and the MacArthur Foundation for the financial support for the development of this chapter, as well as the many ExpandNet members and colleagues whose scaling-up learning and experience are reflected in this chapter.

- Chapter 12 – Savannah Alexander for her assistance with formatting, figures, and references, as well as Dr. Mary Ann Scheirer for the inspiration she has provided us in her foundational work on sustainability.
- Chapter 13 – Drs. David Au and Christine Hartmann, and the VA Quality and Safety QUERI team for providing the intellectual dialogue and scholarship that underpins this chapter, Dr. Diana Naranjo for work on the case studies, and the editors, for their support, and more than a little forbearance.

Finally, we editors wish to express our profound gratitude to Elspeth Nolen for her editorial assistance and keen appreciation of the needs and preferences of the Millennial and Gen Z students for whom this textbook is intended.

Bryan J. Weiner
Cara C. Lewis
Kenneth Sherr

[illegible]

[illegible]

INSTRUCTOR RESOURCES

Practical Implementation Science includes quality resources for the instructor. Faculty who have adopted the text may gain access to these resources by emailing textbook@springerpub.com.

Instructor resources include:

- Sample Course Syllabus
- Instructor's Manual
- PowerPoint Presentations for Lecture

1

Introducing Implementation Science

Bryan J. Weiner, Cara C. Lewis, and Kenneth Sherr

Learning Objectives

By the end of this chapter, readers will be able to:

- Define implementation and implementation science
- Distinguish implementation science from related fields
- Discuss the similarities and differences in implementation science in the United States and in global health
- Argue the case that implementation matters
- Recognize core concepts and key features of implementation science

CASE STUDY 1.1 IMPLEMENTING UNIVERSAL SOCIAL RISK SCREENING

Savannah M., MPH, Associate Director of the Patient-Centered Care Program of Big Lake Health System, has been tasked to support the implementation of universal social risk screening of patients receiving care in the health system's primary care clinics. Social risk screening identifies social and material risks that affect health and well-being, the results of which can be used to personalize care plans, called "social risk-informed care." It is also a critical first step in linking patients experiencing social risks to interventions or community-based resources to address them. These two approaches to using social risk data are emerging evidence-based social health interventions. Although Big Lake Health System's leadership is committed to universal social risk screening, Savannah anticipates many implementation challenges lie ahead; so many, in fact, she is not sure where to begin. At a recent Learning Health System conference, she heard panelists talk about "implementation science," which the panelists described as a newer scientific field that offers frameworks, processes, tools, and guidance to support implementation. Savannah wonders: What exactly is implementation science? Can it help her address the practical issues of implementing universal social risk screening? How does it complement quality improvement approaches like the one her health system typically uses?

INTRODUCTION

Savannah M. faces a problem all too common in public health. There are now hundreds, if not thousands, of interventions proven effective for preventing, detecting, and treating disease, injury, illness, substance use, and other conditions affecting health and mental health. Indeed, many argue that we could address the world's most pressing health challenges if we simply implemented widely and effectively the evidence-based interventions (EBIs) we already have in hand. EBI is a shorthand phase referring to "programs, practices, principles, procedures, products, pills, and policies that have been found to be effective at improving health behaviors, health outcomes, or health-related environments in one or more well-designed research studies" (Leeman et al., 2017, p. 3). For example, some estimate that cervical cancer deaths could be reduced by 90%, colorectal cancer deaths by 70%, and lung cancer deaths by 95% if existing EBIs were widely and effectively implemented (Blue Ribbon Panel et al., 2016). Others estimate that maternal and infant mortality could be reduced by 40% or more if existing EBIs for preventing and managing life-threatening complications were widely and effectively implemented (Gülmezoglu et al., 2016). Still others note that death, disability, and suffering from opioid use disorder could drop dramatically if existing EBIs were implemented to restrict supply, alter prescribing practices, reduce demand, and reduce harm (Health and Medicine Division et al., 2017). The potential gains in public health that could be achieved by implementing existing EBIs are so great that some health policy experts have argued we would see a higher return on investment if we spent less on developing medical advances and more on improving systems for delivering care (Woolf & Johnson, 2005).

This still leaves Savannah with the problem: How to effectively implement an EBI? We now have a rapidly growing body of scientific knowledge and associated tools to support effective EBI implementation. For a long time, though, implementation was not considered a subject worthy of scientific inquiry. The prevailing model of biomedical research, which governed the investment of hundreds of billions of dollars over several decades, simply assumed that developing evidence that a clinical intervention was efficacious was sufficient to generate public health impact (Bauer & Kirchner, 2020), when in fact, it was not sufficient. Investment in biomedical research produced an ever-greater number of EBIs; yet the "translation" of these EBIs into practice remained slow, uneven, and haphazard (Balas & Boren, 2000; Chalmers & Glasziou, 2009; Wolfenden et al., 2015). The hoped-for improvements in public health were modest and slow to materialize (Bauer et al., 2015; Colditz & Emmons, 2017). Worse still, **know-do gaps**—that is, gaps between what we know works and what we do in practice—persisted (Walker et al., 2017; Yang et al., 2020) and in some cases widened (Petersen et al., 2019; Singh et al., 2015), contributing to racial/ethnic, socio-economic, and other disparities in health outcomes. To close these know-do gaps and realize the public health impact of EBIs, a new science was created. This new science, implementation science, seeks to accelerate the translation of research into practice by identifying the barriers that slow or impede the adoption, implementation, sustainability, and scale-up of EBIs, and by developing, testing, and deploying strategies to integrate and sustain EBIs. This book represents the first systematic attempt to make accessible and practical the wealth of scientific knowledge and associated tools that this field of implementation science has produced.

DEFINING IMPLEMENTATION AND IMPLEMENTATION SCIENCE

Before we delve into implementation science, let us consider its subject for a moment. What is "implementation"? When users of the English language say they are implementing something, they typically mean they are putting that something into practice or into use. This is consistent with the formal definition found in most dictionaries. There are three aspects of the everyday use of the term "implementation" that are noteworthy. First, implementation is purposeful. There is an aim involved; namely, to put something into practice or into use. Second, implementation involves action. It might be a simple, straightforward act that one person could do, or it might be a complicated series of acts that only many people working in concert could do. Third, implementation is temporally bounded. The action involved in implementation is bounded on the side by the intention or decision to put something into practice or into use and on the other side by the successful putting of that something into practice or into use. As the term is ordinarily used in the English language, implementation focuses on initial use or early use. Once something is "in practice" or "in use," English language users will often employ the past tense of the verb to convey that the something in question has been implemented.

Putting this together, and recognizing that the something of interest in implementation science is typically an EBI, **implementation** refers to purposeful actions taken to put an EBI into practice or into use. Moreover, implementation can be viewed as a stage or phase of activity that is preceded by the decision to make use of an EBI (often referred to as *adoption*) and followed by continued use of an EBI (sometimes referred to as *sustainment*). Thinking about implementation as a stage is useful, as we will see in subsequent chapters, although it is not always easy to delineate when the implementation stage begins and when it ends. Decisions to make use of an EBI, for example, are sometimes but not always discrete events. Intentions to use an EBI can change over time. Implementation itself can be a continuous and seemingly never-ending process, especially for dynamic EBIs that are frequently updated or upgraded. And the point in time in which an EBI can be considered "in practice" or "in use" can be, and often is, difficult to determine precisely.

For implementation science, the fuzziness of stage boundaries poses several methodological problems that researchers are still working through. For implementation practice, however, stage models of implementation offer a useful heuristic for assessment, diagnosis, and action.

The U.S. National Academy of Science defines "science" as "the use of evidence to construct testable explanations and predictions of natural phenomena, as well as the knowledge generated through this process" (National Academy of Sciences, 2017). **Implementation science** is a multidisciplinary field designed to generate evidence to explain and predict translation of research results and EBIs into practice settings to improve public health, and to yield effective methods uncovered through this process. Scholars from all over the world and numerous disciplines (e.g., public health, anthropology, psychology, sociology, informatics, computer science, systems dynamics, policy, social work) are contributing to this field. Together they are trying to make sense of how, when, where, and why research results and EBIs are, or are not, being used. The field casts a wide net in terms of what is "in scope." Examples of issues that are in the scope of implementation science are: How can we efficiently and effectively integrate EBIs into specific settings? How can we help the public understand available research results and request or even demand EBIs over commonly available interventions? What are the most effective mechanisms for designing policies based on research results that simultaneously consider implementation processes? Important to note is that this broad field has been referred to in at least 29 ways across nine countries, including the terms that follow and knowledge translation, the latter of which is commonly used in Canada (Odeny et al., 2015).

Implementation research is a bit narrower in its definition. The U.S. National Institutes of Health (NIH) defines implementation research as "the scientific study of the use of strategies to adopt and integrate EBIs into clinical and community settings to improve individual outcomes and benefit population health," (NIH, 2021). Put simply, implementation research focuses on the question: How can we effectively and efficiently get people to use research results and EBIs in a consistent, high quality way? Complementary to implementation research is dissemination research, which NIH has defined as "the scientific study of targeted distribution of information and intervention materials to a specific public health or clinical practice audience" (NIH, 2021). Put simply, dissemination research focuses on the question: How can we use theory and evidence to best communicate and integrate knowledge and EBIs into new settings? This book covers both implementation and dissemination research, as both are critical in most practical implementation endeavors.

Low- and middle-income country (LMIC) settings are notably different from the United States in terms of disease burden, population demographics, sources and levels of resources for implementing EBIs, and the design and culture of health systems. In many LMICs, the majority of healthcare services are delivered through the public sector and are organized through more centralized and less fragmented systems that enable scale-up of EBIs to meet population-level health needs. Recognizing these differences, we offer a definition of implementation science for LMIC settings, where implementation science asks and answers the fundamental question: How do we get "what works" to people who need it with greater speed, fidelity, efficiency, sustainability, and relevant coverage? This definition focuses attention on expediting the delivery of EBIs to improve health at a population level. It also emphasizes that to achieve population-level impact, the "active ingredients" of an EBI must be maintained, costs contained, and implementation sustained. As in the United States, implementation science in the LMIC settings applies the tools and approaches of multiple disciplines to improve the delivery of EBIs. Although not comprehensive, we have identified 10 methods that are most relevant for improving the implementation and scale-up of EBIs in LMIC settings (Figure 1.1).

As an emerging field that is still under development, there are a number of areas of inquiry adjacent to implementation science. These fields—such as operations research, improvement science, knowledge translation, scale-up science, and program science (to name a handful)—share the intent of improving the implementation of EBIs. However, there is utility in differentiating implementation science from these other fields. Operations research and improvement science focus on identifying and addressing barriers to delivery of EBIs at the local level (e.g., in one clinic or ward of a hospital). While results from these efforts may be transferrable to other settings, the principal motivation is to drive change in a specific setting. Knowledge translation—a term broadly used in Canada—focuses on efforts to enhance the use and usefulness of research among decision-makers and implementers to improve the implementation of EBIs. Scale-up science focuses on processes to improve the spread and/or scale up of EBIs. Finally, program science describes an approach to bring together program leaders and implementers with researchers to improve the design, implementation, and evaluation of public health programs. We recognize that the distinctions between implementation science and these related fields are not always clear or agreed upon. However, we are optimistic that boundaries will be further clarified as the state of the fields matures.

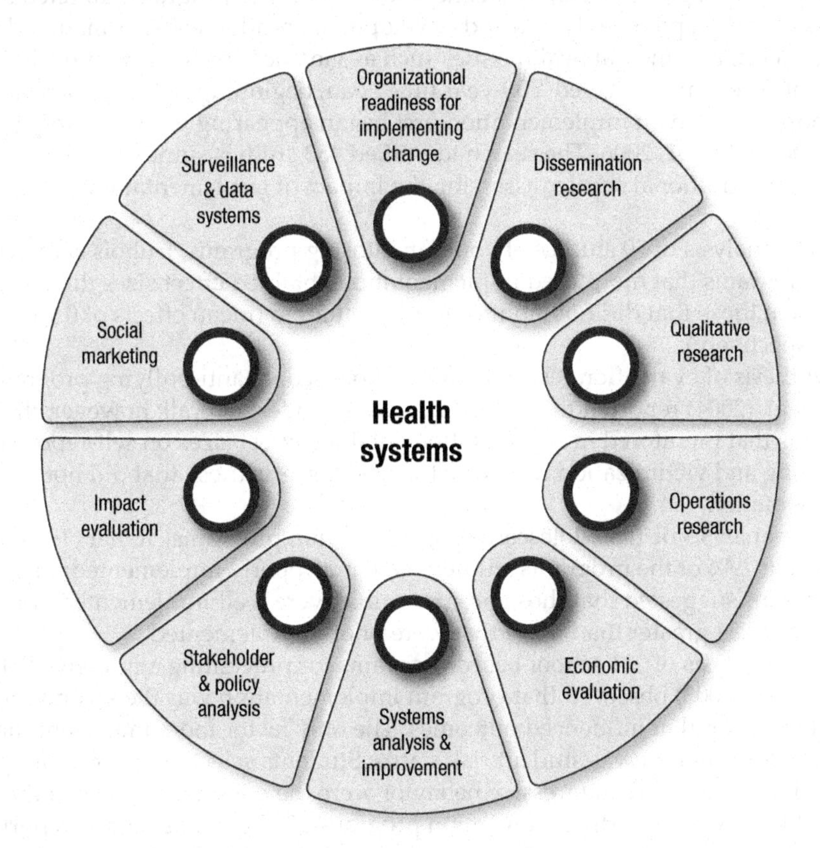

FIGURE 1.1 Ten methods for improving the implementation and scale-up of evidence-based interventions (EBIs) in low- and middle-income country (LMIC) settings.

Making the Case That Implementation Matters

It might seem obvious that implementation matters. Interventions that are poorly implemented—or not implemented at all—do not produce expected health benefits, including EBIs. At best, partial implementation yields partial benefits, assuming some minimally necessary level of implementation is achieved. Do we have evidence, though, that implementation influences outcomes? This question was raised early in the history of implementation science (described in the following) as skeptics of the newly emerging field wondered whether scientific study of implementation was necessary, desirable, or even feasible. In 2008, Durlak and DePre answered this critically important question through a review of research on the implementation and outcomes of prevention and promotion programs targeting children and adolescents (Durlak & DuPre, 2008). The review is now several years old; the studies included are older still. Yet, despite its age, the review remains noteworthy not only for its conclusion—spoiler alert: implementation matters—but also for the sheer number of studies included and the breadth of prevention and promotion programs examined. Importantly, the review focused on programs implemented in real-world settings by non-researchers. A brief summary follows.

Durlak and DuPre (2008) searched multiple electronic bibliographic databases using various search terms to locate both published and unpublished studies of prevention and health promotion programs for children and adolescents. The programs targeted a variety of concerns including physical health and development, academic performance, drug use, and various social and mental health issues such as violence, bullying, and positive youth development. The search covered a 30-year time span, beginning in 1976 when, according to the authors, research on implementation first began appearing with any frequency, and ending on December 31, 2006. The search identified 483 studies summarized in five meta-analyses and 59 additional studies assessing the impact of implementation on outcomes.

- In a meta-analysis of 59 studies of youth mentoring programs, Dubois et al. (2002) found programs that monitored implementation obtained effect sizes three times larger than those that did not monitor implementation (mean effects of 0.18 versus 0.06, respectively).
- In a synthesis of evaluation research on 14 whole-school anti-bullying programs, Smith et al. (2004) reported that effect sizes were modest overall; however, those programs that monitored implementation obtained effect sizes on self-reported rates of bullying and victimization that were twice as large as those that did not monitor implementation.
- In a meta-analysis of 143 adolescent drug prevention programs, Tobler (1986) reported that 29% of the programs studied were improperly implemented; further, comparisons suggested that those programs that were well-implemented obtained effect sizes 0.34 greater than those that were poorly implemented.
- In a meta-analysis of 221 school-based programs for preventing aggressive behavior, Wilson et al. (2003) observed that program implementation was the second most important factor that influenced outcomes. The only factor more important than program implementation was student risk status: Students selected for program participation due to their early aggressive behavior were the ones that improved the most.
- In a meta-analysis of 46 drug-prevention programs, Derzon et al. (2005) reported the mean effect size on drug use was nearly zero (0.02, specifically) and not statistically significant. Worse still, 21 of the 46 sites obtained negative effect sizes, meaning youth in the comparison condition engaged in *less* drug use than did program participants. They observed, however, three factors with strong effects on outcomes.

> Two were related to implementation: the degree to which program objectives and procedures were put into everyday practice, and the intensity of program delivery. The third related to the control group: Some students in the comparison condition were exposed to alternative drug prevention programs. The authors re-estimated program outcomes adjusting for these factors, essentially asking how the results would have differed if students in the comparison condition had received no alternative drug prevention programs and if the programs of interest had been implemented consistently and with sufficient intensity. In synthetic projections, mean effect size for the 46 programs rose from 0.02 to 0.24 and achieved statistical significance. Only one program still had a negative effect size.

Durlak and DuPre (2008) examined 59 additional studies of prevention and promotion programs for children and adolescents and reported the following results. A significant positive relationship was observed in 76% (45 out of 59) of the studies between the level of implementation and at least half of all observed program outcomes. Moreover, minimal variation in the level of program implementation could explain the non-significant relationship between implementation and outcomes observed in eight of the remaining 14 studies. Finally, the significant positive relationships observed in most of the studies did not depend on how implementation was assessed.

MAKING THE CASE FOR IMPLEMENTATION SCIENCE

Although statistics are hard to come by, it is widely acknowledged that EBI implementation often produces suboptimal results and implementation failure occurs all too frequently. This is not surprising. EBI implementation is complex and challenging, even when the effort is well-resourced. Few naturalistic studies of "implementation as usual" exist, but anecdotal reports indicate that implementation efforts are often guided by organizational inertia (i.e., "we've always done it this way"), personal preferences (i.e., "let's do it my way"), or the ISLAGIATT principle (i.e., "it seemed like a good idea at the time"). What is needed is evidence-based implementation of EBIs. The overriding purpose of implementation science is to improve the practice of implementation by generating a robust body of knowledge and set of associated tools to address the problems that commonly arise in "implementation as usual." Four such problems are described in the following.

Adapting EBIs. EBIs usually require adaptation to better fit the needs, resources, values, and constraints of the setting in which they are delivered or those of the population served by the setting. In implementation as usual, adaptations are often made with good intentions, out of convenience, and without careful consideration of how those adaptations might alter the effectiveness of the intervention. Implementation science has developed systematic approaches and tools to guide decision-making about adaptation, engage stakeholders in the adaptation process, monitor and document adaptations, and evaluate the effects of adaptations. Use of these approaches and tools increases the likelihood that adaptations will enhance the adoption, implementation, effectiveness, and sustainability of the EBI.

Identifying and prioritizing determinants. A critical task before and during implementation is to assess the setting or context to identify factors that assist or impede implementation. These factors, commonly referred to as barriers and facilitators, are called "determinants" in implementation science. In implementation as usual, determinant assessment, when it occurs, tends to be informal and brief. Important determinants may go undetected, increasing the likelihood of implementation challenges and the risk of implementation failure. Implementation science has produced a growing body of knowledge about determinants of implementation and a set of methods and tools for identifying them. Systematic use of these tools often reveals more determinants than can be addressed with available resources. Implementation science has developed practical methods for prioritizing determinants that, while not perfect, can focus attention on those determinants that have greatest potential to undermine or support implementation.

Selecting and matching strategies to determinants. In implementation as usual, strategies are often selected without knowledge of the critical determinants operating in the setting in which implementation will occur. That is, many organizations and technical assistance teams have familiar or favorite "go to" implementation strategies, such as training (e.g., online Continuing Medical Education modules), audit and feedback (common for quality improvement teams working in health systems), or learning collaboratives (bringing together community-based organizations). Although these strategies can be effective, their effectiveness is neither absolute nor universal. Rather, their effectiveness depends on the EBI, the local context, and the stakeholders involved, for example. Implementation science has identified and categorized dozens of implementation strategies beyond the "usual suspects," developed evidence about the effectiveness of commonly used strategies, created tools for selecting and matching strategies to determinants, and generated guidance for implementation planning. Use of these approaches and tools increases the likelihood that the implementation effort is well conceived, designed, and planned.

Monitoring and evaluating implementation efforts. Too often, implementation as usual does not include robust monitoring and evaluation. Monitoring is important for assessing progress or delay and for making adjustments along the way. Adjustments could include modifying the pace of implementation, adapting the EBI to better fit the local context or population served, or adding implementation strategies to address emergent determinants. Evaluation is important for assessing implementation success and outcomes achieved, as well as determining what did or did not happen during implementation. Implementation science offers several frameworks, methods, and tools that can be used to monitor, improve, evaluate, and report an implementation effort and inform future implementation efforts.

KEY CONCEPTS AND FEATURES OF IMPLEMENTATION SCIENCE

Every field of study, perhaps every specialized field of human activity, develops its own vocabulary so that those working in the field can communicate complex ideas with each other efficiently and with some precision. Implementation science is no exception. To make implementation science accessible, the authors of this textbook have agreed to use as little field-specific jargon as possible and, when using the field's specialized terms, to do so as consistently as possible. However, some mastery of the vocabulary of implementation science is necessary to fully comprehend the scientific knowledge accumulated and fully use the associated tools developed. Table 1.1 lists and defines key concepts in implementation science that will appear in many chapters. Additional, nuanced concepts are defined in the chapters that follow and are collated in the glossary at the end of the textbook.

To aid those new to the field, as well as others needing a brief and plain language introduction to key concepts in implementation science, Curran (2020) developed a slide (reproduced in Figure 1.2) that provides simple, jargon-free definitions of implementation science, implementation strategies, and implementation outcomes, and describes how implementation research relates to effectiveness research.

Implementation science endeavors to be a practical science, one that is useful for those seeking to implement EBIs in real-world settings. Implementation science possesses three inter-related features that work together to keep it real. First, implementation science

TABLE 1.1 Key Implementation Science Concepts and Definitions

CONCEPT	DEFINITION
Acceptability	The perception among implementation stakeholders that an EBI is agreeable, palatable, or satisfactory (Proctor et al., 2011).
Adaptation	A process of thoughtful and deliberate alteration to the design or delivery of an intervention, with the goal of improving its fit or effectiveness in a given context (Wiltsey Stirman et al., 2017).
Adoption	The intention, initial decision, or action to make use of an EBI. Also referred to as "uptake" (Proctor et al., 2011).
Appropriateness	The perceived fit, relevance, or compatibility of the EBI for a given practice setting, provider, or consumer (Proctor et al., 2011).
Coverage	The extent to which people in need actually receive important health interventions (Boerma et al., 2014).
Deimplementation	Reducing or stopping the use or delivery of services or practices that are ineffective, unproven, harmful, overused, or inappropriate (Norton et al., 2017).
Determinants	Factors that obstruct or enable adoption, institutionalization, or scale up of EBIs in target settings (Krause et al., 2014).
Dissemination	The targeted distribution of information and intervention materials to a specific public health, clinical practice, or public audience (National Institutes of Health, 2021).
Evidence-based intervention	Programs, practices, principles, procedures, products, pills, and policies that have been found to be effective at improving health behaviors, health outcomes, or health-related environments in one or more well designed research study (Leeman et al., 2017).
External validity	The extent that findings from one study can be generalized to other groups of people and/or different contexts.
Feasibility	The extent to which an EBI can be successfully used or carried out within a given agency or setting (Proctor et al., 2011).
Fidelity	The degree to which an EBI was implemented as it was prescribed in the original testing or as it was intended by its developers (Proctor et al., 2011).
Framework	An analytical tool that groups concepts into larger categories and depicts relations among those categories.
Implementation	Purposeful actions to put an EBI into use.
Implementation outcomes	The effects, intended or unintended, of deliberate and purposive actions to implement EBIs (Proctor et al., 2011).
Implementation strategy	Methods or techniques used to support the adoption, integration, and sustainability of an EBI (Proctor et al., 2011).
Internal validity	The level of confidence that any causal relationship tested is not impacted by additional factors or variables.

(*continued*)

TABLE 1.1 Key Implementation Science Concepts and Definitions (*continued*)

CONCEPT	DEFINITION
Know-do gap	The gap between what we know works and what we do in practice. Used to describe practice gaps for which an EBI exists.
Modification	A broad concept that encompasses any changes made to interventions, whether deliberately and proactively (i.e., adaptation), or in reaction to unanticipated challenges that arise in a given session or context (Wiltsey Stirman et al., 2017).
Penetration	The integration of an EBI within a service setting and its subsystems (Proctor et al., 2011).
Process model	An analytical tool for describing or guiding the process of translating research into practice or implementing EBIs, often denoting a temporal order of phases and activities.
Scale-up	Deliberate efforts to increase the impact of EBIs so as to benefit more people and to foster policy and program development on a lasting basis (Simmons et al., 2010).
Scale-up strategy	The operationalized steps required to embed the EBI in existing programs, services, and formal practices.
Sustainability	After a defined period of time, the EBI continues to be delivered and/or individual behavior change (i.e., clinician, patient) is maintained; the program and individual behavior change may evolve or adapt while continuing to produce benefits for individuals/system (Moore et al., 2017).

EBI, evidence-based intervention.

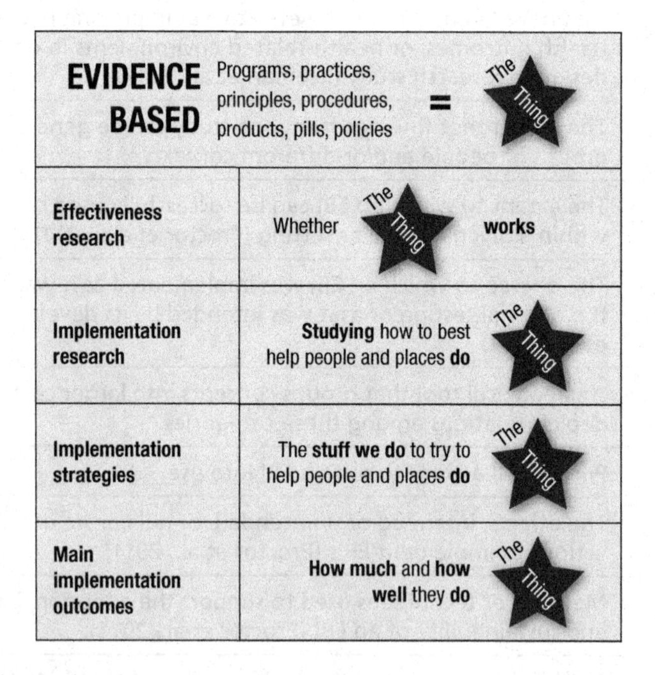

FIGURE 1.2 The basics of implementation science.
Source: Adapted from Curran, G. M. (2020). Implementation science made too simple: A teaching tool. *Implementation Science Communications*, *1*, 27. https://doi.org/10.1186/s43058-020-00001-z. Courtesy of BioMed Central.

involves multiple stakeholders in planning, execution, and evaluation. To inform and support implementation in practice, implementation science must be responsive to stakeholders' priorities, attentive to stakeholders' constraints, knowledgeable of stakeholders' working conditions (especially those implementing the EBIs), and sensitive to stakeholders' accountabilities. Second, implementation science embraces pragmatism. To be useful, implementation science has to be *usable.* The knowledge that implementation science generates has to be relevant and actionable, the implementation strategies tested have to be feasible and affordable, and the assessment tools and methods developed have to be accessible and easy to use. Third, implementation science recognizes that context matters. Implementation is context-sensitive. What works well in one setting might not work well or work at all in another. Rather than attempting to isolate the effects of interventions or implementation strategies from context, implementation science explicitly examines the effects of context so that implementers can adapt interventions and tailor strategies to achieve desired outcomes.

Finally, health equity has emerged as a focal concern in implementation science, particularly in light of ongoing social protest for racial justice, renewed attention to structural racism's pernicious effects on health, and disparate impacts of the COVID-19 pandemic and response on oppressed communities. In fact, a recently published commentary by leaders in the field called for "making health equity the highest priority in implementation science and thus a central indicator of the field's success" (Brownson et al., 2021, p. 2). Recommendations include: increasing diversity in study samples and settings where interventions and implementation strategies are tested (Baumann & Cabassa, 2020); designing interventions for vulnerable populations and low-resource settings and packaging them with implementation strategies (Baumann & Cabassa, 2020; Galaviz et al., 2020); adapting implementation science frameworks to better account for the historical, cultural, economic, and political forces that contribute to inequities in access to, receipt of, quality of, and outcomes of EBIs (Brownson et al., 2021); developing implementation strategies that target the factors that contribute to these inequities (Brownson et al., 2021); and evaluating implementation efforts for their impact on equity (Baumann & Cabassa, 2020).

OUTLINE OF THE TEXTBOOK

Social psychologist Kurt Lewin, founder of the concept of action research, claimed, "There is nothing as practical as a good theory" (Lewin, 1952, p. 169). Implementation science has generated many theories, models, and frameworks, some of which are useful for both implementation research *and* implementation practice. An early review identified 61 theories, models, and frameworks used in dissemination and implementation research (Tabak et al., 2012). A recent review found more than twice that number (Strifler et al., 2018). To help implementation researchers and implementers select a theory, model, or framework appropriate for their needs, implementation scientists have devised several schemes to categorize and organize them. Nilsen (2015), for example, identified three overarching aims for the use of theories, models, and frameworks in implementation science: (a) describing or guiding the process of implementing EBIs, (b) understanding or explaining what influences implementation success or failure, and (c) evaluating implementation efforts. Other chapters in this book will describe and illustrate the use of theories, models, and frameworks for the last two aims. Here we will focus on those useful for the first aim, recognizing that: (a) theories, models, and frameworks are terms sometimes used interchangeably in implementation science even though there are important distinctions among these concepts; and (b) some theories, models, and frameworks can be used for more than one of the three aims that Nilsen (2015) identifies.

Nilsen (2015) labels as "process models" those theories, models, and frameworks that are useful for describing or guiding the process of implementing EBIs. **Process models** identify steps, stages, or phases that characterize the process of translating research into practice generally or implementing EBIs specifically. Some process models, like the Knowledge-to-Action framework (Wilson et al., 2011), are largely descriptive, depicting the research-to-practice process in terms of stages or phases, beginning with the discovery and production of scientific knowledge and concluding with the implementation and use of research findings in various settings. Other process models are more prescriptive in nature. They delineate various steps or actions that should be followed in the process of implementing EBIs and offer "how to" guidance for planning and managing implementation efforts. There are many process models available to facilitate implementation. Here we focus on the Quality Implementation Framework, or QIF (Meyers et al., 2012).

The QIF was generated by synthesizing information from 25 implementation frameworks about the procedures or strategies thought to be critical for achieving "quality implementation," defined by the authors as "putting an innovation into practice in such a way that it meets the necessary standards to achieve the innovation's desired outcomes" (Meyers et al., 2012, p. 465). The QIF identifies 14 critical actions organized into four temporal phases: initial considerations regarding the host setting for the EBI, creating a structure for implementation, ongoing structure once implementation begins, and improving future application. The 14 critical actions are themselves ordered temporally into steps (see Table 1.2), some of which occur or should occur before implementation begins (steps 1–10), others during implementation (steps 11–13), and still others when implementation is far along or complete (step 14).

Critical steps in the first phase involve assessments of organizational needs, EBI-organization fit, and organizational capacity or readiness. These assessments inform decisions about EBI adaptation and actions to build organizational capacity for implementation, including securing buy-in from key stakeholders. Critical steps in the second phase include developing an implementation plan and creating implementation teams that will carry out the plan and take responsibility for implementation. Critical steps in the third phase, when implementation begins, involve providing technical assistance, coaching, and supervision to providers delivering the EBI; monitoring ongoing implementation; and providing feedback to involved parties to keep them apprised of implementation progress and create opportunities to make timely adjustments as needed. The last critical step, which occurs in the fourth phase, focuses on learning from experience through evaluation, analysis, and reflection to glean lessons for enhancing future implementation efforts.

The QIF informs the organizational structure of this book. The eight chapters that follow delve into the critical steps described in the QIF. Each chapter seeks to make accessible and practical the wealth of scientific knowledge and associated tools that implementation science has produced about these steps. The chapters follow the temporal order of the four phases of the QIF, although some early critical steps are covered in a later chapter because it made sense to discuss them in conjunction with later critical steps. Also included are five chapters on topics of practical importance related to implementing EBIs: disseminating EBIs, scaling up EBIs, sustaining EBIs, de-implementing practices that are no longer effective or never were, and implementation science in policy. Given the broad applicability of implementation science, and the wide-ranging interests of those seeking to learn about it and apply it, each chapter includes some discussion of research findings, examples, and tools from implementation science conducted in LMICs. In addition, each chapter attends to the issue of health equity, a rapidly rising concern and focus of implementation science.

Chapter 2 focuses on a key initial consideration in implementation: identifying and documenting a gap between actual and expected performance in access, quality, or outcomes. In implementation science, such gaps are sometimes referred to as care gaps or

TABLE 1.2 Quality Implementation Framework and Organization of this Book

PHASE 1: INITIAL CONSIDERATIONS REGARDING THE HOST SETTING	
Assessment strategies	
1. Conducting a needs and resource assessment	Chapter 2, 3
2. Conducting a fit assessment	Chapter 4
3. Conducting a capacity/readiness assessment	Chapter 5
Decisions about adaptation	
4. Possibility for adaptation	Chapter 4
Capacity-building strategies	
5. Obtaining explicit buy-in from critical stakeholders and fostering a supportive community/organizational climate	Chapter 5
6. Building general/organizational capacity	Chapter 6
7. Staff recruitment/maintenance	Chapter 8
8. Effective pre-innovation staff training	Chapter 8
PHASE 2: CREATING A STRUCTURE FOR IMPLEMENTATION	
9. Creating implementation teams	Chapter 7
10. Developing an implementation plan	Chapter 7
PHASE 3: ONGOING STRUCTURE ONCE IMPLEMENTATION BEGINS	
11. Technical assistance/coaching/supervision	Chapter 8
12. Process evaluation	Chapter 8, 9
13. Supportive feedback mechanism	Chapter 8
PHASE 4: IMPROVING FUTURE APPLICATIONS	
14. Learning from experience	Chapter 9

quality gaps; in this book, a broader term—practice gaps—is used. A best practice in implementation is to focus on those problems or conditions for which there is clear evidence that a gap exists and for which there is sufficient room for improvement to warrant an implementation effort. Drawing on the Knowledge Translation perspective, this chapter focuses on how to identify a practice gap, select or develop indicators to assess the gap, develop a strategy to measure the gap, and develop a plan to understand why the gap exists.

Practice gaps become know / do gaps when one or more EBIs exist that, if implemented, would close the gap. Chapter 3 focuses on identifying, appraising, and selecting EBIs to reduce practice gaps. After defining and describing types of EBIs, the chapter discusses how to assess the evidence in support of an EBI's effectiveness, the strengths and limitations of the evidence of effectiveness with respect to subpopulations and specific settings, and the evidence in support of an EBI's potential to be implemented in practice. The chapter also discusses how to search for and locate EBIs, evaluate the credibility of the sources of EBIs, and select EBIs that have the strongest evidence of effectiveness and the best fit with one's objectives, service population, and delivery setting. The value of modeling EBI impact, and the methods for doing so, are also discussed.

Chapter 4 focuses on another key initial consideration: whether or not, and how, to adapt the EBI. Implementing EBIs evokes a tension between delivering the EBI as closely as it was in the research studies that generated the evidence of its effectiveness so that the same benefits result, on the one hand, and on the other, modifying the EBI to better fit the needs, resources, values, and constraints of the setting in which it will be delivered, and the population served by the setting. The chapter examines the need for both fidelity and adaptation when implementing an EBI, especially in low-resource settings and particularly to address health equity. The chapter describes how to assess the fit of EBIs in varying contexts, how to decide whether or not to adapt an EBI, and how to adapt an EBI using a conceptual framework when adaptation is warranted. The chapter also describes taxonomies for documenting and classifying adaptations, as well as reasons and methods for evaluating the effects of adaptations on implementation outcomes and health outcomes.

A key insight in implementation science is that context matters. When it comes to implementation, what works in one context often does not work in another. Chapter 5 focuses on assessing context, capacity, and readiness to implement the EBI. The chapter explores how context is defined and conceptualized and explains how contextual factors at multiple levels influence implementation. Recalling the three overarching aims for the use of theories, models, and frameworks in implementation science (Nilsen, 2015), the chapter explains how theories, models, and frameworks can be used prior to implementation to identify contextual factors that function as barriers or facilitators to implementation. Methods for applying these theories, models, and frameworks and conducting a capacity or readiness assessment are discussed. So, too, are methods for prioritizing which contextual factors to address to improve implementation.

Implementing EBIs to improve health is inherently a social enterprise. An important initial consideration, therefore, is to engage stakeholders to obtain their input, secure their buy-in, and mobilize their expertise, influence, and resources to support the implementation effort. Chapter 6 clarifies the meaning of the terms "stakeholder" and "engagement," describes the types of stakeholders commonly involved in implementation efforts, and discusses the levels of engagement that stakeholders could have across multiple critical steps in the QIF. The chapter also discusses how to conduct a stakeholder analysis, how to identify potential challenges to engaging stakeholders, and how to select strategies to engage stakeholders.

Chapter 7 jumps ahead to the second phase of the QIF: creating a structure for implementation. The chapter focuses on the critical steps of developing an implementation plan and creating implementation teams that will carry out the plan and take responsibility for implementation. In addition, it delves into a critical step not mentioned, although implied, in the QIF: selecting and matching implementation strategies to address the barriers and facilitators identified through context, capacity, and readiness assessment. The chapter describes tools for planning and communicating about an implementation effort, as well as approaches for building and managing effective implementation teams. All too often, implementation strategies are mismatched to implementation barriers, resulting in suboptimal implementation. The chapter explains why this occurs and describes several methods for ensuring a good fit between the implementation strategies selected and the implementation challenges that must be addressed.

After assessment, planning, and preparation, implementation begins. Chapter 8 focuses on the critical steps depicted in the third phase of the QIF: providing technical assistance, supervision, and coaching to front-line providers delivering the EBI; monitoring ongoing implementation; and creating feedback mechanisms so that those involved in implementation know how implementation is going. The chapter reintroduces process models and explains how their usefulness for guiding the implementation effort. Several process models are described and compared, but particular attention is given to the Stages of Implementation Completion, or SIC. In addition to the critical steps already mentioned, earlier critical steps in the QIF concerning recruiting, training, and retaining staff are also discussed. The chapter explores common pitfalls that arise in implementing EBIs and examines the risks of rushing through or skipping over the stages of implementation.

Chapter 9 covers the fourth and final phase of the QIF: improving future implementation efforts through evaluation and learning. Whereas the QIF emphasizes informal methods of learning from experience, such as feedback assessment and self-reflection, the chapter focuses on formal evaluation approaches that balance rigor and practicality. The chapter discusses the basics of implementation evaluation including how to develop evaluation questions appropriate for different stages of implementation, how to apply evaluation frameworks to answer those questions, and how to select implementation, service, and health outcomes for assessing success. The chapter describes several evaluation study designs, illustrating their use, and discussing their relative strengths and weaknesses for answering implementation research questions.

Although implementation is the central concern of implementation science, the field has also generated scientific knowledge and associated tools about matters of practical importance that precede or follow implementation. Chapter 10 focuses on disseminating information and intervention materials to public health and clinical practice audiences to promote widespread uptake of EBIs. The chapter describes how dissemination is both distinct from and related to diffusion, implementation, health communication, and consumer marketing and advertising. The chapter then discusses how to apply dissemination theories, models, frameworks, and strategies to change a target audience's knowledge, attitudes, skills, self-efficacy, and social norms related to an EBI. The chapter also covers how to design, execute, and evaluate a dissemination campaign.

To realize improvements in population health, EBIs must be implemented, and implemented well, in dozens, hundreds, or even thousands of settings and communities across wide geographic regions. Yet implementing an EBI "at scale" is challenging. There are many examples of scale-up efforts that failed or proved only partially successful. Chapter 11 clarifies the meaning of scale-up, describes different types of scale-up, and introduces key concepts common to scale-up frameworks. The chapter then describes the ExpandNet/WHO framework, a systematic approach to scale-up. The chapter covers key elements of the framework and offers practical guidance on how to design a demonstration project or pilot study with scale-up in mind, how to develop a systematic scale-up strategy, and how to manage the scale-up process. A discussion follows of common pitfalls and lessons learned in scaling up EBIs in LMICs across a range of health and development issues.

Implementing EBI effectively is challenging. Sustaining EBI delivery and outcomes in practice settings may be even more difficult. Chapter 12 defines sustainability, distinguishes it from implementation, explains its importance from the perspectives of various stakeholders, and examines its dynamic relationship with adaptation. Following a discussion of practical considerations and common challenges in sustaining EBIs, the chapter describes how to use theories, models, and frameworks to assess factors at multiple levels that affect sustainability; how to use tools to plan for sustainability; and how to develop strategies to sustain the delivery and outcomes of EBIs. The chapter examines the challenges of measuring, monitoring, and evaluating sustainability efforts when resources and in-house evaluation capabilities are limited. The chapter then discusses how to address these challenges using existing evaluation frameworks and pragmatic assessment approaches.

Many interventions used in practice are ineffective (little evidence that they work), contradicted (new evidence indicates they do not work), mixed (evidence is unclear that they work), or untested (no evidence whatsoever). Others have been superseded by more effective interventions or are no longer needed or desired. Interventions falling into any of these categories are candidates for de-implementation, or removal. Chapter 13 focuses on an emerging topic in implementation science: de-implementing low-value practices in healthcare and public health. The chapter defines and describes various types of low-value practices, characterizes the extent and cost of low-value practices, and explains why low-value practices exist and persist. The chapter then delves into the challenges that make de-implementing low-value practices difficult and different than the challenges of implementing EBIs. A discussion follows of the strategies that could be used at the patient (public), provider, and systems levels to de-implement low-value practices and concludes with practical advice for adapting strategies for various low-value practices.

The final chapter in the book focuses on another emerging topic in implementation science: the use of research evidence in the formulation and implementation of public policy. Although policy implementation research has a long and storied history, implementation scientists have only recently begun to examine how policy implementation and EBI implementation intersect. Chapter 14 discusses what implementation means from a policy perspective and describes how public policy is made using the heuristic model of the policy cycle. The chapter then examines how and when research evidence can inform the policy agenda, inform policy options, inform policy implementation, and provide policy feedback. The chapter concludes by describing how to apply a framework to conduct a policy analysis in support of implementation planning and how to support evidence-informed policy processes.

CASE STUDY 1.2 IMPLEMENTING UNIVERSAL SOCIAL RISK SCREENING

Intrigued to learn more about implementation science and how it might help her implement universal social risk screening, Savannah M. contacted an implementation scientist working at a local university. The scientist encouraged Savannah to take a systematic approach like that recommended in the QIF, pointed her to a variety of implementation science resources and tools available on several websites, and offered to advise her along the way through periodic check-in calls. Savannah's first stop was the university library, where a librarian searched the literature for answers to the following questions: (a) What do we know about the impact of universal social risk screening on patient care in primary care settings?; (b) What social risk screening tools are available and how good are they for use in health systems?; and (c) What barriers or facilitators have other health systems encountered in implementing universal screening into primary care? The literature indicated that screening is effective at surfacing social risks that are highly correlated with physical health and that patients generally found screening acceptable; however, those who reported prior experience of discrimination in healthcare reported lower acceptability. Patients underscored the importance of screening with empathy and compassion and introducing screening in ways that reduce suspicion that patients are being selectively screened based on their race/ethnicity, English proficiency, and other factors. Several screening tools are available; although none have been rigorously tested, several appear to be comparable in how well they perform. Finally, providers see the importance of screening in principle but report skepticism about its value in primary care given constraints on their ability to take action and the additional time it would take in their visit.

(continued)

CASE STUDY 1.2 IMPLEMENTING UNIVERSAL SOCIAL RISK SCREENING *(continued)*

With this information in hand, Savannah convened an implementation team, shared the findings of the literature search, recommended a social risk screening tool rated highly for its practicality (brief, no cost, easy to administer, easy to interpret, available in English and Spanish), and initiated a context assessment to identify barriers and facilitators to implementing universal social risk screening. Her implementation scientist advisor recommended using a "determinants" framework sensitive to the equity concerns noted in the literature in addition to provider concerns and health system considerations. The assessment highlighted three key potential barriers to implementation: Patients were indeed concerned about how screening is introduced and conducted, providers were indeed concerned about what they can do if screening reveals unmet social needs, and clinic managers were concerned about how the screening could be integrated into clinic workflow with minimal disruption or loss of efficiency. Consulting the implementation science resources mentioned by the implementation scientist advisor, Savannah and the implementation team selected implementation strategies to address these barriers, developed an implementation plan, and engaged with clinic managers, providers, and staff to increase readiness for implementation.

Implementation proceeded smoothly, although not entirely without hiccups. Front desk staff were provided patient-friendly brochures in various languages to distribute to patients to introduce the notion of social risk screening, explain why the clinic was doing it and what it would do with the information, and emphasize the screening was universal, not selective. Provider and staff training in universal social risk screening included implicit bias training, communication scripts for addressing frequently asked questions, and rehearsals to reinforce empathy and compassion. The implementation team engaged the clinic managers in mapping clinic workflow and conducting small tests of change to optimally integrate screening that integrated medical assistants in flagging those at risk directly in the electronic health record. The team also worked with clinic managers to strengthen current referral systems to social service agencies and community-based organizations and developed a follow-up system to "close the loop" in referral. These strategies—coupled with a Continuing Medical Education training on social risk-informed care—increased providers' confidence that they could take meaningful action to address patients' social needs. With encouragement from her implementation scientist advisor, Savannah and the implementation team provided ongoing coaching to reinforce training, monitored implementation, and provided feedback to clinic managers. She and her team also developed an evaluation plan to assess not only the effectiveness of universal social risk screening in addressing patients' social needs, but also implementation outcomes like the following: care plan adjustments made in response to documented social risk, patient and provider acceptability, percentage of providers using the screening tool, percentage of patients screened, and, through periodic observations, fidelity to the screening approach (e.g., screening with empathy and compassion). The evaluation plan included an assessment of whether the implementation of universal social risk screening had a positive or negative impact on equity.

One year later, Savannah reflected on the implementation of universal social risk screening that she supported. By all accounts, the implementation was a success. Savannah received positive feedback from clinic managers, providers, and staff on how well she and her team managed the implementation process and avoided the problems that they had experienced in previous implementation efforts.

SUMMARY

This chapter introduced the field of implementation science, highlighted its potential for improving public health, made the case that implementation matters, and described the field's historical development, core concepts, and key features. The chapter also provided an overview of the textbook's subsequent chapters.

KEY POINTS FOR PRACTICE

1. Take a systematic approach to implementation. Many of the problems that result in suboptimal implementation in practice can be avoided by viewing implementation as a process and by making use of the scientific knowledge and associated tools that implementation science has produced.
2. Context matters. When it comes to implementing EBIs, what works in one context might not work in another. Use an implementation science framework to assess the local context in which implementation will occur to identify features that could serve as facilitators or barriers to EBI implementation. Using a framework reduces the risk of overlooking contextual features that might not seem salient or important, but in fact are.
3. Practitioners often need implementation support. Implementing EBIs successfully requires a combination of expertise and experience that many people do not have because implementation is not the main thing they do. Seek out training to acquire implementation knowledge and skills. Participate in learning collaboratives or engage in peer learning. Find an implementation scientist at a local university or seek technical assistance from an implementation support organization.
4. Look for opportunities to reduce inequity when implementing EBIs. When conducting a context assessment, for example, pay attention to broader, structural factors like social determinants of health that contribute to disparities in access to, receipt of, quality of, or outcomes from an EBI. Employ implementation strategies that address the factors that generate these disparities. Use implementation science frameworks to monitor and evaluate whether EBI implementation is increasing, decreasing, or leaving unchanged disparities in access, receipt, quality, or outcomes.

COMMON PITFALLS IN PRACTICE

1. Many people find the specialized language of implementation science to be unfamiliar and off-putting. This can pose a significant barrier to accessing the scientific knowledge and associated tools that implementation science has generated or seeking out implementation support from an implementation scientist. It is the responsibility of implementation scientists to make the field's knowledge and resources accessible and useful for implementation practice. If we do not, we will fail to achieve our goals. In the meantime, Curran's (2020) simple, plain language description of key implementation science concepts can serve as a touchstone.
2. Implementation science means different things to different people. As a result, people can think they understand each other when in fact they are talking past one another. Consensus has yet to emerge on what implementation science is and what it is not. A key distinction to keep in mind is that implementation and implementation science are not the same thing. One is doing; the other is studying the doing. An overarching

goal of implementation science is to develop scientific knowledge and tools to support more effective implementation.

3. Implementation science is often confused with process evaluation, leading many to believe that they are doing implementation science when they are not. Process evaluation can take several forms, some of which resemble implementation science. There are at least two features that distinguish implementation science from process evaluation: (a) the testing of implementation strategies for effectiveness using experimental or quasi-experimental study designs, and (b) the use of implementation science frameworks to explain, not simply describe, implementation processes and outcomes (e.g., fidelity or dosage).
4. When implementing EBIs, the pressures to act quickly and move fast are hard to resist. Yet, evidence is growing that rushing or skipping critical implementation activities can prove detrimental to implementation success. The adage of measure twice, cut once applies when implementing EBIs. Perhaps that is why the QIF, like other process models, lists many critical steps in the assessing and planning phases.

DISCUSSION QUESTIONS

1. Implementation science emerged in the United States in the late 1990s and early 2000s to address the long delay that typically occurs in research into practice. Its emergence in the United States coincided with its emergence in global health, focusing initially on tropical disease and accelerating with the launch of large-scale efforts to combat the high burden of HIV/AIDS in LMICs. How have historical, institutional, and cultural forces influenced the development and trajectory of implementation science as a field? How have these forces shaped both the common and distinctive features of implementation science in the United States and in global health?
2. Why has health equity emerged only recently as a key concern in implementation science? How might implementation science address disparities and improve equity? What challenges might arise?
3. How is implementation science similar or different from quality improvement? Could the two be combined? If so, in what ways?
4. What are some common challenges in "implementation as usual" beyond those mentioned herein? How might implementation science help practitioners address those challenges? What scientific knowledge or associated tools would prove helpful?

REFERENCES

Balas, E. A., & Boren, S. A. (2000). Managing clinical knowledge for health care improvement. *Yearbook of Medical Informatics, 09*(01). https://doi.org/10.1055/s-0038-1637943

Bauer, M. S., Damschroder, L., Hagedorn, H., Smith, J., & Kilbourne, A. M. (2015). An introduction to implementation science for the non-specialist. *BMC Psychology, 3*(1), 1–12. https://doi.org/10.1186/S40359-015-0089-9

Bauer, M. S., & Kirchner, J. A. (2020). Implementation science: What is it and why should I care? *Psychiatry Research, 283*. https://doi.org/10.1016/j.psychres.2019.04.025

Baumann, A. A., & Cabassa, L. J. (2020). Reframing implementation science to address inequities in healthcare delivery. *BMC Health Services Research, 20*(1). https://doi.org/10.1186/s12913-020-4975-3

Blue Ribbon Panel, Jacks, T., Jaffee, E., & Singer, D. (2016). *Cancer Moonshot Blue Ribbon Panel Report 2016*. https://www.cancer.gov/research/key-initiatives/moonshot-cancer-initiative/blue-ribbon-panel/blue-ribbon-panel-report-2016.pdf

Boerma, T., AbouZahr, C., Evans, D., & Evans, T. (2014). Monitoring intervention coverage in the context of universal health coverage. *PLoS Medicine, 11*(9). https://doi.org/10.1371/journal.pmed.1001728

Brownson, R. C., Kumanyika, S. K., Kreuter, M. W., & Haire-Joshu, D. (2021). Implementation science should give higher priority to health equity. *Implementation Science, 16*(1). https://doi.org/10.1186/s13012-021-01097-0

Chalmers, I., & Glasziou, P. (2009). Avoidable waste in the production and reporting of research evidence. *The Lancet, 374*(9683). https://doi.org/10.1016/S0140-6736(09)60329-9

Colditz, G. A., & Emmons, K. M. (2017). The promise and challenge of dissemination and implementation research. In R. C. Brownson, G. A. Colditz, & E. K. Proctor (Eds.), *Dissemination and implementation research in health: Translating science to practice* (2nd ed., pp. 1–18). Oxford University Press. https://books.google.com/books?id=ycM9DwAAQBAJ

Curran, G. M. (2020). Implementation science made too simple: A teaching tool. *Implementation Science Communications, 1*(1). https://doi.org/10.1186/s43058-020-00001-z

Derzon, J. H., Sale, E., Springer, J. F., & Brounstein, P. (2005). Estimating intervention effectiveness: Synthetic projection of field evaluation results. *Journal of Primary Prevention, 26*(4). https://doi.org/10.1007/s10935-005-5391-5

Dubois, D. L., Holloway, B. E., Valentine, J. C., & Cooper, H. (2002). Effectiveness of mentoring programs for youth: A meta-analytic review. *American Journal of Community Psychology, 30*(2). https://doi.org/10.1023/A:1014628810714

Durlak, J. A., & DuPre, E. P. (2008). Implementation matters: A review of research on the influence of implementation on program outcomes and the factors affecting implementation. *American Journal of Community Psychology, 41*(3–4), 327–350. https://doi.org/10.1007/s10464-008-9165-0

Galaviz, K. I., Breland, J. Y., Sanders, M., Breathett, K., Cerezo, A., Gil, O., Hollier, J. M., Marshall, C., Wilson, J. D., & Essien, U. R. (2020). Implementation science to address health disparities during the coronavirus pandemic. *Health Equity, 4*(1). https://doi.org/10.1089/heq.2020.0044

Gülmezoglu, A. M., Lawrie, T. A., Hezelgrave, N., Oladapo, O. T., Souza, J. P., Gielen, M., Lawn, J. E., Bahl, R., Althabe, F., Colaci, D., & Hofmeyr, G. J. (2016). Interventions to reduce maternal and newborn morbidity and mortality. In M. Temmerman, N. Walker, R. Laxminarayan, & R. Black (Eds.), *Reproductive, maternal, newborn, and child health* (Vol. 2, pp. 115–136). World Bank Publications. https://doi.org/10.1596/978-1-4648-0348-2_ch7

Health and Medicine Division, National Academies of Sciences Engineering and Medicine (US) Committee on Pain Management and Regulatory Strategies to Address Prescription Opioid Abuse, Board on Health Sciences Policy. (2017). In J. K. Phillips, M. A. Ford, & R. J. Bonnie (Eds.), *Pain management and the opioid epidemic: Balancing societal and individual benefits and risks of prescription opioid use* (). National Academies Press. https://books.google.com/books?id=baA4DwAAQBAJ

Krause, J., Van Lieshout, J., Klomp, R., Huntink, E., Aakhus, E., Flottorp, S., Jaeger, C., Steinhaeuser, J., Godycki-Cwirko, M., Kowalczyk, A., Agarwal, S., Wensing, M., & Baker, R. (2014). Identifying determinants of care for tailoring implementation in chronic diseases: An evaluation of different methods. *Implementation Science, 9*(1), 1–12. https://doi.org/10.1186/s13012-014-0102-3

Leeman, J., Birken, S. A., Powell, B. J., Rohweder, C., & Shea, C. M. (2017). Beyond "implementation strategies": Classifying the full range of strategies used in implementation science and practice. *Implementation Science, 12*(1), 1–9. https://doi.org/10.1186/s13012-017-0657-x

Lewin, K. (1952). *Field theory in social science: Selected theoretical papers by Kurt Lewin*. Tavistock.

Meyers, D. C., Durlak, J. A., & Wandersman, A. (2012). The Quality Implementation Framework: A synthesis of critical steps in the implementation process. *American Journal of Community Psychology, 50*(3–4), 462–480. https://doi.org/10.1007/s10464-012-9522-x

Moore, J. E., Mascarenhas, A., Bain, J., & Straus, S. E. (2017). Developing a comprehensive definition of sustainability. *Implementation Science, 12*(1). https://doi.org/10.1186/s13012-017-0637-1

National Academy of Sciences. (2017). *Definitions of evolutionary terms*. National Academy of Sciences. http://www.nas.edu/evolution/Definitions.html

National Institutes of Health. (2021). *Dissemination and implementation research in health (R01 Clinical Trial Optional) PAR-19-274*. https://grants.nih.gov/grants/guide/pa-files/PAR-19-274.html

Nilsen, P. (2015). Making sense of implementation theories, models and frameworks. *Implementation Science, 10*(1), 1–13. https://doi.org/10.1186/s13012-015-0242-0

Norton, W. E., Kennedy, A. E., & Chambers, D. A. (2017). Studying de-implementation in health: An analysis of funded research grants. *Implementation Science, 12*(1), 144. https://doi.org/10.1186/s13012-017-0655-z

Odeny, T. A., Padian, N., Doherty, M. C., Baral, S., Beyrer, C., Ford, N., & Geng, E. H. (2015). Definitions of implementation science in HIV/AIDS. *The Lancet HIV*. https://doi.org/10.1016/S2352-3018(15)00061-2

Petersen, E. E., Davis, N. L., Goodman, D., Cox, S., Syverson, C., Seed, K., Shapiro-Mendoza, C., Callaghan, W. M., & Barfield, W. (2019). Racial/ethnic disparities in pregnancy-related deaths — United States, 2007–2016. *MMWR. Morbidity and Mortality Weekly Report, 68*(35). https://doi.org/10.15585/mmwr.mm6835a3

Proctor, E., Silmere, H., Raghavan, R., Hovmand, P., Aarons, G., Bunger, A., Griffey, R., & Hensley, M. (2011). Outcomes for implementation research: Conceptual distinctions, measurement challenges, and research agenda. *Administration and Policy in Mental Health and Mental Health Services Research, 38*(2), 65–76. https://doi.org/10.1007/s10488-010-0319-7

Scribbr, & Streefkerk, R. (2020). *Internal vs external validity*. Scribbr. https://www.scribbr.com/methodology/internal-vs-external-validity/

Simmons, R., Ruth S., Ghiron, L., Fajans, P., Newton, N., Research., W. H. O. R. H., & ExpandNet. (2010). *Nine steps for developing a scaling-up strategy*. World Health Organization.

Singh, G. K., Siahpush, M., Azuine, R. E., & Williams, S. D. (2015). Widening socioeconomic and racial disparities in cardiovascular disease mortality in the United States, 1969–2013. *International Journal of MCH and AIDS, 3*(2), 106–118. https://pubmed.ncbi.nlm.nih.gov/27621991

Smith, J. D., Schneider, B. H., Smith, P. K., & Ananiadou, K. (2004). The effectiveness of whole-school antibullying programs: A synthesis of evaluation research. *School Psychology Review, 33*(4). https://doi.org/10.1080/02796015.2004.12086267

Strifler, L., Cardoso, R., McGowan, J., Cogo, E., Nincic, V., Khan, P. A., Scott, A., Ghassemi, M., MacDonald, H., Lai, Y., Treister, V., Tricco, A. C., & Straus, S. E. (2018). Scoping review identifies significant number of knowledge translation theories, models, and frameworks with limited use. *Journal of Clinical Epidemiology, 100*. https://doi.org/10.1016/j.jclinepi.2018.04.008

Tabak, R. G., Khoong, E. C., Chambers, D. A., & Brownson, R. C. (2012). Bridging research and practice: Models for dissemination and implementation research. *American Journal of Preventive Medicine, 43*(3), 337–350. https://doi.org/10.1016/j.amepre.2012.05.024

Tobler, N. S. (1986). Meta-analysis of 143 adolescent drug prevention programs: Quantitative outcome results of program participants compared to a control or comparison group. *Journal of Drug Issues, 16*(4). https://doi.org/10.1177/002204268601600405

Walker, T. Y., Elam-Evans, L. D., Singleton, J. A., Yankey, D., Markowitz, L. E., Fredua, B., Williams, C. L., Meyer, S. A., & Stokley, S. (2017). National, regional, state, and selected local area vaccination coverage among adolescents aged 13–17 years — United States, 2016. *MMWR. Morbidity and Mortality Weekly Report, 66*(33). https://doi.org/10.15585/mmwr.mm6633a2

Wilson, K. M., Brady, T. J., Lesesne, C., & NCCDPHP Work Group on Translation. (2011). An organizing framework for translation in public health: The Knowledge to Action Framework. *Preventing Chronic Disease, 8*(2), A46. http://ovidsp.ovid.com/ovidweb.cgi?T=JS&CSC=Y&NEWS=N&PAGE=fulltext&D=medl&AN=21324260

Wilson, S. J., Lipsey, M. W., & Derzon, J. H. (2003). The effects of school-based intervention programs on aggressive behavior: A meta-analysis. *Journal of Consulting and Clinical Psychology, 71*(1). https://doi.org/10.1037/0022-006X.71.1.136

Wiltsey Stirman, S., Gamarra, J. M., Bartlett, B. A., Calloway, A., & Gutner, C. A. (2017). Empirical examinations of modifications and adaptations to evidence-based psychotherapies: Methodologies, impact, and future directions. *Clinical Psychology: Science and Practice, 24*(4). https://doi.org/10.1111/cpsp.12218

Wolfenden, L., Ziersch, A., Robinson, P., Lowe, J., & Wiggers, J. (2015). Reducing research waste and improving research impact. *Australian and New Zealand Journal of Public Health, 39*(4). https://doi.org/10.1111/1753-6405.12467

Woolf, S. H., & Johnson, R. E. (2005). The break-even point: When medical advances are less important than improving the fidelity with which they are delivered. *Annals of Family Medicine, 3*(6), 545–552. https://doi.org/10.1370/afm.406

Yang, K. G., Rodgers, C. R. R., Lee, E., & Lê Cook, B. (2020). Disparities in mental health care utilization and perceived need among Asian Americans: 2012–2016. *Psychiatric Services, 71*(1). https://doi.org/10.1176/appi.ps.201900126

2

Assessing the Practice (Know-Do) Gap

Christine Fahim and Sharon E. Straus

Learning Objectives

By the end of this chapter, readers will be able to:

- Identify the know-do gap as the starting point of knowledge implementation
- Use an integrated knowledge translation approach to involve relevant stakeholders in the process of identifying the know-do gap
- Apply principles of intersectionality in an assessment of the know-do gap
- Determine how to identify gaps in practice
- Select or develop quality indicators to assess identified gaps
- Develop a strategy to measure the practice gaps
- Understand why gaps may exist

CASE STUDY 2.1 IDENTIFYING THE PRACTICE GAP

Jessie is a nurse manager at a long-term care home (LTCH). She has been tasked with ensuring the LTCH at which she works minimizes the spread of COVID-19 infections among LTCH staff and residents. Jessie's first task is to create a plan to determine what needs to be done in the LTCH to minimize the risk of infections. To do so, she must work with LTCH stakeholders to compare infection prevention and control evidence to the practices currently happening at her LTCH. She must select relevant indicators and measurement strategies to determine the scope of the problem and to create her knowledge implementation plan.

In this chapter, we will discuss the knowledge to practice gap and will outline how this gap can be identified, measured, and understood. At the end of the chapter, we will return to this vignette to demonstrate how Jessie identified the know/do gap related to infection prevention and control of COVID-19 cases at her LTCH.

WHAT IS A GAP AND WHO SHOULD IDENTIFY IT?

Knowledge Translation (KT) is the science and practice of disseminating and implementing evidence into practice (Straus et al., 2009). The first step to implementing knowledge is to determine what the evidence says versus what is actually done in practice. This gap between evidence and practice is sometimes referred to as the **"know-do" gap** (Graham et al., 2006).

It is important to involve relevant stakeholders when identifying and assessing the know-do gap. **Integrated knowledge translation** is the process of involving stakeholders (such as decision-makers, clinicians and practitioners, policy makers, patients and members of the public) throughout the lifecycle of an implementation project (Gagliardi et al., 2015; Kothari & Wathen, 2013; Straus et al., 2013). In an integrated KT approach, stakeholders work closely with practitioners to guide the project from inception (i.e., identifying the problem or research question) to data analysis, interpretation, and support of the creation, evaluation, and dissemination of implementation plans (Gagliardi et al., 2015; Kothari & Wathen, 2013; Straus et al., 2013). The goal of integrated KT is to promote co-creation and collaborative decision-making to ensure the needs of end-users are being appropriately addressed. The use of an integrated KT approach can improve buy-in for implementation efforts, thereby improving evidence uptake, and may result in reduced research waste in the form of both time and resources (Gagliardi et al., 2015; Kothari & Wathen, 2013; Straus et al., 2013). Integrated KT is also sometimes referred to as collaborative research, action-oriented research, or co-produced research (Gagliardi et al., 2015; Jull et al., 2017).

It is important to consider the types of stakeholders that should be included in the identification and assessment of the know-do gap. In this context, we refer to **stakeholders** as individuals who have an interest in the project, either because it relates to them directly, impacts their practices, or because they are involved in the administration, finances or policies that may impact/be impacted by the project (Government of Canada, 2007). End-users are one type of stakeholder who will be directly impacted by the intervention (e.g., healthcare providers who will implement the intervention, patients, caregivers, family members who will be impacted by the intervention; Government of Canada, 2007).

Often, the know-do gap can (and should) be identified and assessed by integrating multiple stakeholder perspectives, including the patient/public, organization/administration, healthcare provider, or policy maker perspectives to determine project priorities and needs (Kitson & Straus, 2010). Therefore, it is important to take time to consider which stakeholders should be included in the identification of the gap. As we consider engaging stakeholders, we should also ensure they reflect the diversity of the population or populations whom implementation will impact. Later in this chapter, we will present concrete steps on how to identify and assess the know-do gap.

Considering Equity When Identifying the Practice Gap

It is important for practitioners to identify their "blind spots" when assessing the know-do gap and reflect on how individual, organizational, and cultural factors impact stakeholder experiences and perceptions of the gap. Such considerations are necessary to ensure that interventions implemented to close the practice gap do not result in disadvantages or drive inequity among certain populations (Bowen et al., 2011). Building on the example presented in Case Study 2.1, as a nurse manager aiming to reduce infection spread in a LTCH, Jessie may be focused on identifying operational gaps in infection prevention and control (e.g., improper hand hygiene, improper use of personal protective equipment). However, by focusing on this practice gap, she may overlook other important problems such as staff burnout during the pandemic, the latter of which may be of greater priority to LTCH staff. If Jessie only addresses infection prevention practices in her know-do gap, she may develop solutions that fail to address stakeholder-important problems or may exacerbate existing problems. For instance, if she aims to reduce infections by minimizing entry into LTCH, she may preclude essential care partners (i.e., families and other caregivers) from supporting the care of residents in the home. This in turn might increase personal support workers' workloads, leading to increased staff burnout and, ultimately, reduced compliance with infection prevention and control practices.

Intersectionality is a concept rooted in Black feminist thought and the advocacy work of Black feminists in the 1980s (Collins, 2002; Crenshaw, 1989, 1991, 1998). Intersectionality underscores that an individual's experience is shaped by a combination of individual factors (e.g., gender, age, ability, race/ethnicity, social capital, religion) occurring within connected systems, cultures, and structures of power (e.g., sexism, ageism, racism; Collins, 2002; Crenshaw, 1989, 1991, 1998; Hankivsky et al., 2014; *Issue 15: Intersectionality—Learning Network—Western University,* 2015). At the beginning of a project, it is important for the research and implementation team to consider which intersecting categories compose their identity within a context of structures of power and oppression, and how these categories may impact their ideologies, internal biases, and overall perceptions of society. With respect to identifying the know-do gap, it is important to consider how identities relate to the project area, and how they may impact work on the implementation project. See **Exhibit 2.1** for an example of a reflective exercise that the implementation and stakeholder team can conduct prior to initiating a project. For more information on how to consider intersecting factors when planning KT work, see the Intersectionality and KT workbook available via the Knowledge Translation Program: https://knowledgetranslation.net/portfolios/intersectionality-and-kt/

When selecting stakeholders to involve in your identification and assessment of the know-do gap, consider the following questions: *What is this person's stake in the implementation process? What is their viewpoint? Can they affect implementation? Are they affected by implementation?*

EXHIBIT 2.1 Intersectionality Reflection Worksheet

Where Am I Situated?

- What intersecting categories make up your identity?[1]
- Reflecting on your response to the preceding question, how do your intersecting categories impact your place in society?[1]
- How do your identities relate to the project's topic area? How might your place in society impact your work on this project?[1]

Who Is on the Implementation Team?

- What does an inclusive approach mean to you?[1]
- What inclusive approaches have been used on your team, in your organization, or in other organizations? What is good or bad about these approaches? Note that not all teams or organizations take an inclusive approach.[1]
- Who is the patient, healthcare provider, and community population affected by the project topic area? What would they want to get out of the project topic area? How do you plan to get them involved?[2]
- What are the real and perceived power differences on the team?[2,3]
- Reflect on whether everyone who could be on the team has been asked if and how they would like to be involved. Think about how different perspectives that represent a range of intersecting categories have been examined.
- Does your team reflect the makeup of the patient, community, and healthcare providers that experience the project topic?[2]

Identifying the Problem

- Whose point of view is reflected when defining the problem? For example, is it the chief executive officer or the nurse who has prioritized a specific problem as the focus of the KT project?
- What are the information gaps in the problem area? How can these gaps be filled? Information gaps are areas where you do not have complete knowledge.

Defining the Evidence-to-Practice Gap

- Who decides which evidence-to-practice gap is prioritized?

Selecting the Practice Change

- Of the practice changes under consideration, who is expected to change their behavior and "do" the practice changes? This "who" could be a health professional, the patient, the community, and/or another group.
- Think about the group expected to change their behavior (e.g., nurses). What intersecting categories of group members can we reflect on? Think about the group affected by the practice change (e.g., patients). What intersecting categories of group members can we reflect on?

(*continued*)

EXHIBIT 2.1 Intersectionality Reflection Worksheet (*continued*)

Appraising Evidence

- What information do I have? What information do I wish I had? Who might have this information? Who should I talk to about this?
- Critically assess the data.

1. Hankivsky, O., Grace, D., Hunting, G, Ferlatte, O., Clark, N., Fridkin, A., Giesbrecht, M., Rudrum, S., & Laviolette, T. (2012). *Intersectionality-based policy analysis. An intersectionality-based policy analysis framework* (pp. 33–45). Institute for Intersectionality Research & Policy.
2. Arthritis Research Canada. (2018). *Workbook to guide the development of a patient engagement in research (PEIR) plan.* https://www.arthritisresearch.ca/wp-content/uploads/2018/06/PEIR-Plan-Guide.pdf
3. Shimmin, C., Wittmeier, K., Lavoie, J., & Sibley, K. (2017). Moving towards a more inclusive patient and public involvement in health research paradigm. *BMC Health Services Research, 17*(1), 539. https://doi.org.10.1186/S12913-017-2463-1

Reproduced with permission from the Knowledge Translation Program.

Who Should Identify Gaps in Practice?

When defining the know-do gap, it is important to consider whose point of view is reflected in the definition. For instance, Jessie's perception of the problem may be quite different than the perception of Claire, a personal support worker. Personal support workers are often racialized women living in multigenerational households, and their perspectives are not typically included in LTCH intervention planning, which may result in inequities (Chamberlain et al., 2019; Estabrooks et al., 2015, 2020; Tannenbaum et al., 2016). It is also important to think about who gets to decide *which* know-do gap is prioritized. The implementation team should aim to ensure relevant and diverse stakeholders are invited to the planning table. Ideally, stakeholders should be selected to reflect the diversity and perceptions of the target population impacted by the know-do gap and targeted by the implementation interventions. This can help reduce information gaps, or "blind spots," which occur when one does not hold complete knowledge. Typically, the **implementation team** leads the process of identifying and assessing the know-do gap; this team will also be responsible for the day-to-day accountability, implementation, and scale up of the evidence-based practices identified. The implementation team is typically composed of a small group of individuals who have dedicated time to support the process of implementing evidence-based practices in response to the know-do gap (*Module 3: Implementation Teams, NIRN*, 2013). The implementation team should also involve additional stakeholders to provide insight throughout the process of identifying and assessing the know-do gap and implementing corresponding evidence-based practice. The key to engagement is ensuring the approach is tailored to stakeholder needs and circumstances.

How Do We Assess the Know-Do Gap?

Step 1: In partnership with your stakeholders, determine the priority practice gap areas.

The implementation team should consider key questions when determining whether the identified gap is a priority to stakeholders, and whether other priority gaps exist. Such questions could include, *Is this an issue of concern? If yes, who is it of concern to? Is there evidence that can be used to determine what should be done? Are there available data to demonstrate what is currently in practice?* In **Exhibit 2.2**, we present a worksheet that can be used to prioritize gaps identified by stakeholders. For this exhibit, the focus is on clinical topic areas and provider practice know-do gaps, however the questions can be adapted to prioritize organizational or system gaps.

EXHIBIT 2.2 Questions to Consider When Prioritizing a Gap in Clinical Practice

Instructions: For each clinical topic area/problem your stakeholder group has identified as a practice gap, go through the following questions and answer either Yes, No, or N/A (not applicable). When all questions have been answered, identify the top five topics with the most "yes" responses. Next, critically reflect on whose opinions the top responses reflect—is there representation of diverse stakeholder opinions? If not, discuss with your team how the topic areas could be defined to ensure they also address the needs of these populations.

QUESTIONS

1. Is the area/problem of clinical concern to patients and/or their families?
2. Is the area/problem of concern to healthcare providers and other stakeholders?
3. Do clinical practice guidelines/evidence exist that you could use to identify best practices to address this area/problem?
4. Are there baseline data available to demonstrate what the practice currently is (at your site, or at the sites you wish to intervene)?
5. Is there sufficient interest from your stakeholders to work on this area/problem?
6. Is there sufficient interest from the frontline/end-users impacted by this area/problem for this implementation work?
7. Is there a local champion that can work on this area/problem?
8. Is there support from management for this area/problem?
9. Does this initiative align with other organizational, regional or national initiatives?
10. Would doing something about this area/problem be:
    a. Feasible?
    b. Practical?
    c. Desirable?
    d. Impactful?

Sources: Straus S.E., Tetroe, K., Graham, I. (2013) *Knowledge translation in health care: Moving from evidence to practice.* John Wiley and Sons; Kitson, A., Straus, S.E. (2010). The knowledge to action cycle: Identifying the gaps. *Canadian Medial Association Journal, 182*(2), E73–77. https://doi.org/10.1503/cmaj.081231

Step 2: In partnership with your stakeholders, identify the best available evidence.

Once priority practice gap areas have been determined, move to identify the best available research evidence for the practice/policy that will be used to address the gap (Graham et al., 2006). Aim to identify research evidence summarized in clinical practice guidelines and best practice recommendations. For instance, the Canadian Task Force on Preventive Health Care (Task Force) synthesizes available evidence to create guidelines for preventive healthcare (e.g., cancer screening; *Canadian Task Force on Preventive Health Care, Published Guidelines*, n.d.; *Recommendation Topics, United States Preventive Services Taskforce*, n.d.). The Task Force first invites key stakeholders, such as professional societies, health organizations, policy makers, and academics to work collaboratively to identify the priority gaps in an area of preventive health (Step 1). Next, the Task Force conducts a comprehensive systematic evidence review to inform the preventive health guideline. Throughout

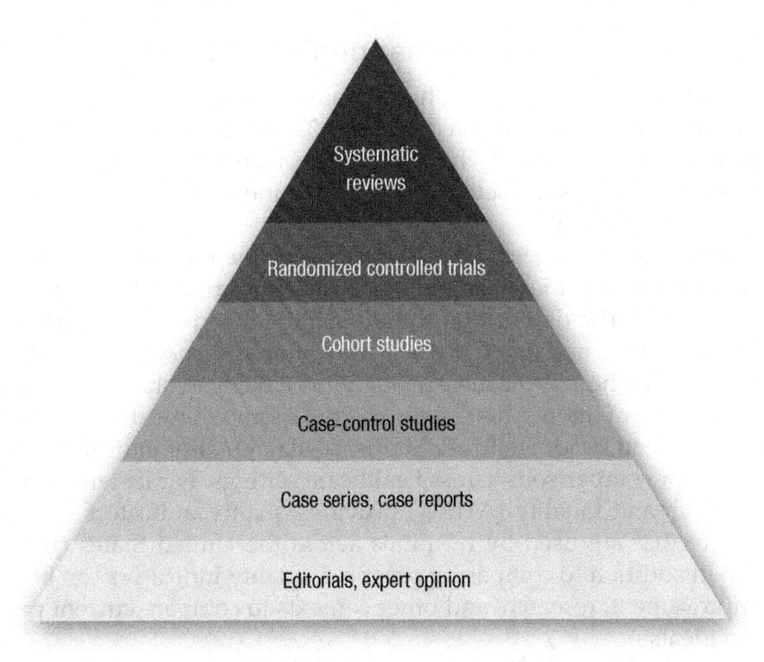

FIGURE 2.1 Evidence pyramid.
Source: Reproduced with permission from Centre for Evidence-Based Medicine. CEBM, Levels of Evidence (2014). https://www.cebm.net/wp-content/uploads/2014/06/CEBM-Levels-of-Evidence-2.1.pdf

the process of reviewing the evidence, the Task Force involves patients and other key stakeholders to select the outcomes and priorities that are of utmost importance to them (*Canadian Task Force on Preventive Health Care, Methods*, 2014). Following the evidence review, patients and other stakeholders (such as clinical experts and peer reviewers) are once again consulted to draft recommendations based on the identified evidence—these recommendations are used to draft and refine the guideline. Finally, the guideline and practice recommendations are disseminated using a variety of formats (e.g., manuscripts, evidence briefs, infographics) to target audiences such as practitioners, patients, or policy makers. Using the example from our case study, Jessie may want to review the World Health Organization (WHO) guidance on infection prevention and control for long-term care facilities in the context of COVID-19 to determine evidence-based practice recommendations for her site (*Infection prevention and control guidance for long-term care facilities in the context of COVID-19*, 2020).

Ideally, evidence to inform the practice/policy will come from high quality clinical practice guidelines, recommendations, or systematic reviews/meta analyses. However, sometimes such evidence is not readily available. In this case, it is important to use the **evidence pyramid** (see Figure 2.1) to determine which evidence is considered high quality. The evidence pyramid underscores that not all evidence is of the same strength; weaker evidence (e.g., expert opinions, case reports) are placed at the bottom of the pyramid while higher quality evidence (e.g., meta analyses, systematic reviews) placed at the top of the pyramid.

The goal is to ensure that only practices/policies with robust supporting evidence are implemented. If such evidence does not exist, or if the evidence-based intervention must be adapted to fit the context/setting, then proceed cautiously with your implementation efforts. It is important not to incorrectly utilize financial, time, or human resources to implement interventions that are not evidence based. If strong evidence does not exist to support the policy or practice, it is critical to plan for a robust process and outcome evaluation at project onset to learn about "what works" within different settings and "why."

Step 3: Assess what is currently happening in practice or policy.

In Step 2, practitioners aim to identify high-quality evidence to determine the practice ideal, or what "should" be implemented. In Step 3, practitioners complete the know-do gap by describing what is currently happening in practice or policy within the project context. This process requires the selection of quality indicators that will be measured to determine the scope of the gap.

A **quality indicator** is a process or healthcare outcome measure that provides a clear description on the measure of interest and how data should be collected and reported for this measure of interest. The description should include the ideal timing and frequency of data collection (how often, and when the measure of interest should be assessed), population of interest (among whom is the measure of interest being evaluated), method of analysis (how is the measure of interest assessed), and the format of results (how is the measure of interest presented and used; Stelfox & Straus, 2013a). Quality indicators are often standardized to allow for comparisons across healthcare settings. For instance, the Agency for Healthcare Research and Quality (AHRQ) provides quality indicators on inpatient care and patient safety that are used by hospitals across the United States (*AHRQ—Quality Indicators*, n.d.). In addition to comparing practices, quality indicators can be used in various quality improvement, research, and other contexts to compare current processes with evidence-based ideals.

It is often helpful to use a **quality improvement** or **implementation science** framework or model to guide the process of measuring the know-do gap. The Donabedian model is a commonly cited framework in the context of quality improvement (Donabedian, 2002). Donabedian highlighted that structures, processes, and outcomes are the three core components of quality as related to healthcare. *Structures* include the organizational and environmental contexts in which care is provided, *processes* refer to the channels and methods of providing care by providers to patients in the system, and *outcomes* refer to patient-important health measures. Donabedian outlined that structures impact processes, which in turn impact outcomes. As such, quality indicators and improvement efforts ought to focus on all three aspects (patient outcomes, processes impacting these outcomes, and the structures impacting these processes) when aiming to improve patient care. In implementation science, process models are descriptive overviews that aim to simplify a phenomenon. One commonly cited model in implementation science is the **Knowledge to Action cycle**, which outlines the iterative process of generating and synthesizing evidence to create evidence-based recommendations and then adapting, implementing, and evaluating that evidence to fit the implementation context, stakeholder needs, and implementation challenges. Notably, the first step in the Knowledge to Action implementation cycle is to connect knowledge syntheses (know) to the practice (do) gap (Graham et al., 2006).

While the origin of the fields of quality improvement and implementation science differs, there are many intersections with the ultimate shared goal of identifying gaps in order to improve patient outcomes (Koczwara et al., 2018). One key distinguishing factor between quality improvement and implementation science is that the latter aims to bring about the implementation of evidence-based interventions using theoretical approaches, while quality improvement aims to evaluate processes as related to structures and outcomes in order to optimize efficiency and quality (Kao, 2014). Yet, when conducting either quality improvement or implementation science, it is important to (a) have the buy-in of end users in order to identify stakeholder-important issues; (b) assess the organizational, environmental, and structural factors that, in addition to human behavior, impact behaviors, processes, and outcomes; and (c) iteratively measure and evaluate efforts to ensure the ideal/evidence-based practice is implemented as intended, over time.

How Do We Select a Quality Indicator?

When selecting a quality indicator, it is important to first review the evidence to identify existing indicators and then subsequently examine the strength and evidence of these indicators. Indicators can be identified using knowledge syntheses that include both peer-reviewed, published evidence (Campbell et al., 2003; Stelfox & Straus, 2013b; e.g., manuscripts, guidelines in academic journals) and the grey literature (e.g., websites such as *AHRQ—Quality Indicators,* n.d.) and established databases such as the Society of Thoracic Surgeons National Database for cardiothoracic surgery (n.d.). Quality indicators can undoubtedly be used to measure patient outcomes, but can also be used to assess organizational, system processes, and outcomes. For instance, using the example in our case study, Jessie could choose to focus on patient (i.e., LTCH resident) outcomes such as number of COVID-19–related infections, hospitalizations and deaths, and/or organizational outcomes such as rate of compliance with infection prevention and control recommendations such as entrance screening or masking.

When selecting an indicator, it is important to consider whether the measure is reliable (reproducible) and valid (whether it measures what it is intended to measure), but also acceptable to the needs of the project stakeholders and the goals of the gap assessment (Stelfox & Straus, 2013a). Creating a valid quality indicator is not simple, and practitioners are strongly encouraged to first ensure there are no existing indicators that can be used or enhanced/adapted to assess the gap. In the event that a valid indicator is not identified, one can be developed using high-quality evidence and a rating process (Monica & California, 1967; Turoff & Linstone, 1975). Developing a new indicator begins with a knowledge synthesis (e.g., via a systematic, scoping, or rapid review) to identify the factors that impact a measure of interest (Core Library of Qualitative Synthesis Methodology, 2021; Morton et al., 2018; *Research guides: Knowledge syntheses…,* n.d.; Tricco et al., 2017, 2018). *The Joanna Briggs Institute Manual for Evidence Synthesis* can be used to guide the conduct and reporting of scoping reviews (Peters et al., 2020). Rapid reviews are a form of knowledge synthesis that streamline components of the systematic review process, allowing stakeholders such as patients, clinicians, and policy makers timely access to evidence-based health information (Tricco et al., 2017). Tools such as Tricco et al.'s *What Review Is Right for You* web-based tool can guide practitioners to select the form of knowledge synthesis that may be most appropriate for their project (available at: https://whatreviewisrightforyou.knowledgetranslation.net).

Once potential process or outcome measures are identified during knowledge synthesis, a rating process such as a Delphi technique can be used to rank the importance of identified measures to inform the development of quality indicators. A Delphi study provides consensus on a topic by a group of experts (Hasson et al., 2000; Okoli & Pawlowski, 2004). Typically, Delphi studies put forth multiple rounds (at least 2–3) of questionnaires canvassing expert opinion, aiming to generate a minimum level of consensus (e.g., 70%) and allowing for discussions and revisions of answers following each round. Delphi studies can be used to prioritize, rate, or select topics and indicators for implementation. The Delphi panel should include relevant stakeholder experts (e.g., patients or individuals with lived experience) in addition to content experts. Once the Delphi process is used to create the quality indicator, the indicator should be piloted in a practice setting to ensure acceptability, feasibility, validity, and reliability. See **Box 2.1,** adapted from Stelfox's work (2013b), for key considerations when selecting a quality indicator (Stelfox, 2013). Practitioners may also choose to use a real-time Delphi as an alternative approach to the traditional Delphi method that aims to improve efficiency by forgeoing the use of multiple "rounds"

BOX 2.1 Considerations for Selecting Quality Indicators

When selecting a quality indicator, first determine if one already exists. If not, an indicator can be developed using knowledge syntheses, consensus generating processes, and evaluation of the indicator for implementation.

When selecting or developing an indicator, consider whether the indicator is:

- Important (will be of relevance to the target stakeholders, end users)?
- Evidence-based (the measure is reliable and valid)?
- Feasible (can be implemented in the project context)?
- Usable (the stakeholders and end-users understand the data and can use them to inform decision-making, intervention planning)?

Source: Adapted from Stelfox, H. T. (2013). *How to develop quality indicators?* (p. 28). Institute for Public Health: Innovation for Health and Health Care

of consensus ratings (Gnatzy, 2011; Gordon & Pease, 2006). Practitioners may also consider use of a Nominal Group Technique, during which a skilled facilitator presents questions, ideas, or options to participants and asks participants to share their ideas and reflections on these items. Following a group discussion, participants rank items using a Likert scale and multiple rounds of ranking are held until the top items emerge (Hugé & Mukherjee, 2018).

How Can We Measure the Know-Do Gap?

Once relevant quality indicators have been selected, assessors can proceed to measure the gap between current and ideal practice (which is informed by evidence). This assessment can be informed by a wide range of data sources including needs assessments with key stakeholders (e.g., interviews, in-depth discussions, focus groups), patient-level or clinical-level administrative datasets, direct observation, competency assessments, or chart/audit data. For questions to consider when beginning a chart audit, see **Exhibit 2.3**. Assessors should select quality indicators suitable to the goal of the assessment and the topic of interest (Kitson & Straus, 2010; Strifler et al., 2018). Additionally, different sources should be used to measure gaps at the population, organization, or care provider levels. If possible, multiple sources of data can be collected and triangulated to obtain a holistic understanding of the practice gap.

EXHIBIT 2.3 Questions to Consider When Beginning a Chart Audit

Questions About Comparing Actual and Desired Clinical Practice	Yes/No/Not sure
Before you measure: ▪ Have you secured sufficient stakeholder interest and involvement? ▪ Have you selected an appropriate topic? ▪ Have you identified the right sort of people, skills, and resources? ▪ Have you considered ethical issues?	

(continued)

EXHIBIT 2.3 Questions to Consider When Beginning a Chart Audit (*continued*)

Questions About Comparing Actual and Desired Clinical Practice	Yes/No/Not sure
What to measure: ■ Should your criteria be explicit or implicit? ■ Should your criteria relate to the structure, process or outcomes of care? ■ Do your criteria have sufficient impact to lead to improvements in care? ■ What level of performance is appropriate to aim for?	
How to measure: ■ Is the information you need available? ■ How are you identifying an appropriate sample of patients? ■ How big should your sample be? ■ How to choose a representative sample? ■ How will you collect the information? ■ How will you interpret the information?	

Reproduced from NorthStar (www.rebeqi.org) and taken from Kitson and Straus. Reprinted with permission from *Canadian Medical Association Journal.*

Table 2.1 provides an overview of considerations, including strengths and limitations, on using various data sources to measure gaps at the population, organization, and care provider levels.

TABLE 2.1 Data Sources to Measure Practice Gaps

DATA SOURCE	EXAMPLE	STRENGTHS	LIMITATIONS	LEVEL OF GAP
Administrative/ clinical database	Health insurance claims databases (e.g., CMS, OHIP), DHIS2 platform commonly used in low-and-middle income countries	Objective measures Large sample, population-level trends	May not have information needed for the quality indicator Databases may have incomplete data, incorrectly coded data Database may not include all members of the population (specifically underrepresented groups—e.g., uninsured patients)	Can be used to assess the gap at the population level

(*continued*)

TABLE 2.1 Data Sources to Measure Practice Gaps (*continued*)

DATA SOURCE	EXAMPLE	STRENGTHS	LIMITATIONS	LEVEL OF GAP
Patient database	Database of patients in a certain organization, health authority, hospital and so forth	Objective measures Typically, a large sample Can be used to identify trends in certain populations (e.g., a hospital, a division)	May not have information needed for the quality indicator Databases may have incomplete data, incorrectly tracked data Database may not include all members of the population (specifically underrepresented groups—e.g., uninsured patients)	Can be used to assess the gap at the population or organizational level
Chart audit/local audit data	Paper-based or electronic patient record audit to identify documentation on patient outcomes (e.g., delirium in acute care hospitals) or process measures (e.g., clinician documentation of falls risk for frail, older adults admitted to acute care hospitals)	Can provide detailed, granular patient-related information Electronic patient records facilitate extraction of such data	Data may not be complete or legible (e.g., handwritten notes in paper charts) Require significant time to complete (particularly for paper charts)	Can be used to assess the gap at the organizational or care-provider level
Direct observation	Direct observations or recordings on routine processes or via simulation to demonstrate skills (e.g., standardized patients)	Objective assessment Can be tailored to assess the topic of interest	Resource intensive May be subject to Hawthorne bias May not capture actual practice	Can be used to assess the gap at the care-provider level

(*continued*)

TABLE 2.1 Data Sources to Measure Practice Gaps ***(continued)***

DATA SOURCE	EXAMPLE	STRENGTHS	LIMITATIONS	LEVEL OF GAP
Competency assessment	Multiple choice examination to assess knowledge	Objective assessment Can be tailored to assess the topic of interest	May be resource intensive May not capture actual practice	Can be used to assess the gap at the care-provider level
Needs assessments with key stakeholders	In-depth discussions, key informant interviews or focus groups with stakeholders and/or end users	Can be used to elicit perceptions of participants. Can be used to contextualize the problem/ needs and tailor solutions to these contexts.	May be resource intensive Limitations include subjectivity of participant perceptions	Can be used to assess gaps at the care-provider, organizational or system level (based on participant perceptions)

CMS, Centers for Medicare & Medicaid Services; DHIS2, District Health Information Software; OHIP, Ontario Health Insurance Plan.

Adapted from Kitson, A., & Straus, S. E. (2010). The knowledge-to-action cycle: Identifying the gaps. *CMAJ*, *182*(2), E73–E77. https://doi.org/10.1503/cmaj.081231

See **Case Study 2.2** for an example of how Jessie can identify practice gaps in LTCH at both the organizational and population levels.

CASE STUDY 2.2 IDENTIFYING GAPS AT THE ORGANIZATIONAL LEVEL

Jessie, a nurse manager at a LTCH, has been tasked with ensuring the LTCH at which she works minimizes the spread of COVID-19 infections among LTCH staff and residents. First, Jessie reviews the literature and identifies a current, WHO-developed, evidence-based guideline on how to prevent and control infectious disease outbreaks in LTCHs. Additionally, Jessie is able to identify corresponding KT tools to support the implementation of this guideline (e.g., a LTCH COVID-19 infection prevention and control [IPAC] checklist). Next, Jessie assembles a project steering committee and stakeholder panel, which includes various LTCH staff (e.g., physicians, nurses, personal support workers, housekeeping, and kitchen staff), resident family members and essential care givers, and the leadership of the LTCH. Together, they prioritize the IPAC practices that require immediate implementation, using a ranking exercise. The team selected the following practices:

- Improving screening assessments and entry into the LTCH
- Ensuring proper use of personal protective equipment (e.g., masking, gloves, gowns) and hand hygiene

(*continued*)

CASE STUDY 2.2 IDENTIFYING GAPS AT THE ORGANIZATIONAL LEVEL (*continued*)

- Improving processes of physical distancing while maintaining staff wellness and daily activities
- Implementing wellness initiatives to reduce burnout and improve morale among frontline LTCH staff, particularly personal support workers

The team worked together with implementation practitioners from the local university to identify appropriate quality indicators to assess the preceding areas and conducted direct observations, documentation audits using LTCH internal records and administrative databases to compare current practice gaps (e.g., related to behaviors, supplies, knowledge, and so forth) to guideline recommendations.

When determining which quality indicators to select, the team considered the following questions:

DEFINING THE PROBLEM

1. What local data do we have that tell us that we have a problem?
2. What do colleagues think about the problem?
3. How are we currently managing the issue?
4. What do our end-users and stakeholders think about this problem?
5. What research evidence exists about what best practice is?
6. Describe what "success" would look like if we addressed this problem.
7. What indicators are available for us to assess the problem?
8. How reliable are the sources of data?
9. Who needs to be on the team to make this work? Who else needs to provide buy-in?
10. Who is on the team? What skills do they have? What biases do they hold? Are there other perspectives/individuals that should be brought on to the team?
11. How will we keep team members and stakeholders interested in the work for the duration of the project?
12. What sources of funding do we have to conduct this work?
13. What is a reasonable timeline to implement the intervention(s)?
14. How can we begin to plan for sustainability of the intervention(s)?

Adapted from Kitson, A. L., Wiechula, R., Salmons, S., & Jordan, Z. (2012). *Knowledge translation in healthcare.* Lippincott Williams & Wilkins.

Why Do Gaps Exist?

Gaps may exist because new evidence needs to be implemented, de-implemented, or processes need to be improved. When assessing a gap, it is important to assess not only *what* is being done compared to the ideal practice, but also to assess *why* these actions exist. In addition to individual-level factors that determine behavior, there are organizational- and systems-level factors that impact why (or why not) evidence is implemented or de-implemented. A plethora of implementation science determinant frameworks, as found in Strifler et al. (2018), and Nilsen (2020), such as the Theoretical Domains Framework (Cane et al., 2012; Michie & Prestwich, 2010), and the Consolidated Framework for Implementation Research (Damschroder et al., 2009) can be used to assess these barriers and identify facilitators. Barriers and facilitators at the individual, organizational, systems, and policy levels can be assessed to understand the "why"; these factors can be mapped to corresponding strategies to mitigate barriers and leverage facilitators.

In quality improvement, the Donabedian model similarly highlights that both structure and process factors can ultimately impact outcomes (Damschroder et al., 2009). Methods such as root cause analysis may be used to identify upstream problems leading to negative outcomes. Root cause analysis, while commonly used in science and engineering (e.g., aviation industry) has also been used in medicine (*Root Cause Analysis*, 2019). For instance, root cause analysis has been used to assess negative outcomes in surgery and use an "upstream" approach to identify and mitigate potentially preventive complications (Johna et al., 2012). Methods on the conduct of root cause analysis in a clinical context are provided by Charles et al. in *Patient Safety in Surgery* (2016). Another example is cascade analysis, which can be performed to evaluate the impact of various interventions that may have a cumulative impact on outcomes (for instance, evaluating the intensity of a treatment/intervention for HIV in the testing and/or treatment and/or follow up period). Through cascade analysis, practitioners can aim to assess the impact of the intervention at different stages to optimize strategies. Indicators in cascade analysis are often longitudinal or cross-sectional, to demonstrate impact over time. The WHO provides methodological guidance on cascade analysis methods using a 10-step approach (World Health Organization, Regional Office for the Eastern Mediterranean, 2017).

Practitioners should aim to clearly define challenges to identifying and addressing know-do gaps. For instance, lack of relevant or patient-important quality indicators or insufficient data to assess gaps are barriers to conducting a know-do gap analysis. Further, methods on how to incorporate an equity and intersectionality lens in the process of identifying, measuring, and assessing the gap is an area that requires additional research and development.

EXAMPLES OF KNOW-DO GAPS

Below are real-world examples of know-do gaps. Each of the following examples generally follows the same structure. First, the priority practice gap area (i.e., the problem) is identified in collaboration with key stakeholders. Next, evidence to inform these practice gaps is identified—where possible, use high-quality evidence (e.g., high-quality guidelines, systematic reviews, and meta analyses) to inform practice (the "know"). Finally, an assessment of what is currently happening in practice is completed (the "do"). This is often followed by a barriers and facilitators assessment to better understand why a practice gap exists and to identify strategies to close the gap.

Use of Misoprostol to Prevent Postpartum Hemorrhage in Low- and Middle-Income Countries

Postpartum hemorrhage (PPH), or extreme blood loss following childbirth, is the leading cause of maternal death and morbidity worldwide (Bazirete et al., 2021). In partnership with four low- and middle-income (LMIC) countries, the Guideline-driven, Research priorities, Evidence Synthesis, Application of evidence, and Transfer of knowledge (GREAT) Network used KT methods to implement evidence-based guidelines aimed at preventing maternal morbidity and mortality (Puchalski Ritchie et al., 2016; Vogel et al., 2016). First, local stakeholders (including frontline healthcare workers, senior administrators, researchers, and policy makers) from four target LMIC countries were engaged in a priority-setting exercise to identify key priorities related to maternal health. During this exercise, stakeholders identified prevention and management of PPH as a key priority. The GREAT network team used the WHO guidelines on the prevention and perinatal management of PPH to provide evidence-based recommendations related to PPH in LMICs. The team held workshops and focus groups with stakeholders to determine (a) what was currently being done in practice to prevent and manage PPH, and (b) to prioritize PPH prevention guideline recommendations for implementation based on feasibility, importance and acceptability (*GREAT Network, Products*, 2011). This assessment demonstrated an underuse of misoprostol, a medication recommended in several WHO maternal health guidelines to prevent PPH (WHO, 2012). A barriers and facilitators assessment revealed that stakeholders were hesitant to use this drug out of fear that it would be misused to unsafely terminate pregnancy or induce labor; therefore, the medication was not approved for use in some countries (Puchalski Ritchie et al., 2016). In others, supply chain gaps created significant barriers, resulting in a lack of misoprostol availability to healthcare providers. To address the know-do gap of underuse of misoprostol to prevent PPH, the GREAT network focused on implementing strategies at the policy level (ensuring availability of misoprostol in the supply chain); organizational level (approval of misoprostol use for PPH in healthcare settings); and provider level (providing education about the medication, task shifting to determine whose role it is to prescribe misoprostol and when; *GREAT Network, Products*, 2011).

Mobilizing Older Adults in Hospitals

Typically, older adults admitted to hospitals are immediately put to bed, leading them to spend significant amounts of time lying down. This immobility is directly related to functional decline, leading to loss of muscle strength, increased inflammation, and decreased functional and cognitive status (Brown et al., 2004, 2009). An implementation team composed of clinicians, patient advocates, healthcare managers, and researchers conducted a study entitled *Mobilization of Vulnerable Elders (MOVE) to improve mobilization of older adults in 16 university-affiliated Canadian hospitals* (Moore et al., 2019). The research team identified the following evidence-based recommendations in which their implementation efforts were rooted: (a) all patients over 65 should be assessed for mobility within 24 hours of admission; (b) patients should be mobilized at least 3 times/day; and (c) mobilization should be progressive and scaled to each individual patient's ability (Callen et al., 2004; Liu et al., 2013, 2018). These recommendations were informed using randomized trial evidence and a Cochrane systematic review on use of exercise interventions for hospitalized older patients. The evidence demonstrated reduced hospital length of stay, functional decline, and reduced healthcare costs when patients were mobilized (de Morton et al., 2007). Despite this strong evidence, surveys across Canadian hospitals showed an underuse of early mobilization among older adults in various hospital units including cardiology, medical stepdown, orthopedics, and surgery (Finely et al., 2011; Liu et al., 2013). The MOVE team conducted a barriers and facilitators assessment among hospitals in Ontario, Canada, and identified barriers to mobilization at the patient ("I'm scared to fall if I move while in the hospital"), provider ("It's not my job as the physician to mobilize patients"), and organizational ("Where in the hospital should patients be mobilized?") levels. Facilitators that could be leveraged to support older adult mobilization were also identified during the assessment ("Once I encouraged my patients to move, many did it on their own and I saw improvements so quickly"). Therefore, to address the know-do gap of low rates of older adult mobilization while in the hospital, the MOVE team implemented education sessions and materials for patients and providers and used reminders and mobility champions to increase rates of mobilization (*MOVEs Canada: Getting Ready*, 2011). These efforts were scaled up in a subsequent intervention called MOVE-ON across the country (Moore et al., 2014; *MOVEs Canada: Getting Ready*, 2011).

Discontinuation of Tight Blood Glucose Control in ICU Patients

The first two examples describe scenarios where evidence-based recommendations (e.g., use of misoprostol to prevent PPH, mobilization of older adults when in the hospital to reduce functional decline) were not being implemented into practice. However, the know-do gap can also arise when current implemented practices are not aligned with evidence-based recommendations—and efforts to address this are known as de-implementation (Norton & Chambers, 2020). Low-value or inappropriate care is a growing concern among the research and healthcare community; the discontinuation of low-value or potentially harmful medications is an example of an evidence-based de-implementation effort. For instance, clinical trials have shown the risks of using medications to achieve tight glycemic control in older adults with type II diabetes (ACCORD Study Group et al., 2011; Action to Control Cardiovascular Risk in Diabetes Study Group et al., 2008; ADVANCE Collaborative Group et al., 2008; Canadian Diabetes Association Clinical Practice Guidelines Expert Committee & Cheng, 2013; Duckworth et al., 2009; *Geriatrics—Choosing Wisely*, 2013). The hemoglobin A1c test can provide an indicator of a person's blood sugar, as people who have diabetes typically have A1c levels of 6.5% or higher. Physicians often use medications to bring glycated hemoglobin levels (i.e., blood sugar levels) down to below 7%. However, data show that among most older adults, tight glycemic control results in higher rates of hypoglycemia (low blood sugar), which can cause harm or mortality (*Geriatrics—Choosing Wisely*, 2013). This is especially true among adults with comorbidities or shorter life expectancies, such as patients in ICUs. Therefore, the know-do gap is that tight glucose control should be reduced among most older adults in hospital, particularly those in ICU (the "know"); however, providers continue to use medications to achieve this tight control, despite evidence of potential harm to patients (the "do"). Researchers are currently in the process of assessing the factors that prevent de-implementation of this low-value practice as well as evaluating the impact of strategies to guide de-implementation and promote appropriate medication use (Nilsen, 2020; Niven, 2015).

SUMMARY

This chapter reviews various approaches to identifying the "know-do" gap in practice including the use of relevant quality indicators. While understanding what the gap is, it is also critically important to understand why this gap exists to ensure that relevant implementation strategies are developed.

KEY POINTS FOR PRACTICE

1. Identifying gaps in practice compared to evidence (know-do gap) is the first step to knowledge implementation.

2. The process of identifying, assessing, and addressing know-do gaps should always be done in consultation with project stakeholders, keeping in mind an intersectionality

lens or other similar conceptual approach that allows reflection on biases and systems of privilege and oppression to facilitate emphasis on equity and inclusion.

3. Quality indicators to assess practice gaps should be rooted in high-quality evidence and should be assessed for validity, reliability, and appropriateness to stakeholder need and feasibility within the implementation context. If quality indicators are not readily available, they can be developed using evidence synthesis (e.g., scoping review, rapid review) and consensus processes (e.g., Delphi methodology).
4. Various data sources can be used to assess quality indicators to inform the gap assessment. Consider the advantages and disadvantages of each source and, when possible, aim to triangulate the gap assessment using multiple sources of data.
5. In addition to understanding *what* the gap is, it is also important to understand *why* the gap exists to develop corresponding implementation strategies. Various theoretically rooted implementation science determinant frameworks and/or quality improvement methodologies can be used to identify and address the *why.*

COMMON PITFALLS IN PRACTICE

1. Project stakeholders may prioritize gaps differently than the project team. It is important to include a diverse set of stakeholders at project onset and use an equitable and collaborative approach to determine which gaps will be prioritized for assessment and evidence implementation.
2. Quality indicators must be evidence based, valid, and reliable to provide an objective assessment of actual versus ideal practice. Taking time to select high-quality indicators at project onset is important to overall success.
3. Sometimes it is difficult to keep stakeholders and end-users engaged throughout a project. Develop trust by co-establishing regular communication and engagement strategies for the duration of the project period. Ensure sufficient funds are dedicated to support engagement and compensation for stakeholder/end-user time.
4. Be mindful that it takes time to build trust, navigate institutional/institutional review board processes, and implement an intervention. Ensure your timelines are appropriate and plan for sustainability from project onset.

DISCUSSION QUESTIONS

1. Who are the project stakeholders, and what perspectives do they bring to the table? Reflect on your own project team: Are any perspectives missing from the target population, healthcare provider, or administration/management team that should be included?
2. How do you tailor engagement of stakeholders to their needs across the duration of the project?
3. What quality indicators are appropriate for your intervention and will facilitate your assessment of the know-do gap? Is it feasible for your team to develop quality indicators using established methods?

FINAL NOTE

Identifying gaps in actual practice as compared to evidence-based ideals is the starting point for implementation. Often, we rush to implementation without spending sufficient time understanding "what" it is that we are implementing. If we don't spend time clarifying this, our implementation efforts will fail. Practitioners should use evidence-based quality indicators and appropriate data sources to assess the practice gap, recognizing the limitations and advantages of each data source. Practitioners should also consider rooting their know-do gap assessment in an implementation science or quality improvement conceptual framework. Prioritization and assessment of the gap should be done in constant collaboration with project stakeholders who should reflect the diversity and perspectives of the target population or populations. Determinant frameworks to understand why practice gaps exist can be used to develop corresponding theoretically rooted, evidence-based solutions.

ACKNOWLEDGMENT

The authors thank Sarah Deshpande for supporting the formatting and references for this chapter.

REFERENCES

ACCORD Study Group, Gerstein, H. C., Miller, M. E., Genuth, S., Ismail-Beigi, F., Buse, J. B., Goff, D. C., Probstfield, J. L., Cushman, W. C., Ginsberg, H. N., Bigger, J. T., Grimm, R. H., Byington, R. P., Rosenberg, Y. D., & Friedewald, W. T. (2011). Long-term effects of intensive glucose lowering on cardiovascular outcomes. *The New England Journal of Medicine, 364*(9), 818–828. https://doi.org/10.1056/NEJMoa1006524

Action to Control Cardiovascular Risk in Diabetes Study Group, Gerstein, H. C., Miller, M. E., Byington, R. P., Goff, D. C., Bigger, J. T., Buse, J. B., Cushman, W. C., Genuth, S., Ismail-Beigi, F., Grimm, R. H., Probstfield, J. L., Simons-Morton, D. G., & Friedewald, W. T. (2008). Effects of intensive glucose lowering in type 2 diabetes. *The New England Journal of Medicine, 358*(24), 2545–2559. https://doi.org/10.1056/NEJMoa0802743

ADVANCE Collaborative Group, Patel, A., MacMahon, S., Chalmers, J., Neal, B., Billot, L., Woodward, M., Marre, M., Cooper, M., Glasziou, P., Grobbee, D., Hamet, P., Harrap, S., Heller, S., Liu, L., Mancia, G., Mogensen, C. E., Pan, C., Poulter, N., ... Travert, F. (2008). Intensive blood glucose control and vascular outcomes in patients with type 2 diabetes. *The New England Journal of Medicine, 358*(24), 2560–2572. https://doi.org/10.1056/NEJMoa0802987

AHRQ—Quality Indicators. (n.d.). Retrieved May 18, 2021, from https://www.qualityindicators.ahrq.gov/

Bazirete, O., Nzayirambaho, M., Chantal, U., Umubyeyi, A., & Marilyn, E. (2021). Factors affecting the prevention of postpartum hemorrhage in Low-and Middle-Income Countries: A scoping review of the literature. *Journal of Nursing Education and Practice, 11*. https://doi.org/10.5430/jnep.v11n1p66

Bowen, S., Botting, I., & Roy, J. (2011). *Promoting action on equity issues: A knowledge-to-action handbook*. School of Public Health, University of Alberta. http://www.publichealth.ualberta.ca/research/research_publications.aspx

Brown, C. J., Friedkin, R. J., & Inouye, S. K. (2004). Prevalence and outcomes of low mobility in hospitalized older patients. *Journal of the American Geriatrics Society, 52*(8), 1263–1270. https://doi.org/10.1111/j.1532-5415.2004.52354.x

Brown, C. J., Redden, D. T., Flood, K. L., & Allman, R. M. (2009). The underrecognized epidemic of low mobility during hospitalization of older adults. *Journal of the American Geriatrics Society, 57*(9), 1660–1665. https://doi.org/10.1111/j.1532-5415.2009.02393.x

Callen, B. L., Mahoney, J. E., Grieves, C. B., Wells, T. J., & Enloe, M. (2004). Frequency of hallway ambulation by hospitalized older adults on medical units of an academic hospital. *Geriatric Nursing (New York, N.Y.), 25*(4), 212–217. https://doi.org/10.1016/j.gerinurse.2004.06.016

Campbell, S. M., Braspenning, J., Hutchinson, A., & Marshall, M. N. (2003). Research methods used in developing and applying quality indicators in primary care. *BMJ (Clinical Research Ed.), 326*(7393), 816–819. https://doi.org/10.1136/bmj.326.7393.816

Canadian Diabetes Association Clinical Practice Guidelines Expert Committee, & Cheng, A. Y. Y. (2013). Canadian Diabetes Association 2013 clinical practice guidelines for the prevention and management of diabetes in Canada. Introduction. *Canadian Journal of Diabetes, 37*(Suppl. 1), S1–S3. https://doi.org/10.1016/j.jcjd.2013.01.009

Canadian Task Force on Preventive Health Care | Published Guidelines. (n.d). Canadian Task Force on Preventive Health Care. https://canadiantaskforce.ca/guidelines/published-guidelines/

Canadian Task Force on Preventive Health Care | Methods. (2014). Canadiantaskforce.ca. Retrieved May 19, 2021, from https://canadiantaskforce.ca/methods/

Cane, J., O'Connor, D., & Michie, S. (2012). Validation of the theoretical domains framework for use in behaviour change and implementation research. *Implementation Science*, *7*(1), 37. https://doi.org/10.1186/1748-5908-7-37

Chamberlain, S. A., Hoben, M., Squires, J. E., Cummings, G. G., Norton, P., & Estabrooks, C. A. (2019). Who is (still) looking after mom and dad? Few improvements in Care Aides' Quality-of-Work Life. *Canadian Journal on Aging / La Revue Canadienne Du Vieillissement*, *38*(1), 35–50. https://doi.org/10.1017/S0714980818000338

Charles, R., Hood, B., Derosier, J. M., Gosbee, J. W., Li, Y., Caird, M. S., Biermann, J. S., & Hake, M. E. (2016). How to perform a root cause analysis for workup and future prevention of medical errors: A review. *Patient Safety in Surgery*, *10*(1), 20. https://doi.org/10.1186/s13037-016-0107-8

Collins, P. H. (2002). *Black feminist thought: Knowledge, consciousness, and the politics of empowerment*. Routledge.

Core Library of Qualitative Synthesis Methodology. (2021). *Cochrane methods: Qualitative and implementation*. Retrieved May 18, 2021, from /qi/core-library-qualitative-synthesis-methodology

Crenshaw, K. (1989). *De-marginalizing the intersection of race and sex: A black feminist critique of antidiscrimination doctrine, feminist theory and antiracist politics*. University of Chicago Legal Forum.

Crenshaw, K. (1991). Mapping the margins: Intersectionality, identity politics, and violence against women of color. *Stanford Law Review*, *43*(6), 1241–1299. https://doi.org/10.2307/1229039

Crenshaw, K. (1998). A Black feminist critique of antidiscrimination law and politics. In *The politics of law: A progressive critique* (3rd ed., 752 pp. [p. 195]). Basic Books.

Damschroder, L. J., Aron, D. C., Keith, R. E., Kirsh, S. R., Alexander, J. A., & Lowery, J. C. (2009). Fostering implementation of health services research findings into practice: A consolidated framework for advancing implementation science. *Implementation Science*, *4*(1), 50. https://doi.org/10.1186/1748-5908-4-50

de Morton, N. A., Keating, J. L., & Jeffs, K. (2007). Exercise for acutely hospitalised older medical patients. *The Cochrane Database of Systematic Reviews*, *1*, CD005955. https://doi.org/10.1002/14651858.CD005955.pub2

Donabedian, A. (2002). *An introduction to quality assurance in health care*. Oxford University Press.

Duckworth, W., Abraira, C., Moritz, T., Reda, D., Emanuele, N., Reaven, P. D., Zieve, F. J., Marks, J., Davis, S. N., Hayward, R., Warren, S. R., Goldman, S., McCarren, M., Vitek, M. E., Henderson, W. G., Huang, G. D., & VADT Investigators. (2009). Glucose control and vascular complications in veterans with type 2 diabetes. *The New England Journal of Medicine*, *360*(2), 129–139. https://doi.org/10.1056/NEJMoa0808431

Estabrooks, C. A., Squires, J. E., Carleton, H. L., Cummings, G. G., & Norton, P. G. (2015). Who is looking after mom and dad? Unregulated workers in Canadian long-term care homes. *Canadian Journal on Aging / La Revue Canadienne Du Vieillissement*, *34*(1), 47–59. https://doi.org/10.1017/S0714980814000506

Estabrooks, C. A., Straus, S. E., Flood, C. M., Keefe, J., Armstrong, P., Donner, G. J., Boscart, V., Ducharme, F., Silvius, J. L., & Wolfson, M. C. (2020). Restoring trust: COVID-19 and the future of long-term care in Canada. *Facts*, *5*(1). https://doi.org/10.1139/facets-2020-0056

Finely, E., McCarthy, E., & Borrie, M. (2011). *A Summary of Senior Friendly Care in South West LHIN Hospitals* (p. 41). Ontario South West Local Health Integration Network. https://www.rgptoronto.ca/wp-content/uploads/2018/03/SFH_Summary_of_SW_LHIN_2011-1.pdf

Gagliardi, A. R., Berta, W., Kothari, A., Boyko, J., & Urquhart, R. (2015). Integrated knowledge translation (IKT) in health care: A scoping review. *Implementation Science*, *11*(1), 1–12.

Geriatrics—Meds for type 2 diabetes control | Choosing Wisely. (2013, February 21). https://www.choosingwisely.org/clinician-lists/american-geriatrics-society-medication-to-control-type-2-diabetes/

Gordon, T., & Pease, A. (2006). RT Delphi: An efficient, "round-less" almost real time Delphi method. *Technological Forecasting and Social Change*, *73*(4), 321–333. https://doi.org/10.1016/j.techfore.2005.09.005

Government of Canada, C. I. of H. R. (2007, May 14). *Glossary of funding-related terms—CIHR*. https://cihr-irsc.gc.ca/e/34190.html

Graham, I. D., Logan, J., Harrison, M. B., Straus, S. E., Tetroe, J., Caswell, W., & Robinson, N. (2006). Lost in knowledge translation: Time for a map? *Journal of Continuing Education in the Health Professions*, *26*(1), 13–24. https://doi.org/10.1002/chp.47

GREAT Network | Products. (2011). Retrieved May 19, 2021, from https://greatnetworkglobal.org/products/

Hankivsky, O., Grace, D., Hunting, G., Giesbrecht, M., Fridkin, A., Rudrum, S., Ferlatte, O., & Clark, N. (2014). An intersectionality-based policy analysis framework: Critical reflections on a methodology for advancing equity. *International Journal for Equity in Health*, *13*(1), 119. https://doi.org/10.1186/s12939-014-0119-x

Hasson, F., Keeney, S., & McKenna, H. (2000). Research guidelines for the Delphi survey technique. *Journal of Advanced Nursing*, *32*(4), 1008–1015. https://doi.org/10.1046/j.1365-2648.2000.t01-1-01567.x

Hugé, J., & Mukherjee, N. (2018). The nominal group technique in ecology & conservation: Application and challenges. *Methods in Ecology And Evolution*, *9*(1), 33–41. https://doi.org/10.1111/2041-210x.12831

Infection prevention and control guidance for long-term care facilities in the context of COVID-19. (2020, March). World Health Organization. https://www.who.int/publications-detail-redirect/WHO-2019-nCoV-IPC-long-term-care-2020-1

Issue 15: Intersectionality—Learning Network—Western University. (2015, October). Western Education Centre for Research & Education on Violence against Women and Children Learning Network. http://www.vawlearningnetwork.ca/our-work/issuebased_newsletters/issue-15/index.html

Johna, S., Tang, T., & Saidy, M. (2012). Patient safety in surgical residency: Root cause analysis and the surgical morbidity and mortality conference—Case series from clinical practice. *The Permanente Journal, 16*(1), 67–69. https://doi.org/10.7812/tpp/11-097

Jull, J., Giles, A., & Graham, I. D. (2017). Community-based participatory research and integrated knowledge translation: Advancing the co-creation of knowledge. *Implementation Science, 12*(1), 1–9. https://doi.org/10.1186/s13012-017-0696-3

Kao, L. S. (2014). Implementation science and quality improvement. In J. B. Dimick & C. C. Greenberg (Eds.), *Success in academic surgery: Health services research* (pp. 85–100). Springer. https://doi.org/10.1007/978-1-4471-4718-3_8

Kitson, A., & Straus, S. E. (2010). The knowledge-to-action cycle: Identifying the gaps. *Canadian Medial Association Journal, 182*(2), E73–E77. https://doi.org/10.1503/cmaj.081231

Koczwara, B., Stover, A. M., Davies, L., Davis, M. M., Fleisher, L., Ramanadhan, S., Schroeck, F. R., Zullig, L. L., Chambers, D. A., & Proctor, E. (2018). Harnessing the synergy between improvement science and implementation science in cancer: A call to action. *Journal of Oncology Practice, 14*(6), 335–340. https://doi.org/10.1200/JOP.17.00083

Kothari A., & Wathen, C. N. (2013). A critical second look at integrated knowledge translation. *Health Policy, 109*(2):187–191. https://doi.org/10.1016/j.healthpol.2012.11.004

Liu, B., Almaawiy, U., Moore, J. E., Chan, W.-H., Straus, S. E., & The MOVE ON Team. (2013). Evaluation of a multisite educational intervention to improve mobilization of older patients in hospital: Protocol for mobilization of vulnerable elders in Ontario (MOVE ON). *Implementation Science, 8*(1), 76. https://doi.org/10.1186/1748-5908-8-76

Liu, B., Moore, J. E., Almaawiy, U., Chan, W.-H., Khan, S., Ewusie, J., Hamid, J. S., & Straus, S. E. (2018). Outcomes of Mobilisation of Vulnerable Elders in Ontario (MOVE ON): A multisite interrupted time series evaluation of an implementation intervention to increase patient mobilisation. *Age and Ageing*. https://doi.org/10.1093/ageing/afx128

Michie, S., & Prestwich, A. (2010). Are interventions theory-based? Development of a theory coding scheme. *Health Psychology, 29*(1), 1–8. https://doi.org/10.1037/a0016939

Module 3: Implementation Teams | NIRN. (2013). Nirn.fpg.unc.edu. Retrieved 19 May 2021, from https://nirn.fpg.unc.edu/module-3.

Monica, & California 90401-3208. (1967). *Delphi method*. Retrieved May 18, 2021, from https://www.rand.org/topics/delphi-method.html

Moore, J. E., Liu, B., Khan, S., Harris, C., Ewusie, J. E., Hamid, J. S., & Straus, S. E. (2019). Can the effects of the mobilization of vulnerable elders in Ontario (MOVE ON) implementation be replicated in new settings: An interrupted time series design. *BMC Geriatrics, 19*(1), 99. https://doi.org/10.1186/s12877-019-1124-0

Moore, J. E., Mascarenhas, A., Marquez, C., Almaawiy, U., Chan, W.-H., D'Souza, J., Liu, B., Straus, S. E., & MOVE ON Team. (2014). Mapping barriers and intervention activities to behaviour change theory for Mobilization of Vulnerable Elders in Ontario (MOVE ON), a multi-site implementation intervention in acute care hospitals. *Implementation Science, 9*, 160. https://doi.org/10.1186/s13012-014-0160-6

Morton, S. C., Murad, M. H., O'Connor, E., Lee, C. S., Booth, M., Vandermeer, B. W., Snowden, J. M., D'Anci, K. E., Fu, R., Gartlehner, G., Wang, Z., & Steele, D. W. (2018). *Quantitative synthesis—An update*. Agency for Healthcare Research and Quality (AHRQ). https://doi.org/10.23970/AHRQEPCMETHGUIDE3

MOVEs Canada: Getting Ready. (2011). MOVEs Canada. Retrieved May 19, 2021, from https://www.movescanada.ca/resources-for-hospitals/getting-ready/

Nilsen, P. (2020). Making sense of implementation theories, models, and frameworks. In B. Albers, A. Shlonsky, & R. Mildon (Eds.), *Implementation science 3.0* (pp. 53–79). Springer International Publishing. https://doi.org/10.1007/978-3-030-03874-8_3

Niven, D. (2015). *The de-adoption of low-value clinical practices in adult critical care medicine*. https://doi.org/10.11575/PRISM/28042

Norton, W. E., & Chambers, D. A. (2020). Unpacking the complexities of de-implementing inappropriate health interventions. *Implementation Science, 15*(1), 2. https://doi.org/10.1186/s13012-019-0960-9

Okoli, C., & Pawlowski, S. D. (2004). The Delphi method as a research tool: An example, design considerations and applications. *Information & Management, 42*(1), 15–29. https://doi.org/10.1016/j.im.2003.11.002

Peters, M., Godfrey, C., McInerney, P., Munn, Z., Trico, A., & Khalil, H. (2020). Chapter 11: Scoping reviews. In E. Aromataris & Z. Munn (Eds.), *JBI manual for evidence synthesis*. JBI. https://doi.org/10.46658/JBIMES-20-12

Puchalski Ritchie, L. M., Khan, S., Moore, J. E., Timmings, C., van Lettow, M., Vogel, J. P., Khan, D. N., Mbaruku, G., Mrisho, M., Mugerwa, K., Uka, S., Gülmezoglu, A. M., & Straus, S. E. (2016). Low- and middle-income countries face many common barriers to implementation of maternal health evidence products. *Journal of Clinical Epidemiology, 76*, 229–237. https://doi.org/10.1016/j.jclinepi.2016.02.017

Recommendation Topics | United States Preventive Services Taskforce. (n.d.). https://www.uspreventiveservicestaskforce.org/uspstf/recommendation-topics

Research guides: Knowledge syntheses: Systematic & scoping reviews, and other review types: Different types of knowledge syntheses. (n.d.). University of Toronto Libraries. Retrieved May 18, 2021, from https://guides.library.utoronto.ca/c.php?g=713309&p=5083157

Root Cause Analysis. (2019). https://psnet.ahrq.gov/primer/root-cause-analysis

Stelfox, H. T. (2013). *How to develop quality indicators?* (p. 28). Institute for Public Health: Innovation for Health and Health Care.

Stelfox, H. T., & Straus, S. E. (2013a). Measuring quality of care: Considering measurement frameworks and needs assessment to guide quality indicator development. *Journal of Clinical Epidemiology, 66*(12), 1320–1327. https://doi.org/10.1016/j.jclinepi.2013.05.018

Stelfox, H. T., & Straus, S. E. (2013b). Measuring quality of care: Considering conceptual approaches to quality indicator development and evaluation. *Journal of Clinical Epidemiology, 66*(12):1328–1237. https://doi.org/10.1016/j.jclinepi.2013.05.017

Straus, S., Tetroe, J., & Graham, I. D. (2013). *Knowledge translation in health care: Moving from evidence to practice.* John Wiley & Sons.

Straus, S. E., Tetroe, J., & Graham, I. (2009). Defining knowledge translation. *CMAJ, 181*(3–4), 165–168. https://doi.org/10.1503/cmaj.081229

Strifler, L., Cardoso, R., McGowan, J., Cogo, E., Nincic, V., Khan, P. A., Scott, A., Ghassemi, M., MacDonald, H., Lai, Y., Treister, V., Tricco, A. C., & Straus, S. E. (2018). Scoping review identifies significant number of knowledge translation theories, models, and frameworks with limited use. *Journal of Clinical Epidemiology, 100*, 92–102. https://doi.org/10.1016/j.jclinepi.2018.04.008

STS National Database | STS. (n.d.). The Society of Thoracic Surgeons. Retrieved May 18, 2021, from https://www.sts.org/registries/sts-national-database

Tannenbaum, C., Greaves, L., & Graham, I. D. (2016). Why sex and gender matter in implementation research. *BMC Medical Research Methodology, 16*(1), 145. https://doi.org/10.1186/s12874-016-0247-7

Tricco, A. C., Langlois, E. V., & Straus, S. E. (2017). *Rapid reviews to strengthen health policy and systems: A practical guide.* World Health Organization. https://www.who.int/alliance-hpsr/resources/publications/rapid-review-guide/en/

Tricco, A. C., Lillie, E., Zarin, W., O'Brien, K. K., Colquhoun, H., Levac, D., Moher, D., Peters, M. D. J., Horsley, T., Weeks, L., & Hempel, S. (2018). PRISMA Extension for Scoping Reviews (PRISMA-ScR): Checklist and explanation. *Annals of Internal Medicine. 169*(7): 467–473. https://doi.org/10.7326/M18-0850

Turoff, M., & Linstone, H. A. (1975). *The Delphi method-techniques and applications.* Addison-Wesley.

Vogel, J. P., Moore, J. E., Timmings, C., Khan, S., Khan, D. N., Defar, A., Hadush, A., Terefe, M. M., Teshome, L., Ba-Thike, K., Than, K. K., Makuwani, A., Mbaruku, G., Mrisho, M., Mugerwa, K. Y., Ritchie, L. M. P., Rashid, S., Straus, S. E., & Gülmezoglu, A. M. (2016). Barriers, facilitators and priorities for implementation of WHO Maternal and Perinatal Health Guidelines in four lower-income countries: A GREAT Network Research Activity. *PLoS One, 11*(11), e0160020. https://doi.org/10.1371/journal.pone.0160020

World Health Organization. (2012). *WHO recommendations for the prevention and treatment of postpartum haemorrhage.* http://www.myilibrary.com?id=1003393

World Health Organization, Regional Office for the Eastern Mediterranean. (2017). *HIV test-treat-retain cascade analysis: Guide and tools 2017.* Author. https://apps.who.int/iris/handle/10665/259856

3

Selecting Evidence-Based Interventions to Reduce Practice Gaps

Jennifer Leeman, Mary Wangen, and Cam Escoffery

Learning Objectives

By the end of this chapter, readers will be able to:

- Define evidence-based interventions (EBIs)
- Search for EBIs that address a defined health problem
- Apply criteria to assess evidence in support of an EBI's:
  - effectiveness
  - potential for implementation in real-world practice
  - potential to promote health equity
- Discuss the value of simulation modeling and cost-effectiveness analysis
- Execute a multi-step, stakeholder-engaged process to select one or more EBIs

CASE STUDY 3.1 SELECTING EVIDENCE-BASED INTERVENTIONS TO ADDRESS A DEFINED HEALTH PROBLEM

Stacey S. is a health educator in her region's health department. She has been asked to advise health department leadership on the best ways to address increasing rates of overweight and obesity among the region's 2- to 5-year-old children. A preliminary assessment of the problem determined that many of these children were in daycare and were living in low-income households. The assessment also found that most low-income households got their healthcare at either the health department or the community health center. To advise health department leadership, Stacey engaged a workgroup to help her select one or more evidence-based interventions (EBIs) that would have the greatest potential to prevent overweight and obesity among 2- to 5-year-old children in her region. The workgroup included parents of young children from low-income households and representatives from childcare centers, the regional health authority, and community health centers. Stacey now needs to develop a list of potential EBIs and present it to the workgroup.

DEFINING EVIDENCE-BASED INTERVENTIONS

The primary goal of implementation science is to speed the translation of **evidence-based interventions** (EBIs) into practice. The term "intervention" encompasses a broad range of activities that are intended to improve the health of individuals or populations. These activities may include programs, practices, principles, procedures, policies, and the use of new pills and products (Hendricks-Brown et al., 2017). An intervention is considered "evidence-based" when it has been tested in one or more well-designed research studies and found to be effective at improving health-related outcomes (Leeman et al., 2017).

EBIs improve health-related outcomes by targeting one or more of the multilevel factors that contribute to those outcomes. As illustrated in Figure 3.1, EBIs may target factors at the individual, interpersonal (e.g., family), organization, community, and public policy levels. For example, an EBI to improve colorectal cancer screening rates may target individual-level beliefs about the importance of screening, organization-level systems to remind providers when it is time for their patients to be screened, and/or public policy to provide funding for colorectal cancer screening and follow-up. Figure 3.1 illustrates a range of EBIs that target different levels of the socioecological model with the goal of reducing overweight and obesity among low-income 2- to 5-year-old children.

Both the number of EBIs and the amount of information about those EBIs may seem overwhelming. Peer-reviewed journals have produced millions of publications and numerous organizations disseminate information through their websites, newsletters, and listservs. As one public health practitioner working in obesity prevention reported, "Honestly, the frustration right now for me is you've got Robert Wood Johnson, Policy Link, CDC, Convergence Partnership. You name it and every day somebody is coming out with something" (Leeman et al., 2014, p. 193). This chapter provides guidance on feasible approaches that can be used to search for and select EBIs that best fit local priorities and to ensure the selected EBI has the greatest potential to improve health. Central to this chapter is an understanding of the three primary formats used to disseminate EBIs: (a) systematic review recommendations, (b) packaged interventions, and (c) reports of intervention studies.

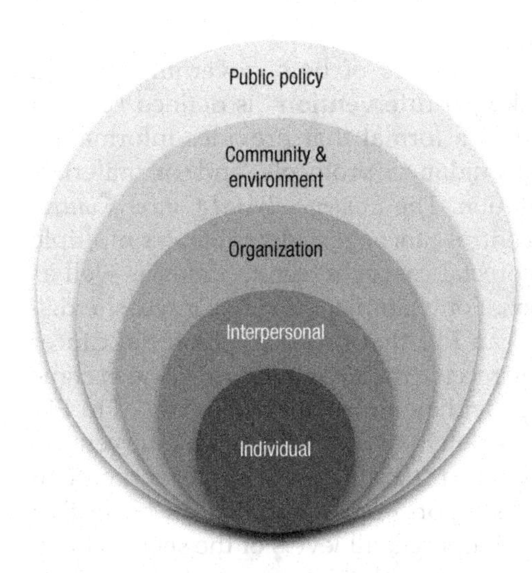

Public policy | Childcare Quality Rating and Improvement System (QRIS): QRIS is a system that state **governments** use to assess, approve, and communicate the quality of childcare programs.

Community & environment | Baltimore Health Stores (BHS): BHS increases the availability of healthier food options and point-of-purchase marketing in small **community stores** to promote customers' selection of healthier foods.

Organization | Nutrition and Physical Activity Self-Assessment for Child Care (NAPSACC): NAPSACC provides tools and training that childcare providers can use to assess and improve their **organization's** nutrition and physical activity policies, environments, and practices.

Interpersonal | High Five for Kids (HFK): HFK uses motivational interviewing and educational sessions to change the health-related and parenting behaviors of **parents of children** who are obese.

Individual | Color Me Healthy (CMH): CMH provides an interactive curriculum that uses color, dance, and play to educate and motivate **children** to be more physically active and eat more fruits and vegetables.

FIGURE 3.1 Evidence-based interventions that target different levels to reduce obesity in 2- to 5-year-olds.
Sources: Data from Administration for Children and Families. (2021). *Child care quality ratings*. https://www.childcare.gov/index.php/consumer-education/child-care-quality-ratings; Center of Excellence for Training and Research, North Carolina State University, & North Carolina Division of Public Health. (2013). *Color me healthy intervention*. http://centertrt.org/content/docs/Intervention_Documents/Intervention_Templates/CMH_research_tested_template.pdf; Center of Excellence for Training and Research Translation, Center for Health Promotion and Disease Prevention, UNC at Chapel Hill, & Division of Public Health, NC Department of Health and Human Services. (2014).*Nutrition and physical activity self-assessment for child-care (NAP SACC)*. Intervention. http://centertrt.org/content/docs/Intervention_Documents/Intervention_Templates/NAPSACC_Template_Updated_April_2014.pdf; Center of Excellence for Training and Research Translation, & Center for Human Nutrition Bloomberg School of Public Health. (2013). *Baltimore healthy stores (BHS). Intervention*. http://centertrt.org/content/docs/Intervention_Documents/Intervention_Templates/Baltimore_Healthy_Stores_template.pdf; National Cancer Institute. (2020c). *High five for kids*. https://ebccp.cancercontrol.cancer.gov/programDetails.do?programId=2539629; National Center on Early Childhood Quality Assurance. (2021). *About QRIS: QRIS resource guide*.

Systematic Review Recommendations

A **systematic review of the literature** involves the use of systematic and explicit methods to identify, select, and appraise reports of research studies and then extract and synthesize their findings with the goal of answering a specific research question (e.g., Is an intervention effective? What types of interventions are effective at achieving specified outcomes?; Moher et al., 2009). Systematic reviews of the literature are disseminated in peer-reviewed journals and on the websites of governmental and non-governmental organizations.

Two types of systematic reviews are important in the selection of EBIs: those that establish clinical practice guidelines and those that identify which broad intervention approaches are effective at improving targeted outcomes. The first type of review establishes what constitutes best practice (e.g., the age at which low-risk adults should be screened for colorectal cancer; Bibbins-Domingo et al., 2016). The second type of review identifies EBIs that may be used to close gaps in achieving those best practices (e.g., create reminder systems to inform healthcare providers that it is time for a patient's cancer screening). Table 3.1 provides a listing of websites that disseminate systematic review recommendations as well as other types of EBIs. This list is not intended to be exhaustive, but rather to provide examples from among the more widely used websites.

Packaged Interventions

Packaged interventions are disseminated on the websites of both governmental and non-governmental organizations. The term "**packaged intervention**" is defined broadly to include any intervention that is disseminated in a format that provides information about the intervention together with additional guidance, protocols, and/or materials to support intervention delivery and implementation. The *Evidence-Based Cancer Control Programs* website (EBCCP; https://ebccp.cancercontrol.cancer.gov) disseminates multiple packaged interventions for use in increasing colorectal cancer screening rates as well as a wide range of other cancer-related interventions. For example, the EBCCP website disseminates the "Flu-FIT and Flu-FOBT Program," an EBI that provides colorectal cancer screening kits and instructions to adults when they receive their annual flu vaccine in clinic (National Cancer Institute, 2020b). In addition to providing information about the "Flu-FIT and Flu-FOBT Program," the EBCCP website links potential adopters to the intervention developers' website where adopters can download the program's logic model and patient education materials along with other materials to support implementation. Websites that disseminate packaged interventions include EBIs that target all levels of the socio-ecological model. This includes websites that disseminate policy EBIs in a format that provides model language and other guidance for use in drafting and enacting policy change. As an example, the *CounterTobacco* website (countertobacco.org) disseminates model language and other guidance to support the enactment of policies to reduce the sale and marketing of tobacco products in the retail environment.

KEY POINT FOR PRACTICE

When possible, look for EBIs that are supported by systematic review findings and also available in a packaged format. Systematic reviews provide strong evidence for the effectiveness of the broad EBI approach while the packaged intervention provides more specific guidance on how to implement the intervention into practice. Some websites help users connect systematic review findings with packaged interventions. For example, for each of its systematic review findings, the *What Works for Health* website provides links to relevant packaged EBIs (countyhealthrankings.org/take-action-to-improve-health/what-works-for-health).

Reports of Intervention Studies

Peer-reviewed journals publish reports of intervention studies that provide another important source of information about EBIs. These reports are available in searchable, online bibliographic databases, including PubMed and The Cumulative Index to Nursing and Allied Health Literature (CINAHL) among others. Intervention developers will often publish multiple articles on a single intervention, including articles describing the intervention and how it was developed, the protocols for the study that tested the intervention, findings from initial pilot studies, and summative findings on the intervention's implementation and effectiveness. For example, Coronado et al. (2018) reported on the effectiveness of an intervention that used electronic health records to identify patients who were due for colorectal screening and then mailed them a screening test kit, followed by a reminder letter. Coronado and her research team have also published articles on the types of adaptations health plans made to the intervention and on factors at the patient, provider, and organizational level that may influence the intervention's effectiveness and/or implementation (Coronado et al., 2020; O'Connor et al., 2020; Petrik et al., 2020; Thompson et al., 2019).

TABLE 3.1 A Partial List of Websites That Disseminate Clinical Practice Guidelines and Evidence-Based Interventions

CLINICAL PRACTICE GUIDELINES	
U.S. Preventive Services Task Force	uspreventiveservicestaskforce.org/uspstf
The National Institute for Health and Care Excellence	nice.org.uk/guidance
World Health Organization Guidelines	who.int/publications/who-guidelines
EVIDENCE-BASED INTERVENTIONS: SYSTEMATIC REVIEW RECOMMENDATIONS	
Cochrane Collaboration	cochrane.org
The National Institute for Health and Care Excellence	nice.org.uk
The Community Guide	thecommunityguide.org
What Works for Health	countyhealthrankings.org/take-action-to-improve-health/what-works-for-health
Health Evidence	health-evidence.ca
Health Systems Evidence	healthsystemsevidence.org
Social Systems Evidence	mcmasterforum.org/find-evidence/social-systems-evidence
HI-5 Health Impact in 5 Years	cdc.gov/policy/hst/hi5/interventions/index.html
Campbell Collaboration	campbellcollaboration.org/better-evidence.html
EVIDENCE-BASED INTERVENTIONS: PACKAGED INTERVENTIONS	
Evidence-Based Cancer Control Programs (formerly Research Tested Intervention Programs)	ebccp.cancercontrol.cancer.gov/searchResults.do
Counter Tobacco	countertobacco.org
Effective Interventions HIV/AIDs	cdc.gov/hiv/effective-interventions/index.html
Evidence-Based Practices Resource Center (Substance abuse and mental health)	samhsa.gov/ebp-resource-center
The California Evidence-Based Clearinghouse for Child Welfare	cebc4cw.org/search

Each of the three EBI formats has both strengths and limitations. ***Systematic reviews*** provide the strongest evidence for an intervention's effectiveness because they synthesize findings across multiple research studies. They offer further advantage in that others have searched and reviewed the literature for you. However, systematic reviews are limited because, while they provide evidence in support of broadly defined intervention approaches, they provide little guidance on how to deliver and implement a specific intervention in practice (Fernandez et al., 2018). ***Packaged interventions*** provide the guidance and materials to support the delivery and implementation of specific interventions in the real world. However, only a limited number of interventions are available in a packaged format, and those that are available have largely been tested in high-resource settings and/or with a specific population or setting. As a result, the packaged interventions that are available may not be feasible in settings with fewer resources, and guidance and materials may not fit new populations or contexts (Castro et al., 2010; Sussman et al., 2006). The third format, ***reports of intervention studies,*** provides the most current information, and may include reports of interventions that were designed for, and therefore best fit, the needs of a specific population and setting. However, searching the peer-reviewed literature is time consuming and, once reports are identified, further expertise and time is required to assess the evidence base in support of the intervention. Furthermore, reports of intervention studies often provide limited detail on how the intervention was delivered and/or implemented.

SEARCHING FOR EVIDENCE-BASED INTERVENTIONS

In this chapter, we recommend a multistep approach to the search for EBIs, with the goal of maximizing the benefits of each EBI format while offsetting their limitations (see Figure 3.2).

Step 1. Start with systematic reviews of intervention studies that address the problem you hope to improve. This will include searching the peer-reviewed literature (e.g., PubMed) and visiting one or more websites that disseminate systematic review findings (see Table 3.1). Systematic review findings provide the strongest evidence for broad intervention approaches that have been tested and found to be effective at addressing a problem. In most cases, these reviews will provide little detail on the design, delivery, or implementation of any specific intervention. Create a menu of the broad EBI approaches identified in the search of systematic review publications and websites. Then, in collaboration with key stakeholders, narrow the list down to the broad EBI approaches that best fit the selected health problem and local context.

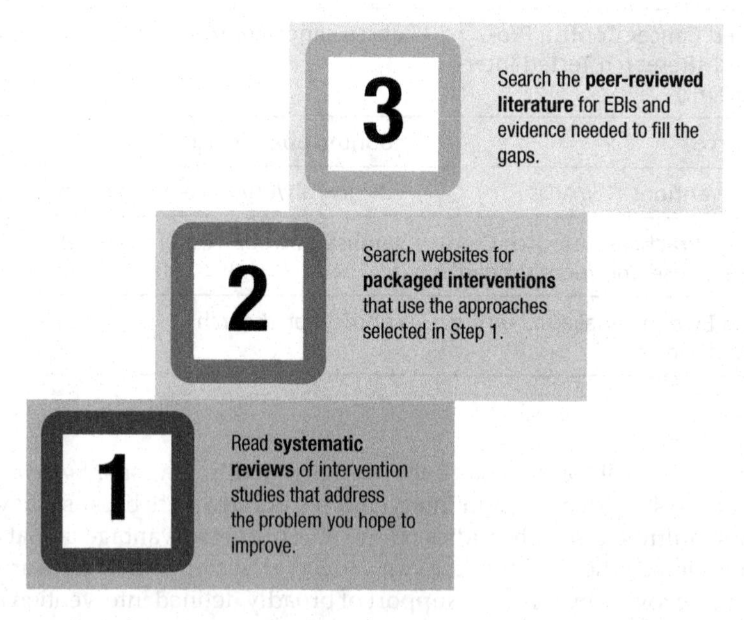
3
Search the peer-reviewed literature for EBIs and evidence needed to fill the gaps.
2
Search websites for packaged interventions that use the approaches selected in Step 1.
1
Read systematic reviews of intervention studies that address the problem you hope to improve.

FIGURE 3.2 The three-step approach to searching for evidence-based interventions (EBIs).

KEY POINT FOR PRACTICE

Partner with a librarian to assist you with Steps 1 and 3. To find a librarian, reach out to a university, college, hospital, public health authority, or health education center. Librarians have both the training and experience needed to search the literature effectively. Furthermore, libraries often provide users with free access to journals and other resources that they would have to pay for if they tried to access them on their own.

Step 2. Search websites for packaged interventions that use one or more of the broad EBI approaches selected in Step 1. The search may include websites that disseminate multiple packaged interventions, such as those listed in Table 3.1. Intervention developers also may create websites where they provide guidance, materials, and other resources to support the implementation of their intervention. During Step 2, the search may identify interventions that use approaches other than those identified in Step 1. If this happens, consider repeating Step 1 to look for systematic reviews that provide evidence in support of the new approach. We recommend searching for packaged interventions because they provide resources to support the implementation of specific interventions. Begin to create a menu of specific EBIs that may fit the selected health problem and local context.

Step 3. Next, search for peer-reviewed journal articles that report on EBIs related to either the broad approaches identified in Step 1 or the more specific approaches identified in Step 2. The purpose of this search is to get the most current information on the EBI, to look for studies that implemented an EBI in a specific population and/or setting, and to find additional EBIs, if needed. Start by looking at the lists of articles included in systematic reviews that recommended the broad EBIs that stakeholders prioritized in Step 1, with a focus on identifying studies that were implemented in settings and populations with key characteristics similar to your own. Search for any papers that were published after the most current systematic review was completed. Findings from more recently published studies may further strengthen (or weaken) support for the effectiveness of an EBI. Next, search the peer-reviewed literature to identify papers reporting on specific EBIs. To find additional reports on an EBI, search the bibliographic database (e.g., PubMed) for other articles published by the intervention developers and do a search using the name of the EBI. A search of the peer-reviewed literature for additional reports on a specific EBI may identify reports that provide guidance on how others have adapted an EBI or its implementation to a specific population or setting. In the case of packaged interventions, the website disseminating the intervention often provides information on journal articles about the intervention. Finally, searching the peer-reviewed literature may identify new EBIs. Add what you learned from Step 3 to the menu that you began creating in Step 2 and then present the findings to your key stakeholders.

This three-step process is rarely linear, and steps may need to be revisited as new EBIs and gaps are identified throughout the process. Many times, Step 2 will not identify any packaged interventions related to a broad EBI identified in Step 1. Packaged interventions may be particularly hard to find for EBIs that target factors at the outer edges of the socio-ecological model (Leeman et al., 2015). In some cases, neither Step 1 nor Step 2 will yield an EBI that addresses a prioritized problem, and reports of intervention studies will need to be the primary source of information about potential EBIs.

COMMON PITFALLS IN PRACTICE

Engaging stakeholders takes time and energy, and this creates the temptation to leave stakeholders out of the selection process and engage them only after the "best" EBIs have been identified. Resist this temptation. Stakeholders have in-depth knowledge of the priority population and can provide input on which EBIs will best fit the local culture, preferences, and needs. Furthermore, engaging stakeholders promotes local ownership and commitment to the EBI and its implementation.

CASE STUDY 3.2 USING THE THREE-STEP PROCESS TO SEARCH FOR EVIDENCE-BASED INTERVENTIONS

Stacey S. engaged her stakeholder group in a multi-step process with the goal of selecting one or more EBIs that would best fit her region's goal of preventing overweight and obesity among 2- to 5-year-old children living in low-income families. Stacey began with a search for systematic review findings on interventions to prevent overweight and obesity in 2- to 5-year-old children, with a focus on interventions that could be implemented in community clinics, health departments, and/or childcare centers (Step 1). She searched several websites that disseminate systematic review findings and partnered with a librarian to identify systematic reviews in the peer-reviewed literature. She then presented a list of broad EBI approaches to the stakeholder workgroup. Based on the health department's assessment findings and stakeholder input, the workgroup decided to focus the search on one EBI approach: nutrition and physical activity interventions in childcare. Stacey then searched websites that disseminate packaged interventions (Step 2), created a list of the specific EBIs, and presented the list to the workgroup. The workgroup decided to move forward with one specific intervention: Nutrition and Physical Activity Self-Assessment for Child Care or NAPSACC. The NAPSACC program is a packaged EBI that provides protocols and an extensive menu of resources for use in improving a daycare program's existing eating and physical activity environment, practices, and policies. Following the selection of NAPSACC, Stacey again worked with a librarian to search the peer-reviewed literature (Step 3) for all papers reporting on the NAPSACC program.

Case Study 3.2 provides a high-level overview of the multi-step process Stacey used to search for EBIs but only tells part of the story. In addition to providing stakeholders with lists of potential EBIs, Stacey also had to provide a summary of the evidence in support of each EBI so that stakeholders could select the EBIs with the greatest potential to reduce obesity rates among 2- to 5-year-old children in their region. We provide a list of criteria that may be applied to assess the evidence in support of an EBI's effectiveness and its potential to be implemented in real-world practice.

CRITERIA FOR ASSESSING EFFECTIVENESS OF AN EVIDENCE-BASED INTERVENTION

In selecting EBIs, the goal is to identify interventions that have been tested and found to improve a priority health behavior and/or health outcome. The terms "efficacy" and "effectiveness" are both used to describe interventions that have been tested and found to improve outcomes. **Efficacy** refers to the impact an intervention has when tested under controlled conditions that limit the influence that factors other than the intervention may have on outcomes. For example, conditions may be controlled through strict criteria for who may participate in the study and the use of study personnel to deliver the intervention. **Effectiveness** refers to the impact an intervention has when delivered in real-world conditions (Singal et al., 2014). Because they are conducted in real-world conditions, studies of intervention effectiveness may yield findings with greater potential for implementation in real-world practice. The following five criteria can be applied to assess the strength of evidence in support of an intervention's efficacy or effectiveness. Table 3.3 illustrates how these criteria might be applied to an assessment of the NAPSACC program.

Effectiveness Criteria #1: Methods Used to Test Intervention Effects on Targeted Outcomes

The strength of the evidence in support of an intervention's effectiveness depends on the methods used to test the intervention's effects on targeted outcomes. A full discussion of the methods used to test interventions is beyond the scope of this chapter. Instead, we provide a brief overview of some of the more important factors, including study design, sample size, and how outcomes were measured. Evidence that an intervention caused an improvement in health-related outcomes (i.e., was effective) is strongest when researchers test the intervention using a randomized controlled trial design (RCT). In an RCT, researchers recruit participants or settings and then randomly assign them to groups that either receive an intervention or not and then determine which group(s) had the best outcomes. RCTs are the gold standard for determining an intervention's efficacy because randomization increases the likelihood that the intervention caused the differences in outcomes rather than other systematic differences between those who did or did not receive the intervention. Table 3.2 provides a brief overview of some of the other designs used to test intervention effectiveness.

TABLE 3.2 A Sampling of Designs Used to Assess Intervention Effectiveness Other Than RCTs

DESIGN	DEFINITION	EXAMPLE
Nonrandomized controlled trials	Used to measure an outcome before and after an intervention in two nonrandomly assigned groups, one that received the intervention and one group that did not	Researchers implement a healthy eating intervention in five elementary schools and measure student consumption of vegetables before and after the intervention in those five schools as compared to five similar schools that did not receive the intervention
One-arm, pre-test/post-test studies	Used to measure an outcome before and after an intervention is implemented, without a control group	A community clinic invites patients to participate in an 8-week diabetes-self management intervention and measures their A1c before and after the intervention
Natural experiments	An event not under the control of researchers divides a population into exposed and unexposed groups; data are collected comparing outcomes across those two groups	Three U.S. states enact a sales tax on soda. Researchers use existing data to study changes in body mass index in those three states before and after enactment of the soda tax as compared to states that did not enact a soda tax

Even though RCTs are the gold standard for establishing an intervention's effectiveness, that type of study design is not always feasible. Using a parachute when jumping from a plane is one example of an intervention for which an RCT would be ill-advised (Verkamp, 2010). Public policy interventions are another example; randomly assigning states to enact a soda tax would be difficult if not impossible. As a result, the strength of evidence for an intervention's effectiveness may vary, particularly for interventions that target the outer levels of the socio-ecological model. In addition to study design, sample size and how outcomes are measured are key to weighing the evidence in support of an intervention's effectiveness. Studies that have large sample sizes and use reliable and valid measures to assess outcomes generally provide stronger evidence than those with small sample sizes (e.g., pilot studies) or that use measures that have not been validated.

Effectiveness Criteria #2: Number of Studies and Consistency of Findings Across Studies

Each study that tests an intervention contributes to the evidence base for that intervention's effectiveness. In addition to the methodological strength of these studies, the number of studies and consistency of findings across studies testing either a specific intervention (e.g., "Flu-FIT/Flu-FOBIT") or an intervention approach (e.g., patient reminders) are important factors in assessing the strength of evidence in support of an intervention's effectiveness. The strength of the evidence in support of an intervention's effectiveness is greatest when there are multiple strong studies that show consistent desired effects.

Effectiveness Criteria #3: Magnitude of Benefits

A study may determine that an intervention has a statistically significant effect on an outcome, which is often designated as a value of $p < .05$ or a probability of less than 5% that the effects were based on chance rather than the intervention. However, the effect of an intervention may be statistically significant and still not be sufficient to justify implementation. For example, a colorectal cancer screening intervention may result in a 3% increase in screening rates that is statistically significant but is too small to justify the effort and resources that would be required to implement the intervention. Therefore, attention should be given to the reported magnitude of benefit that an intervention has achieved in prior studies.

Effectiveness Criteria #4: Effectiveness Across Populations

Interventions may not benefit all populations equally. Members of racial/ethnic minority groups have been under-represented in research studies (Castillo-Mancilla et al., 2014; Evelyn et al., 2001) resulting in limited evidence in support for many interventions' effectiveness in populations at greatest risk for health disparities. Funders are calling for intervention studies to include diverse participants, and as a result the evidence base is increasing regarding intervention effects across populations. In reviewing both research reports and systematic reviews of the literature, it is important to assess the demographic characteristics of the included sample, whether analyses were conducted to assess for differential effects across populations, and what if any differential effects were found. In some cases, websites or publications reporting systematic review findings provide summaries of this information. Particular attention should be given to whether evidence supports the intervention's effectiveness at improving outcomes in populations at greatest risk for health disparities.

Effectiveness Criteria #5: Degree to Which Findings Are Current

Evidence in support of an EBI may have been collected, reviewed, and/or disseminated many years ago. There are no set guidelines for how many years is too many for an EBI to still be current. To assess whether a specific EBI is still current, identify the date that data on the intervention's effectiveness were last collected. If assessing the findings from a systematic review, determine the last publication date for studies included in the review. Then consider whether clinical practice guidelines or the socio-political context has changed since that date and whether those changes raise concerns about the continuing relevance of the intervention. Also consider whether more current data may be available on the intervention's effectiveness and then search for that evidence in the peer-reviewed literature.

COMMON PITFALLS IN PRACTICE

Clinical practice guidelines often change over time. For this reason, it is important not to implement packaged EBIs without first reviewing the patient education and other materials included in the package. Some changes to clinical practice guidelines can be managed by making minor adaptations to intervention materials (e.g., changes to the age at which colorectal cancer screening should start). At other times, the changes required are less feasible (e.g., major changes to guidelines for a heart healthy diet) and another EBI needs to be selected.

TWO ADDITIONAL METHODS FOR ASSESSING INTERVENTION EFFECTIVENESS: SIMULATION MODELING AND COST-EFFECTIVENESS ANALYSIS

Intervention studies are not the only way that researchers evaluate an intervention's effectiveness. They may also use simulation modeling and/or assess an intervention's cost-effectiveness. In the following we provide an overview of these two additional methods for assessing intervention effectiveness.

Simulation Modeling

Modeling methods can be used to simulate how an EBI or multiple EBIs might function within a complex system (Davis et al., 2019). Most EBIs are implemented into complex systems made up of many interacting parts. Within a healthcare system, patients, healthcare providers, and support staff interact with existing care processes and infrastructure across multiple system levels. The introduction of an EBI often changes how providers and staff interact with each other and with existing processes and infrastructure in ways that are both expected and unexpected. In developing simulation models, researchers may start with qualitative approaches that engage diverse stakeholders to develop a model that details the system's parts and how they interact to address a specific healthcare problem (e.g., colorectal cancer screening). These models provide a comprehensive picture that can be used to identify interactions that may influence the implementation and effectiveness of one or more EBIs. Researchers create a model to simulate these actions and then use those models to analyze large amounts of data, with the goal of comparing the effectiveness of alternate EBIs. For example, researchers created a simulation model to compare the effects of colorectal cancer screening EBIs (both alone and in combination) on colorectal cancer screening rates among Medicaid enrollees in Oregon. The model identified the combination of Mailed FIT and patient navigation EBIs as one of the more promising options and projected that, within 5 years, this combination of EBIs would increase screening rates by 20.2% and prevent approximately 77 cancers. Importantly, once researchers develop a simulation model, they can reconfigure it to simulate outcomes for different populations and settings, as was the case for the described model which has also been used to simulate the impact of different EBIs in North Carolina. Another example of a modeling tool is *The Lives Saved Tool* which can be used to estimate the impact that different interventions will have on major causes of neonatal, under-five, and maternal mortality and nutrition outcomes in low and middle income countries (Johns Hopkins School of Public Health & Bill & Melinda Gates Foundation, 2021).

Cost-Effectiveness Analysis

Cost-effectiveness analyses address both the cost and the effectiveness of a new intervention compared with current practice. The results of these analyses are presented as additional dollars in cost per additional unit of health benefit gained (e.g., cost per life year saved; Macones et al., 1999). Cost-effectiveness analyses generate ratios similar to what a grocery store provides as the price per unit of a can of beans (e.g., cost per ounce) to make it easier for consumers to compare prices across items with different quantities. Cost-effectiveness analyses typically calculate costs from the perspective of society rather than the perspective of an implementing organization. For example, in addition to healthcare costs, a cost-effectiveness analysis may include the costs of lost wages due to disability and death. As a result, these analyses often answer questions about which interventions provide the greatest improvement to health outcomes at the societal level rather than questions about how much benefit an implementing organization will gain from implementing an intervention. Reports of cost-effectiveness analyses for some interventions can be found in the peer-reviewed literature (Bajwah et al., 2020) or through a small number of online cost calculators (Harvard T.H. Chan School of Public Health, 2021; RTI International, 2021).

CRITERIA FOR ASSESSING AN EVIDENCE-BASED INTERVENTION'S POTENTIAL FOR IMPLEMENTATION IN REAL-WORLD PRACTICE (RE-AIM)

Even when an EBI has strong evidence in support of its effectiveness, the EBI will not improve health until it is implemented into practice. **RE-AIM**, one of the most widely used frameworks in implementation science, can be used to assess an EBI's potential for implementation in practice (re-aim.org). The letters of RE-AIM each represent one of five elements that are required for an intervention to impact public health. The intervention must **R**each the intended population, be **E**ffective at improving targeted outcomes, and be **A**dopted, **I**mplemented, and **M**aintained over time (Kessler et al., 2013). We have already discussed effectiveness and therefore will focus now on the remaining four components of RE-AIM.

Implementation Criteria #1: Reach

Reach is a measure of the number, proportion, and representativeness of individuals who participated in or were exposed to an intervention (re-aim.org). For example, to assess the reach of the Flu-FIT/Flu-FOBT EBI (National Cancer Institute, 2020b), clinic staff would calculate the number and proportion of eligible clinic patients who received a colorectal cancer screening test kit, with "eligible" defined as patients who were due for screening per current clinical guidelines (Bibbins-Domingo et al., 2016). The measure of reach would also consider the representativeness of the population who received a screening test kit. In other words, were the patients reached representative of the overall population (gender, race/ethnicity, socio-economic status [SES]), or were some groups of patients less likely to receive a screening kit than others? Assessing the representativeness of those reached is one way to guard against the potential for interventions to exacerbate health disparities by disproportionately benefiting low-risk populations (e.g., White, or moderate to high SES). In assessing an EBI's potential reach, review the findings from prior studies of the intervention and solicit key stakeholders' input on the intervention's potential to reach the local population. Reports of intervention studies may include findings on factors that impeded or facilitated the EBI's reach overall or to specific populations (e.g., distrust, low literacy, lack of transportation) that may inform key stakeholders' thoughts about whether an intervention will or will not reach their intended population. If the intervention is likely to have limited or inequitable reach, you may need to select a different EBI or to adapt the intervention and its implementation to address barriers to participation.

Implementation Criteria #2: Adoption

Adoption is a measure of the number, proportion, and representativeness of settings and providers who initiate the implementation or delivery of an intervention (re-aim.org). Measures of adoption parallel those used to measure reach, but with a focus on settings and/or providers. Using the example of the Flu-FIT/Flu-FOBT EBI, measures of adoption might include the number, proportion, and representativeness of community clinics that agree to implement the EBI and/or clinic providers and staff who initiate EBI implementation or delivery. In measuring adoption, representativeness refers to characteristics of settings and providers. For example, research reports may provide evidence that most settings adopting the Flu-FIT/Flu-FOBT EBI have been large, urban clinics but provide little evidence on adoption rates among smaller and more rural clinics. As with reach, in assessing an EBI's potential for adoption, it is important to supplement the information from reports of research studies with stakeholder input on the likelihood that local settings and providers will be willing and able to adopt the EBI.

Implementation Criteria #3: Implementation Fidelity, Cost, and Readiness

Fidelity

Fidelity refers to the extent to which an EBI was delivered or executed as designed (i.e., with fidelity). Measure of fidelity may include (a) adherence to intervention or implementation protocols, (b) dose or amount of the intervention delivered, and (c) quality of intervention delivery (Proctor et al., 2011). Evidence on intervention fidelity may be found in the materials included with a packaged intervention or in reports of intervention studies. The strongest evidence for the potential to maintain fidelity to an intervention in real-world practice will come from studies of an intervention's effectiveness (as opposed to efficacy). In other words, look for evidence that the intervention was delivered with fidelity in studies where the intervention was tested in a practice setting and delivered by the providers and staff who work in that setting (as opposed to members of the research team). In assessing the potential to maintain fidelity to an EBI, it is important to also solicit input from key stakeholders. Ask stakeholders who have experience with the target settings whether they think those settings will be able to deliver the intervention as designed (e.g., with fidelity) and what they see as potential barriers to implementation.

Cost

Two questions related to cost are important criteria for evaluating an EBI's potential for implementation: (a) How much will it **cost** to implement an EBI? and (b) What benefits will an implementing organization gain relative to the money spent? To answer the first question, some packaged interventions and research reports provide details on the resources required to implement and deliver an intervention. This information can be used to estimate the costs of implementing an intervention for a specific number of individuals in a particular setting. Return on investment or business case analyses can be used to answer the second question. In making a business case, analyses are calculated from the perspective of the implementing organization and focus on the health, financial, and other benefits an organization will gain for the dollars spent (Masters et al., 2017). In addition to improving the health of their clients, these benefits may include gaining a competitive advantage over peers and meeting regulatory requirements, among others.

Readiness for Use

EBIs vary in the complexity of their protocols and the number of materials and other guidance required to implement them into practice. For example, a colorectal cancer screening reminder system may be more straightforward to implement than a colorectal cancer screening navigation program. In reviewing EBIs, consider what protocols and materials will be needed to implement the EBI and whether they are available in formats that are ready-to-use. Peer-reviewed reports may provide sufficient information to implement a reminder system, with relatively little additional work required to develop implementation protocols and materials. In contrast, peer-reviewed reports will provide only a small amount of the guidance and materials needed to implement a patient navigation program. Fortunately, packaged interventions are available that provide navigation protocols, downloadable education materials for navigators to use with patients, online trainings to prepare navigators for the role, and other resources to support implementation (National Cancer Institute, 2020a).

Implementation Criteria #4: Maintenance

Maintenance refers to the extent to which the implementation and effectiveness of an intervention are sustained or have the potential to be sustained over time (re-aim.org). Reports of intervention studies and systematic reviews often do not provide information on how well an intervention was maintained more than 1 year following its initiation. In addition to assessing evidence of whether settings were able to maintain an EBI over time, some studies include findings on the degree to which an intervention was integrated into routine practice. This may be referred to as an assessment of the intervention's sustainability or its degree of institutionalization (Proctor et al., 2011). In addition to information gleaned from reports of research studies, it is also important to solicit stakeholder input to review an EBI's potential sustainability prior to implementation (and to begin planning for sustainability early in the implementation process). Tools for engaging stakeholders in sustainability assessments are available at www.sustaintool.org. These measures assess the extent to which leadership support, resources, infrastructure, performance monitoring systems, and other factors are in place to sustain an intervention over time (Luke et al., 2014).

COMMON PITFALLS IN PRACTICE

Stakeholders may select an intervention that is beautifully packaged and ready to implement even when other interventions have stronger evidence of effectiveness and potential for implementation in their setting and population. This is particularly common when stakeholders have heard that others are implementing the selected intervention. Decisions are often influenced by good marketing and the desire to keep up with the latest fad and fashion. The best way to counteract this tendency is to provide clear documentation of the evidence in support of each intervention's effectiveness and potential for implementation.

Applying Criteria to Assess an Evidence-Based Intervention's Potential to Promote Health Equity

Attention to health equity should be incorporated throughout the review of an EBI's effectiveness and potential for implementation. As described, equity is explicitly addressed in the criteria used to assess an EBI's effectiveness and reach across specific populations, with particular attention to populations at greatest risk for the health problem that the EBI is intended to improve. For other implementation criteria, stakeholder input is essential to assessing whether an EBI aligns with the resources, preferences, and existing practice of the settings and providers who serve specific populations, particularly those at greatest risk. See Table 3.3.

TABLE 3.3 Applying Criteria to Assess Evidence in Support of NAPSACC

CRITERIA	FINDINGS
EVIDENCE FOR EFFECTIVENESS	
Methods used to test intervention effects	Tested in four randomized control trials with sample sizes of 17, 26, 31, and 82 childcare centers. Changes to childcare policies and practices were measured using a reliable and valid measure
Consistency of findings across studies	Positive effects on a childcare program's physical and nutrition policies and practices are consistent across most studies. Effects on children's dietary intake and levels of physical activity are mixed
Magnitude of effects	Childcare centers achieved an 11% improvement in their Environment and Policy Assessment and Observation instrument scores following the interventions
Effective-ness across populations	NAPSACC has been tested and shown to be effective in multiple states including North Carolina, Maine, Arizona, and Louisiana and with rural and American Indian populations. NAPSACC has been tested and found to be effective in childcare centers in rural and low-income communi-ties and with populations ranging from 54% to 67% non-White
Degree to which findings are current	The current body of knowledge on NAPSACC was generated from 2008 to 2020
EVIDENCE OF POTENTIAL FOR IMPLEMENTATION IN REAL-WORLD PRACTICE (RE-AIM)	
Reach	In the United States, nearly 75% of children spend time in childcare, giving NAPSACC potential to reach a large number of children
Adoption	In a statewide evaluation study, NAPSACC had an adoption rate of 73% (41/56). The intervention has also been successfully adapted and adopted in multiple states and countries
Implementation	***Fidelity:*** Childcare providers have reported that the intervention was feasible, acceptable and was implemented as planned. NAPSACC has been successfully implemented in multiple state and countries ***Costs*** to implement NAPSACC include: ■ Staff—A healthcare professional (consultant) working 1.5 hr/wk over a 6-mo period is required for each facility in the program. The consultant should attend a virtual, 4-hr training ■ Materials—One tool kit is needed per consultant; material costs per tool kit are approximately $30. Costs of printing additional hand-outs and brochures should be included. Other costs include a laptop, projector, incentives for childcare facilities (i.e., books, classroom supplies), and mileage reimbursement ***Readiness for use:*** NAPSACC provides ready-to-use intervention materi-als and technical support
Maintenance	No information is available on whether childcare facilities have main-tained NAPSACC

NAPSACC, Nutrition and Physical Activity Self-Assessment for Child Care; RE-AIM, Reach, Effectiveness, Adoption, Implementation and Maintenance.

TABLE 3.3 Applying Criteria to Assess Evidence in Support of NAPSACC (*continued*)

Sources: Data from Alkon et al. (2014) Nutrition and physical activity randomized control trial in child care centers improves knowledge, policies, and children's body mass index. *BMC Public Health, 14*(1), 215. https://doi.org/10.1186/1471-2458-14-215; Battista et al., (2014). Improving the physical activity and nutrition environment through self-assessment (NAP SACC) in rural area child care centers in North Carolina. *Preventive Medicine, 67*(S1). https://doi.org/10.1016/j.ypmed.2014.01.022; Benjamin et al., (2007). Reliability and validity of a nutrition and physical activity environmental self-assessment for child care. *International Journal of Behavioral Nutrition and Physical Activity, 4*. https://doi.org/10.1186/1479-5868-4-29; Bonis et al., (2014). Improving physical activity in daycare interventions. *Childhood Obesity, 10*(4). https://doi.org/10.1089/chi.2014.0040; Langford et al., (2019). A physical activity, nutrition and oral health intervention in nursery settings: Process evaluation of the NAP SACC UK feasibility cluster RCT. *BMC Public Health, 19*(1). https://doi.org/10.1186/s12889-019-7102-9 Predy et al., (2021). Examining correlates of outdoor play in childcare centres. *Canadian Journal of Public Health, 112*(2). https://doi.org/10.17269/s41997-020-00404-4; Ward et al., (2008). Nutrition and physical activity in child care. Results from an environmental intervention. *American Journal of Preventive Medicine, 35*(4). https://doi.org/10.1016/j.amepre.2008.06.030; Ward, et al. (2017). Strength of obesity prevention interventions in early care and education settings: A systematic review. *Preventive Medicine, 95*. https://doi.org/10.1016/j.ypmed.2016.09.033

ASSESSING SOURCES OF EVIDENCE: SYSTEMATIC REVIEWS AND WEBSITES

Several factors may influence the strength and reliability of the information provided by different sources of EBIs (i.e., systematic reviews and websites). In addition to the preceding criteria for assessing EBIs, we provide additional guidance on how to assess EBI sources.

Assessing a Systematic Review

Start by identifying the methods used to generate the systematic review findings. Assessing the strength of systematic review methods is beyond the scope of this chapter; however, a few basic criteria can be applied to determine if methods meet the baseline criteria for a systematic review. First, go to the methods section of published reviews or of websites that disseminate reviews. Then, ask the following questions: Did reviewers describe their methods? Did they describe the criteria used to determine which studies were included and which were excluded? Did they assess the quality of included studies and what elements did they assess? Did at least two individuals review each included study? If the answer to any of these questions is no or is unclear, proceed with caution in using the systematic review as a source of EBIs.

In addition, if the systematic review is posted on a website, explore the website to see what other information and resources are available. A growing number of websites are disseminating systematic review findings together with a host of resources to support implementation. For example, in addition to systematic review findings, *The Community Guide* website disseminates tools, in-action stories, and other resources (The Community Guide, 2021).

Assessing Websites

In assessing websites, start by identifying who created the website, often found under a tab labeled "About Us." Consider the credibility of the source and whether there is potential for bias in their presentation of findings. Governmental organizations (e.g., websites ending in .gov for the United States), academic institutions (e.g., websites ending in .edu), and well-established non-profit organizations are among the more reliable sources. In assessing the potential for bias, consider whether an organization has a financial motive (e.g., are they are selling a product?) or an underlying ideological position or agenda (e.g., are they promoting celibacy before marriage?) that may bias their presentation of information on the websites. Websites that disseminate EBIs use a range of terminology to describe the level of evidence in support of a specific intervention or systematic review recommendation (e.g., evidence-based, proven, promising, practice-tested, etc.). They also use diverse criteria to assign interventions to those different levels. Therefore, do not just trust the label that a website gives to an intervention. After establishing who created the website, identify the methods and criteria used to rate interventions. If you cannot identify their methods and criteria, or do not agree with the methods used, proceed with caution in using the website as a source of EBIs.

Some websites disseminate case studies or stories from the field. These may provide useful ideas for how to adapt or implement an EBI in a setting or population similar to your own, as is the case with the "action stories" reported in *The Community Guide* (The Community Guide, 2021).

KEY POINT FOR PRACTICE

Remember that the goal is to implement EBIs, those interventions that have demonstrated effectiveness in one or more research studies (i.e., EBIs). Don't hesitate to use the information in reports of case studies and stories from the field for ideas about how to implement an intervention in real-world practice. However, be sure to identify the EBI that the case study is illustrating, and review research on the EBI in addition to the case study. Doing so will allow you to gain practical guidance from the case study while also maintaining fidelity to the EBI.

SELECTING ONE OR MORE INTERVENTIONS THAT FIT LOCAL PRIORITIES AND ARE SUPPORTED BY EVIDENCE

This chapter has offered multiple criteria for assessing the evidence in support of an EBI's effectiveness and potential to be implemented in real-world practice. As illustrated in the case study at the end of the chapter, these criteria need to be considered alongside criteria for assessing an EBI's fit with local priorities. In other words, to what extent do the candidate EBIs fit the (a) prioritized health problem, (b) specific factors that contribute to that problem, (c) intended population, and (d) settings where the EBI would be implemented? In selecting the best EBIs, stakeholders need to balance information on multiple criteria across multiple EBIs.

COMMON PITFALLS IN PRACTICE

To make an informed decision about the best EBI, stakeholder groups require information about a wide range of EBIs. This is challenging because stakeholders are often busy people with only limited amounts of time, and it is very easy to provide stakeholders with so much information on EBIs that they become overwhelmed.

To avoid overwhelming stakeholders, at each step in the process, it is essential to take the time to meaningfully distill and summarize findings. Rather than presenting findings from each specific criterion (as in Table 3.3), distill that information and present a summary of findings for each category of criteria. At Step 1, a summary of findings might be presented in a table with the following rows (see Table 3.4):

- Brief description of the systematic review recommendations (i.e., broad EBI approaches)
- Names of websites or citations to literature reviews that support each broad EBI
- Evidence of effectiveness
- Reported magnitude of EBI's effect on intended outcomes
- Evidence, if available, on effectiveness in priority populations and settings, with particular focus on those at greatest risk for health disparities
- Additional notes about strengths or limitations of the cited websites and literature reviews (e.g., does the website provide additional tools or resources to support implementation)

In addition, at the end of Steps 2 and 3, the summary table would need to provide more detailed information about specific EBIs, as illustrated in Table 3.4.

KEY POINT FOR PRACTICE

In addition to creating tables of the EBIs that systematic reviews and websites recommend, also keep a list of the names and types of interventions they do not recommend due to insufficient evidence. Stakeholders will often come to meetings with ideas for interventions that they have read about or learned about through their professional networks. As they suggest interventions, you can be prepared to quickly eliminate any that are on your not recommended list and have the evidence to hand to support that decision.

CASE STUDY 3.3 SUMMARIZING THE EVIDENCE NEEDED TO COMPARE EVIDENCE-BASED INTERVENTIONS

Prior to her first meeting with her stakeholder group, Stacey read through multiple systematic reviews on interventions to prevent overweight and obesity in 2- to 5-year-old children (Step 1). As she read the reviews, she took notes on the methods reviewers used to develop their recommendations. She also applied the five recommended criteria to review evidence on effectiveness in support of each review's recommendations. In reviewing websites, she also noted whether they provided tools, case studies, or other resources to support implementation. She then summarized her findings in a report that she presented to stakeholders (see Table 3.4; The Community Guide, 2014, 2017; The University of Wisconsin Population Health Institute and the Robert Wood Johnson Foundation, 2017a, 2017b, 2020a, 2020b). The stakeholders reviewed the list and determined that the broad EBI, "nutrition and physical activity interventions in childcare," was effective at improving children's dietary intake and levels of physical activity. They also determined that the EBI fit their priority population (children from low-income households) and one of their prioritized settings (childcare centers).

Stacey then searched for websites that disseminate packaged interventions that focus on improving nutrition and physical activity in childcare (Step 2). She also revisited one of the websites she searched in Step 1, *What Works for Health* (The University of

TABLE 3.4 Excerpt From a Summary Report on Systematic Review Recommendations (Broad EBIs) to Prevent Obesity in 2- to 5-Year Olds

WEBSITE (WITH RATING)	EVIDENCE OF EFFECTIVENESS	MAGNITUDE OF EFFECTS	EFFECTIVENESS IN PRIORITY POPULATION/ SETTING	ADDITIONAL NOTES
Broad EBI #1. Nutrition and Physical Activity Interventions in Preschool and Childcare				
County Health Rankings: What Works for Health (Scientifically Supported)	Strong evidence of effectiveness in improving children's dietary intake and levels of physical activity. Some evidence of improvement in weight status	The magnitude of effects varied across studies and summarized data were not readily available	Have been tested and found to be effective in childcare settings that serve low-income populations	County Health Rankings use rapid review methods, which are less rigorous than other websites. However, the website includes links to multiple systematic reviews that also support the intervention
Broad EBI #2. Screen Time Interventions for Children				
Community Guide (Strong Evidence) County Health Rankings: What Works for Health (Scientifically Supported)	Strong evidence of effectiveness in reducing recreational sedentary screen time, increasing physical activity, improving diet, and improving or maintaining weight-related outcomes	Time spent on any screen decreased by a median of 26.4 min/day	Have been tested and found to be effective in settings that serve low-income populations and have been conducted in primary care clinics	Studies have also been conducted in schools, homes, communities, and other settings. Interventions were effective regardless of setting
Broad EBI #3. Nutrition: Gardening Interventions to Increase Vegetable Consumption Among Children				
The Community Guide (Sufficient Evidence)	A systematic review of 14 studies found that consumption of vegetables increased in 12 studies; fruit consumption did not change in 10 of the studies	Increase of a median of 0.55 fruits/vegetables per day	Have been tested and found to be effective in low-income populations. Only one study was done in a childcare setting	Most effective when combined with nutrition education

TABLE 3.5 Specific Evidence-Based Interventions That Target the Physical Activity and Nutrition Interventions in Daycare Programs

BRIEF DESCRIPTION	WEBSITE	EFFECTIVENESS	IMPLEMENTATION	FIT WITH PRIORITIZED POPULATION
Specific EBI #1. NAPSACC				
Childcare programs complete a self-assessment of their eating and physical activity environment, practices, and policies. Provides training, tools, and technical assistance to make improvements based on assessment findings	County Health Rankings: What Works for Health: NAPSACC website	Has been tested in multiple RCTs and found to be effective at improving program's physical and nutrition policies and practices. Some evidence of effects on children's dietary intake and physical activity	Many daycare programs have adopted, and childcare providers' report that it is feasible and acceptable. **Resources and costs**. A staff person would need to work 1.5 hr/wk to support each daycare facility over 6 mo. Some costs to purchase toolkits (about $30). Other costs include training, laptop, projector, travel, and classroom supplies **Readiness for use.** Training and materials are available in a ready for use format	NAPSACC has been tested in multiple studies with populations of diverse demographic backgrounds
Specific EBI #2. SHAPES				
Includes four daily components: (a) indoor physical activity, (b) recess, (c) incorporating physical activity into classroom lessons, and (d) enhanced social support and physical environment	NIH EBCCP: SHAPES website	Has been tested in one RCT and found to be effective with a statistically significant but small increase in moderate to vigorous physical activity	Of 16 daycare programs initially invited, 14 adopted the program. **Cost and Resources.** Teachers complete a 90- to 120-min training **Readiness for use.** Training and materials are available in a ready-for-use format	Tested in South Carolina with Caucasian and African American populations

(continued)

TABLE 3.5 Specific Evidence-Based Interventions That Target the Physical Activity and Nutrition Interventions in Daycare Programs *(continued)*

BRIEF DESCRIPTION	WEBSITE	EFFECTIVENESS	IMPLEMENTATION	FIT WITH PRIORITIZED POPULATION
Specific EBI #3. Start for Life				
Provides training and materials to support 30 min of structured physical activity per day	NIH EBCCP: Start for Life	Has been tested in one RCT and found to be effective with a statistically significant but small decrease in obesity and increase in moderate to vigorous physical activity	Little information available concerning reach, adoption, and implementation. **Cost and Resources.** Teacher time to attend training. Costs of training and materials **Readiness for use.** Training manual, slides, observation form, and activity log available from developer. Prices unknown	This intervention has been tested in low-income African American populations

EBI, evidence-based intervention; NAPSACC, Nutrition and Physical Activity Self-Assessment for Child Care; NIH EBCCP, National Cancer Institute Evidence-Based Cancer Control Programs; RCT, randomized control trial; SHAPES, Supporting Health and Activity in Preschool Environments.

Wisconsin Population Health Institute & The Robert Wood Johnson Foundation, 2021), because she had noted that it provided links to intervention websites. She reviewed each website to identify any risk of bias and, for those that rated interventions, she assessed the methods and criteria they applied to do so. She then applied the recommended criteria to review each relevant intervention and documented the evidence in support of its effectiveness and potential for implementation (see Table 3.3 for an example). She also took notes on the populations and settings for whom the intervention was designed. Then she summarized the interventions and presented them to her key stakeholders (see Table 3.5). The workgroup decided to move forward with the NAPSACC intervention because it addresses both physical activity and nutrition and has strong evidence in support of its potential for implementation in real-world practice. Furthermore, the regional health authority was willing to provide the staff needed to coordinate the program, and daycare-program stakeholders were enthusiastic about implementing it.

SUMMARY

In this chapter, a three-step, stakeholder-engaged process was presented for use in locating and selecting EBIs. The chapter also provided detailed guidance on criteria that may be applied to assess an EBI's potential to be effective, to be implemented as intended, and to promote health equity.

KEY POINTS FOR PRACTICE

1. When possible, look for interventions that are supported by systematic review findings and available in a packaged format. The systematic review provides strong evidence for the effectiveness of the broad EBI approach while the packaged intervention provides more specific guidance on how to implement the intervention into practice. Some websites help users connect systematic review findings with packaged interventions. For example, for each of its systematic review findings, the *What Works for Health* website provides links to relevant packaged EBIs (countyhealthrankings.org/take-action-to-improve-health/what-works-for-health).
2. Partner with a librarian to assist you with Steps 1 and 3. To find a librarian, reach out to a university, college, hospital, public health authority, or health education center. Librarians have both the training and experience needed to search the literature effectively. Furthermore, libraries often provide users with free access to journals and other resources that they would have to pay for if they tried to access them on their own.
3. Remember that the goal is to implement EBIs, that is, those interventions that have demonstrated effectiveness in one or more research studies. Don't hesitate to use the information in reports of case studies and stories from the field for ideas about how to implement an intervention in real-world practice. However, be sure to identify the EBI that the case study is illustrating, and review findings from research on the EBI in addition to the case study. Doing so will allow you to gain practical guidance from the case study while also maintaining fidelity to the EBI.
4. In addition to creating tables of the EBIs that systematic reviews and websites recommend, keep a list of the names and types of interventions that are not recommended due to insufficient evidence. Stakeholders will often come to meetings with ideas for interventions that they have read about or learned about through their professional networks. As they suggest interventions, you can be prepared to quickly eliminate any that are on your not recommended list and have the evidence on hand to support that decision.

COMMON PITFALLS IN PRACTICE

1. Engaging stakeholders takes time and energy, and this creates the temptation to leave stakeholders out of the selection process and engage them only after the "best" EBIs have been identified. Resist this temptation. Stakeholders have in-depth knowledge of the priority population and can provide input on which EBIs will best fit the local culture, preferences, and needs. Furthermore, engaging stakeholders promotes local ownership and commitment to the EBI and its implementation.
2. Clinical practice guidelines often change over time. For this reason, it is important not to implement packaged EBIs without first reviewing the patient education and other materials included in the package. Some changes to clinical practice guidelines can be managed by making minor adaptations to intervention materials (e.g., changes to the age at which colorectal cancer screening should start). At other times, the changes required are less feasible (e.g., major changes to guidelines for a heart healthy diet) and another EBI needs to be selected.
3. Stakeholders may select an intervention that is beautifully packaged and ready to implement even when other interventions have stronger evidence of effectiveness and potential for implementation in their setting and population. This is particularly

common when stakeholders have heard that others are implementing the selected intervention. Decisions are often influenced by good marketing and the desire to keep up with the latest fad and fashion. The best way to counteract this tendency is to provide clear documentation of the evidence in support of each intervention's effectiveness and potential for implementation.

4. To make an informed decision about the best EBI, stakeholder groups require information about a wide range of EBIs. This is challenging because stakeholders are often busy people with only limited amounts of time, and it is very easy to provide stakeholders with so much information on EBIs that they become overwhelmed.

DISCUSSION QUESTIONS

1. How do systematic review recommendations, packaged interventions, and reports of intervention studies differ in the strength of the evidence they typically provide for intervention effectiveness?
2. How do systematic review recommendations, packaged interventions and reports of intervention studies differ in the information and resources they typically provide to guide implementation?
3. Why does it make sense to search for systematic review findings before you search for specific interventions?
4. Why might you search for research reports after you and your stakeholders have already selected a packaged intervention as the EBI you plan to implement?
5. Discuss how you would apply at least three criteria to determine the effectiveness of an EBI.
6. Discuss how you would apply at least three criteria to assess an EBI's potential for implementation.

ACKNOWLEDGMENTS

This chapter was supported by the Centers for Disease Control and Prevention of the U.S. Department of Health and Human Services (DHHS) as part of a financial assistance award funded by CDC/DHHS (Cooperative agreement numbers: U48 DP006400, U48 DP006377). The contents are those of the author(s) and do not necessarily represent the official views of, nor an endorsement, by CDC/DHHS, or the U.S. Government.

REFERENCES

Administration for Children and Families. (2021). *Child care quality ratings*. https://www.childcare.gov/index.php/consumer-education/child-care-quality-ratings

Alkon, A., Crowley, A. A., Neelon, S. E. B., Hill, S., Pan, Y., Nguyen, V., Rose, R., Savage, E., Forestieri, N., Shipman, L., & Kotch, J. B. (2014). Nutrition and physical activity randomized control trial in child care centers improves knowledge, policies, and children's body mass index. *BMC Public Health, 14*(1), 215. https://doi.org/10.1186/1471-2458-14-215

Bajwah, S., Oluyase, A. O., Yi, D., Gao, W., Evans, C. J., Grande, G., Todd, C., Costantini, M., Murtagh, F. E., & Higginson, I. J. (2020). The effectiveness and cost-effectiveness of hospital-based specialist palliative care for adults with advanced illness and their caregivers. *Cochrane Database of Systematic Reviews, 9*. https://doi.org/10.1002/14651858.CD012780.pub2

Battista, R. A., Oakley, H., Weddell, M. S., Mudd, L. M., Greene, J. B., & West, S. T. (2014). Improving the physical activity and nutrition environment through self-assessment (NAP SACC) in rural area child care centers in North Carolina. *Preventive Medicine, 67*(S1). https://doi.org/10.1016/j.ypmed.2014.01.022

Benjamin, S. E., Neelon, B., Ball, S. C., Bangdiwala, S. I., Ammerman, A. S., & Ward, D. S. (2007). Reliability and validity of a nutrition and physical activity environmental self-assessment for child care. *International Journal of Behavioral Nutrition and Physical Activity, 4*. https://doi.org/10.1186/1479-5868-4-29

Bibbins-Domingo, K., Grossman, D. C., Curry, S. J., Davidson, K. W., Epling, J. W., García, F. A. R., Gillman, M. W., Harper, D. M., Kemper, A. R., Krist, A. H., Kurth, A. E., Landefeld, C. S., Mangione, C. M., Owens, D. K., Phillips, W. R., Phipps, M. G., Pignone, M. P., & Siu, A. L. (2016). Screening for colorectal cancer: US preventive services task force recommendation statement. *JAMA - Journal of the American Medical Association, 315*(23). https://doi.org/10.1001/jama.2016.5989

Bonis, M., Loftin, M., Ward, D., Tseng, T. S., Clesi, A., & Sothern, M. (2014). Improving physical activity in daycare interventions. *Childhood Obesity, 10*(4). https://doi.org/10.1089/chi.2014.0040

Castillo-Mancilla, J., Cohn, S., Krishnan, S., Cespedes, M., Floris-Moore, M., Schulte, G., Pavlov, G., Mildvan, D., & Smith, K. (2014). Minorities remain underrepresented in HIV/AIDS research despite access to clinical trials. *HIV Clinical Trials, 15*(1). https://doi.org/10.1310/hct1501-14

Castro, F. G., Barrera, M., & Holleran Steiker, L. K. (2010). Issues and challenges in the design of culturally adapted evidence-based interventions. *Annual Review of Clinical Psychology, 6*(1), 213–239. https://doi.org/10.1146/annurev-clinpsy-033109-132032

Center of Excellence for Training and Research, North Carolina State University, & North Carolina Division of Public Health. (2013). *Color me healthy intervention.* http://centertrt.org/content/docs/Intervention_Documents/Intervention_Templates/CMH_research_tested_template.pdf

Center of Excellence for Training and Research Translation, Center for Health Promotion and Disease Prevention, UNC at Chapel Hill, & Division of Public Health, NC Department of Health and Human Services. (2014). *Nutrition and physical activity self-assessment for child-care (NAP SACC). Intervention.* http://centertrt.org/content/docs/Intervention_Documents/Intervention_Templates/NAPSACC_Template_Updated_April_2014.pdf

Center of Excellence for Training and Research Translation, & Center for Human Nutrition Bloomberg School of Public Health. (2013). *Baltimore healthy stores (BHS). Intervention.* http://centertrt.org/content/docs/Intervention_Documents/Intervention_Templates/Baltimore_Healthy_Stores_template.pdf

The Community Guide. (2014). *Obesity: Behavioral interventions that aim to reduce recreational sedentary screen time among children.* https://www.thecommunityguide.org/findings/obesity-behavioral-interventions-aim-reduce-recreational-sedentary-screen-time-among

The Community Guide. (2017). *Nutrition: Gardening interventions to increase vegetable consumption among children.* https://www.thecommunityguide.org/findings/nutrition-gardening-interventions-increase-vegetable-consumption-among-children

The Community Guide. (2021). *The community guide.* https://www.thecommunityguide.org/

Coronado, G. D., Petrik, A. F., Vollmer, W. M., Taplin, S. H., Keast, E. M., Fields, S., & Green, B. B. (2018). Effectiveness of a mailed colorectal cancer screening outreach program in community health clinics the STOP CRC cluster randomized clinical trial. *JAMA Internal Medicine, 178*(9). https://doi.org/10.1001/jamainternmed.2018.3629

Coronado, G. D., Schneider, J. L., Green, B. B., Coury, J. K., Schwartz, M. R., Kulkarni-Sharma, Y., & Baldwin, L. M. (2020). Health plan adaptations to a mailed outreach program for colorectal cancer screening among Medicaid and Medicare enrollees: The BeneFIT study. *Implementation Science, 15*(1). https://doi.org/10.1186/s13012-020-01037-4

Craig, P., Katikireddi, S. V., Leyland, A., & Popham, F. (2017). Natural experiments: An overview of methods, approaches, and contributions to public health intervention research. *Annual Review of Public Health, 38*. https://doi.org/10.1146/annurev-publhealth-031816-044327

Davis, M. M., Nambiar, S., Mayorga, M. E., Sullivan, E., Hicklin, K., O'Leary, M. C., Dillon, K., Hassmiller Lich, K., Gu, Y., Lind, B. K., & Wheeler, S. B. (2019). Mailed FIT (fecal immunochemical test), navigation or patient reminders? Using microsimulation to inform selection of interventions to increase colorectal cancer screening in Medicaid enrollees. *Preventive Medicine, 129*. https://doi.org/10.1016/j.ypmed.2019.105836

Evelyn, B., Toigo, T., Banks, D., Pohl, D., Gray, K., Robins, B., & Ernat, J. (2001). Participation of racial/ethnic groups in clinical trials and race-related labeling: A review of new molecular entities approved 1995-1999. *Journal of the National Medical Association, 93*(Issue 12 suppl.).

Fernandez, M. E., Mullen, P. D., Leeman, J., Walker, T. J., & Escoffery, C. (2018). Evidence-based cancer practices, programs, and interventions. In D. A. Chambers, W. E. Norton, & C. A. Vinson (Eds.), *Advancing the science of implementation across the cancer continuum.* Oxford University Press. https://doi.org/10.1093/med/9780190647421.003.0003

Harvard T.H. Chan School of Public Health. (2021). *Childhood obesity national action kit.* https://choicesproject.org/actionkit/

Hendricks-Brown, C., Curran, G., Palinkas, L. A., Aarons, G. A., Wells, K. B., Jones, L., Collins, L. M., Duan, N., Mittman, Brian, S., Wallace, A., Tabak, R. G., Ducharme, L., Chambers, D. A., Neta, G., Wiley, T., Landsverk, J., Cheung, K., & Cruden, G. (2017). an overview of research andevaluation designs for dissemination and implementation. *Annual Review of Public Health, 38*(March), 1–22.

Johns Hopkins School of Public Health, & Bill & Melinda Gates Foundation. (2021). *The lives saved tool*. https://www.livessavedtool.org

Kessler, R. S., Purcell, E. P., Glasgow, R. E., Klesges, L. M., Benkeser, R. M., & Peek, C. J. (2013). What does it mean to "employ" the RE-AIM model? *Evaluation and the Health Professions, 36*(1). https://doi.org/10.1177/0163278712446066

Langford, R., Jago, R., White, J., Moore, L., Papadaki, A., Hollingworth, W., Metcalfe, C., Ward, D., Campbell, R., Wells, S., & Kipping, R. (2019). A physical activity, nutrition and oral health intervention in nursery settings: Process evaluation of the NAP SACC UK feasibility cluster RCT. *BMC Public Health, 19*(1). https://doi.org/10.1186/s12889-019-7102-9

Leeman, J., Birken, S. A., Powell, B. J., Rohweder, C., & Shea, C. M. (2017). Beyond "implementation strategies": Classifying the full range of strategies used in implementation science and practice. *Implementation Science, 12*(1), 1–9. https://doi.org/10.1186/s13012-017-0657-x

Leeman, J., Myers, A. E., Ribisl, K. M., & Ammerman, A. S. (2015). Disseminating policy and environmental change interventions: Insights from obesity prevention and tobacco control. *International Journal of Behavioral Medicine, 22*(3). https://doi.org/10.1007/s12529-014-9427-1

Leeman, J., Teal, R., Jernigan, J., Reed, J. H., Farris, R., & Ammerman, A. (2014). What evidence and support do state-level public health practitioners need to address obesity prevention. *American Journal of Health Promotion, 28*(3). https://doi.org/10.4278/ajhp.120518-QUAL-266

Luke, D. A., Calhoun, A., Robichaux, C. B., Moreland-Russell, S., & Elliott, M. B. (2014). The program sustainability assessment tool: A new instrument for public health programs. *Preventing Chronic Disease, 11*(2014). https://doi.org/10.5888/pcd11.130184

Macones, G. A., Goldie, S. J., & Peipert, J. F. (1999). Cost-effectiveness analysis: An introductory guide for clinicians. *Obstetrical and Gynecological Survey, 54*(10). https://doi.org/10.1097/00006254-199910000-00024

Masters, R., Anwar, E., Collins, B., Cookson, R., & Capewell, S. (2017). Return on investment of public health interventions: A systematic review. *Journal of Epidemiology and Community Health, 71*(8). https://doi.org/10.1136/jech-2016-208141

Moher, D., Liberati, A., Tetzlaff, J., Altman, D. G., Altman, D., Antes, G., Atkins, D., Barbour, V., Barrowman, N., Berlin, J. A., Clark, J., Clarke, M., Cook, D., D'Amico, R., Deeks, J. J., Devereaux, P. J., Dickersin, K., Egger, M., Ernst, E., ... Tugwell, P. (2009). Preferred reporting items for systematic reviews and meta-analyses: The PRISMA statement. *PLoS Medicine, 6*(7). https://doi.org/10.1371/journal.pmed.1000097

National Cancer Institute. (2020a). *Culturally tailored navigator intervention program for colorectal cancer screening*. https://ebccp.cancercontrol.cancer.gov/programDetails.do?programId=1493683

National Cancer Institute. (2020b). *Flu-FIT and Flu-FOBT program*. https://ebccp.cancercontrol.cancer.gov/programDetails.do?programId=1084580

National Center on Early Childhood Quality Assurance. (2021). *About QRIS: QRIS resource guide*.

O'Connor, E. A., Vollmer, W. M., Petrik, A. F., Green, B. B., & Coronado, G. D. (2020). Moderators of the effectiveness of an intervention to increase colorectal cancer screening through mailed fecal immunochemical test kits: Results from a pragmatic randomized trial. *Trials, 21*(1). https://doi.org/10.1186/s13063-019-4027-7

Petrik, A. F., Green, B., Schneider, J., Miech, E. J., Coury, J., Retecki, S., & Coronado, G. D. (2020). Factors influencing implementation of a colorectal cancer screening improvement program in community health centers: An applied use of configurational comparative methods. *Journal of General Internal Medicine, 35*. https://doi.org/10.1007/s11606-020-06186-2

Predy, M., Holt, N., & Carson, V. (2021). Examining correlates of outdoor play in childcare centres. *Canadian Journal of Public Health, 112*(2). https://doi.org/10.17269/s41997-020-00404-4

Proctor, E., Silmere, H., Raghavan, R., Hovmand, P., Aarons, G., Bunger, A., Griffey, R., & Hensley, M. (2011). Outcomes for implementation research: Conceptual distinctions, measurement challenges, and research agenda. *Administration and Policy in Mental Health and Mental Health Services Research, 38*(2), 65–76. https://doi.org/10.1007/s10488-010-0319-7

RTI International. (2021). *Obesity cost calculator*.

Shadish, W. R., Cook, T. D., & Campbell, D. T. (2002). *Experimental and quasi-experimental designs for generalized causal inference*.

Singal, A. G., Higgins, P. D. R., & Waljee, A. K. (2014). A primer on effectiveness and efficacy trials. *Clinical and Translational Gastroenterology, 5*. https://doi.org/10.1038/ctg.2013.13

Sussman, S., Valente, T. W., Rohrbach, L. A., Skara, S., & Pentz, M. A. (2006). Translation in the health professions: Converting science into action. *Evaluation and the Health Professions, 29*(1). https://doi.org/10.1177/0163278705284441

Thompson, J. H., Schneider, J. L., Rivelli, J. S., Petrik, A. F., Vollmer, W. M., Fuoco, M. J., & Coronado, G. D. (2019). A survey of provider attitudes, beliefs, and perceived barriers regarding a centralized direct-mail colorectal cancer screening approach at community health centers. *Journal of Primary Care and Community Health, 10*. https://doi.org/10.1177/2150132719890950

The University of Wisconsin Population Health Institute, & The Robert Wood Johnson Foundation. (2017a). *Screen time interventions for children: What Works for Health*. https://www.countyhealthrankings.org/take-action-to-improve-health/what-works-for-health/strategies/screen-time-interventions-for-children

The University of Wisconsin Population Health Institute, & The Robert Wood Johnson Foundation. (2017b). *Sugar sweetened beverage taxes: What Works for Health*. https://www.countyhealthrankings.org/take-action-to-improve-health/what-works-for-health/strategies/sugar-sweetened-beverage-taxes

The University of Wisconsin Population Health Institute, & The Robert Wood Johnson Foundation. (2020a). *Healthy food in convenience stores: What Works for Health*. https://www.countyhealthrankings.org/take-action-to-improve-health/what-works-for-health/strategies/healthy-food-in-convenience-stores

The University of Wisconsin Population Health Institute, & The Robert Wood Johnson Foundation. (2020b). *Nutrition and physical activity interventions in preschool & child care: What Works for Health*. https://www.countyhealthrankings.org/take-action-to-improve-health/what-works-for-health/strategies/nutrition-and-physical-activity-interventions-in-preschool-child-care

The University of Wisconsin Population Health Institute, & The Robert Wood Johnson Foundation. (2021). *What Works for Health: County health rankings and roadmaps*.

Verkamp, J. (2010). Why we should stop proving a parachute works in a RCT. *European Archives of Paediatric Dentistry: Official Journal of the European Academy of Paediatric Dentistry*, *11*(5). https://doi.org/10.1007/bf03262749

Ward, D. S., Benjamin, S. E., Ammerman, A. S., Ball, S. C., Neelon, B. H., & Bangdiwala, S. I. (2008). Nutrition and physical activity in child care. Results from an environmental intervention. *American Journal of Preventive Medicine*, *35*(4). https://doi.org/10.1016/j.amepre.2008.06.030

Ward, D. S., Welker, E., Choate, A., Henderson, K. E., Lott, M., Tovar, A., Wilson, A., & Sallis, J. F. (2017). Strength of obesity prevention interventions in early care and education settings: A systematic review. *Preventive Medicine*, *95*. https://doi.org/10.1016/j.ypmed.2016.09.033

4

Adaptation of Evidence-Based Interventions

Heidi La Bash, Fiona C. Thomas, and Shannon Wiltsey Stirman

Learning Objectives

By the end of this chapter, readers will be able to:

- Identify common reasons and goals for adaptation
- Understand the need for a systematic approach to adaptation that retains fidelity to an evidence-based intervention's (EBI) core functions
- Determine if an EBI needs to be adapted
- Apply a conceptual framework to adapt EBIs, when needed
- Describe taxonomies and methods to systematically document and track EBI adaptations and identified outcomes

CASE STUDY 4.1A ADAPTATION OF COGNITIVE PROCESSING THERAPY FOR TREATMENT OF TORTURE SURVIVORS IN KURDISTAN, IRAQ

In the case study presented here, we review the adaptation of cognitive processing therapy (CPT) for posttraumatic stress disorder (PTSD) for a population of torture survivors in Kurdistan, Iraq (Bolton et al., 2014; Kaysen et al., 2013).

OVERVIEW OF COGNITIVE PROCESSING THERAPY

CPT is a 12-session therapy for PTSD that was developed in the United States that incorporates cognitive restructuring with emotional processing of trauma-related content (Resick, Monson et al., 2008). It has been designed for and tested in individual and group therapy settings. Randomized clinical trials of CPT have been conducted primarily in the United States with White participants (Chard, 2005; Monson et al., 2006; Resick, Galovski et al., 2008). More recently, CPT has been adapted for other populations including Bosnian refugees in the United States (Schulz et al., 2006), the Haitian mental health care system (Creed et al., 2019), and for Native American women in the United States (Pearson et al., 2019). This case study was conducted in Kurdistan, Iraq, and is an early example of CPT adaptation for a population outside of the United States.

SETTING AND ADAPTATION PROCESS

Kurdistan is considered an autonomous region of Iraq. The majority of Kurdish people identify as Muslim and have been subjected to political and cultural repression, torture, chemical attacks, ethnic cleansing, and genocide (Rogg & Rimscha, 2007).

An equity lens was integrated by the study team from the outset of CPT adaptation for the Kurdish population. For example, using an equity lens ensured that gender roles were an important consideration in adapting CPT for this context. Women were not always able to independently consent to treatment without approval of a male family member. In such situations, the trainers worked closely with the local members of the study team to negotiate with spouses and families to allow individual access to care or provided alternative solutions (e.g., female relatives would accompany the female client to sessions). Early on, additional barriers to implementation in low-resource settings were identified, such as limited to no access to photocopiers for handouts, lack of access to private rooms for therapy, and concern about male community mental health workers providing treatment to female clients and vice versa. Information pertaining to these and any other culture-related issues was assessed daily with study therapists, so the study team could track and respond to any ripple effects of the EBI adaptation.

INTRODUCTION

Evidence-based interventions (EBIs), in some cases, have been criticized for their perceived inflexibility (e.g., concern that one must rigidly adhere to the treatment protocol) and for not accounting for the demands of real-world settings. For example, EBIs have traditionally been studied in randomized controlled clinical trials, which have been criticized for having less diverse samples, higher levels of provider training, and artificially predetermined parameters (e.g., strict inclusion/exclusion criteria). These concerns gave rise to more practical approaches to evaluating EBIs that better account for the complex variability that can be found in real-world settings. The concerns also led to the development and dissemination of treatment guidelines that aim to reduce disparity in what treatments are delivered and the manner in which they are delivered (American Psychological Association [APA], 2017; International Society for Traumatic Stress Studies [ISTSS], 2018). Treatment guidelines galvanized wide-spread efforts to disseminate and implement EBIs across a range of contexts and populations in which the EBIs were not developed and evaluated (Baumann et al., 2017). In such circumstances, EBI adaptations can have great clinical utility in addressing the needs of a specific population or setting, particularly in helping with issues of health equity. A health equity approach moves us away from the traditional, linear process of EBI development that may result in a disconnect between the EBI and context. Instead of circumstances being viewed as threats to an EBI's feasibility and effectiveness, EBIs can be developed to fit the realities and needs of the population and setting they are intended to serve. From an equity perspective, Baumann and Cabassa (2020) argue that EBIs should be developed with implementation in mind, particularly when it comes to EBIs for vulnerable populations. This means prioritizing implementation outcomes (e.g., acceptability, feasibility, appropriateness, cost) and considering fit between the EBI and context (e.g., population and setting) from the outset (Proctor et al., 2009).

In this chapter, we begin by reviewing the common reasons and goals for EBI adaptation. We then examine key conceptual adaptation frameworks and provide practical guidance for the EBI adaptation process. We discuss these steps in further detail throughout the chapter, reviewing common pitfalls that may occur. We also review key implementation frameworks that guide decision-making regarding which outcomes to prioritize and how to balance between achieving EBI effectiveness and other considerations, such as improving engagement and reach. Finally, we highlight the importance of integrating a health equity lens across all steps of the EBI adaptation process. Throughout the chapter, we revisit the case study introduced at the beginning of the chapter to describe practical ways in which EBI adaptation can occur.

Before delving deeper into the topic of treatment adaptation, it is important to understand conceptual distinctions among several key concepts related to adaptation. **Treatment fidelity** refers to the level at which treatment delivery is consistent with the original EBI protocol or as it was intended by its developers (Dusenbury et al., 2003; Rabin et al., 2008). Treatment fidelity is conceptualized as encompassing the delivery of key elements of a treatment protocol (i.e., adherence) and the skill (i.e., competence) with which the components are delivered (Gearing et al., 2011; Schoenwald et al., 2011). **Treatment modification** is a broad concept that encompasses any changes made to interventions, whether deliberately and proactive (adaptation) or in reaction to unanticipated challenges that arise in a given session or context (Stirman et al., 2019). **Treatment adaptation** is a process of thoughtful and deliberate alteration to the design or delivery of an intervention, with the goal of improving its fit or effectiveness in a given context (Stirman et al., 2017). Ideally, this is done in a data-driven and stakeholder-engaged manner (Miller et al., 2020). Treatment adaptations typically aim to preserve the core functions of a treatment. A treatment's **core functions** are the "active ingredients" of a treatment that make the treatment effective (Stirman et al., 2019). Core functions are also sometime called *core components, core processes,* or *core elements.* In contrast, **peripheral elements** are those that are not essential for the EBI to be effective. (See Table 4.1 for key terms and examples of key terms.)

TABLE 4.1 Glossary of Key Terms

TERM	DEFINITION	EXAMPLE(S)
Treatment modification	A broad concept that encompasses any changes made to interventions, whether deliberately and proactively (i.e., **treatment adaptation**) or in reaction to unanticipated challenges that arise in a given session or context (Stirman et al., 2019)	■ Removing or adding elements of another treatment to an EBI protocol. For example, a protocol with the aim of reducing obesity may be modified to also include elements of a drinking-reduction program, if it is found that high levels of alcohol are contributing to obesity in the target population. ■ Changing where or who delivers an EBI. For example, a protocol may have been developed to be delivered by licensed health professionals. If there are few licensed professionals available to deliver the EBI, the EBI could be modified to be delivered by peers, to increase the target population's access to the treatment
Treatment adaptation	A process of thoughtful and deliberate alteration to the design or delivery of an intervention, with the goal of improving its fit or effectiveness in a given context (Stirman et al., 2017). Treatment adaptations typically aim to preserve the **core functions** of a treatment	■ Changing the format of an intervention but keeping all of the same content. For example, instead of providing psychoeducation material in print format, the protocol is modified for a population with low reading levels by having the information delivered verbally
Core functions (a.k.a. core components, core processes, or core elements)	The "active ingredients" of a treatment that make the treatment effective (Stirman et al., 2019)	■ Socratic questioning is believed to be a core function of CPT, because it has been found to be one aspect of CPT that accounts for symptom improvement in clients who receive this treatment (Farmer et al., 2017)
Peripheral elements	In contrast to **core functions, peripheral elements** are those that are not essential for the EBI to be effective	■ CPT can be delivered with or without the client writing an explicit account of their primary trauma. Even though a client may decide they would like to include this element in their treatment, it is not necessary for symptom reduction (Resick, Galovski et al., 2008)
Fidelity-consistent adaptation	Adaptations that preserve the EBI's core functions	■ Increasing the use of Socratic questioning in CPT for PTSD, when Socratic questioning is believed to be a core function of CPT (Farmer, Mitchell, Parker-Guilbert, & Galovski, 2017)

(continued)

TABLE 4.1 Glossary of Key Terms *(continued)*

TERM	DEFINITION	EXAMPLE(S)
Fidelity-inconsistent adaptation	Adaptations that do not preserve the EBI's core functions	■ Removing Socratic questioning in CPT for PTSD, when Socratic questioning is believed to be a core function of CPT (Farmer, Mitchell, Parker-Guilbert, & Galovski, 2017)
Surface adaptation	Adaptations that are made in response to observable social and behavioral characteristics of the population (Resnicow et al., 1999)	■ Changing examples in an EBI protocol to reflect the culture of the target population
Deep adaption	In **deep adaptations**, emphasis is placed on reflecting how cultural, social, psychological, environmental, and historical factors influence health behaviors differently across racial/ethnic populations and how that will impact desired outcomes for the EBI when applied to the target population (Resnicow et al., 1999). Deep adaptations integrate cultural-specific conceptualizations of the target problem (e.g., explanatory models of illness), social norms (e.g., gender roles, family composition), and cultural beliefs (e.g., stigma related to mental illness) into the EBI to enhance cultural sensitivity and facilitate desired outcomes (Kreuter et al., 2003)	■ An example occurred in Case Study 4.1A, because women were not always able to consent to treatment without approval of a male family member. So the study team negotiated with male family members to allow individual access to care or provided alternative solutions (e.g., female relatives would accompany the female client to sessions)

WHY ADAPT EVIDENCE-BASED INTERVENTIONS?

Implementers (i.e., anyone involved in the decision to modify an EBI and/or the adaptation process; Stirman et al., 2013) have identified a multitude of reasons for why EBIs are adapted. Overall, these reasons are related to barriers that impede progress toward the EBI goals (La Bash et al., 2019). Another consideration for EBI adaptation is the need to integrate an equity lens to address the unique needs of vulnerable populations, communities, and settings (Baumann & Cabassa, 2020). An equity lens explicitly moves us away from a "one-size-fits-all" model, where everyone is treated with the same protocol, regardless of fit. Rather, emphasis is placed on understanding and addressing the unique barriers that vulnerable communities encounter in receiving EBIs, so that implementation strategies and/or the EBI itself can be proactively tailored to address these inequities (Baumann et al., 2017).

Identifying and articulating a clear goal for the adaptation is necessary when thinking about specific changes to the treatment, the expected outcomes of the adaptations, and inclusion of the appropriate assessment tools to measure adaptation success (Roscoe et al., 2019). There are often several interconnected goals for adaptation. For example, goals could include improving treatment feasibility and clinical outcomes and reducing treatment costs. Additional goals for EBI adaptation include: improving fidelity, improving sustainability (i.e., adaptations made to increase the EBI's long-term use), and increasing the likelihood that an EBI will be used at all (i.e., adaptations to improve adoption; Kirk et al., 2020). It may also be the case that modifications are made with no specific goal in mind. This can occur when adaptations are made in an unsystematic and reactive way, without the intention to improve outcomes (Kirk et al., 2020). For instance, consider a provider who ran out of time in a therapy treatment session. The provider does not cover all of the session material (in that session or a later session), and the client leaves the session without a plan to practice any new skills. In this example, the modification was unintentional, and the goal was unrelated to improving outcomes. Although not always possible, we recommend identifying strategies to avoid adaptations without clear goals.

Adaptations ideally occur during the planning phase, so the adapted form of the EBI is implemented from the beginning of delivery and any potential negative "ripple effects" can be mitigated (Kirk et al., 2020). However, it is important to note that despite best efforts, adaptations and their goals may also evolve across the phases of implementation in response to new developments and challenges, as adaptation is fundamentally an iterative, ongoing process (Kirk et al., 2020).

COMMON REASONS AND GOALS FOR EVIDENCE-BASED INTERVENTION ADAPTATION

While it is beyond the scope of this chapter to review all the factors that may prompt EBI adaptation, we focus our review on the most common reasons. Specifically, we review adapting an EBI for a new population or setting, especially to improve cultural fit.

New Target Population

Many EBIs have been adapted to better fit a range of population characteristics, including age (e.g., Cornelius et al., 2008) and sexual orientation (e.g., Reback et al., 2014), and other contextual characteristics. For example, Fasula et al. (2013) adapted an EBI for HIV/sexually transmitted illness (STI) prevention programming for incarcerated women in North Carolina for delivery in prisons. The EBI was originally developed for African American and Mexican American women attending STI clinics in San Antonio, Texas. To adapt the target EBI, the implementers followed a series of steps including stakeholder consultation, formative research, implementation of a randomized controlled clinical trial, and collaborative evaluation (DePue et al., 2010). By following a systematic adaptation process with an equity lens incorporated from the outset, an efficacious EBI is now available for incarcerated women, a historically underserved community.

It is important to consider the influence of culture[1] when deciding if you need to adapt an EBI for a new population. Cultural adaptation can be defined as "the systematic modification of an evidence-based treatment . . . or intervention protocol to consider language,

[1] Culture has been defined as ". . . shared learned behavior which is transmitted from one generation to another to promote individual and group adjustment and adaptation. Culture is represented externally as artifacts, roles, and institutions, and is represented internally as values, beliefs, attitudes, cognitive styles, epistemologies, and conscious patterns" (Marsella, 1988, p. 10).

culture, and context in such a way that it is compatible with the client's cultural patterns, meanings, and values" (Bernal et al., 2009, p. 362). The need to culturally adapt EBIs is rooted in the recognition of the limited availability of culturally specific EBIs with strong empirical support (Marsiglia & Booth, 2015), as historically underserved communities are underrepresented in the development of EBIs (e.g., Santiago & Miranda, 2014). This exclusion not only creates blind spots in research, but also in translating science into practice (Baumann & Cabassa, 2020). For this reason, it is integral to proactively tailor the target EBI, its implementation, and the associated research design approaches to address the unique needs of underrepresented populations, communities, and settings (Baumann et al., 2017). This tailoring can result in improved relevance, acceptability, effectiveness, and sustained delivery of EBIs for a target population (Cabassa & Baumann, 2013).

When considering cultural adaptations of an EBI, there is an important distinction between surface adaptations and deep adaptations. **Surface adaptations** are those made in response to observable social and behavioral characteristics of the population (Resnicow et al., 1999). These may include language translations or customizing metaphors to increase alignment with the target population's culture (Cabassa & Baumann, 2013). As the name suggests, in **deep adaptations** emphasis is placed on reflecting how cultural, social, psychological, environmental, and historical factors influence health behaviors differently across populations and how these intersecting factors will impact desired outcomes for the EBI when applied to the target population (Resnicow et al., 1999). Deep adaptations integrate culture-specific conceptualizations of the target problem (e.g., explanatory models of illness), social norms (e.g., gender roles, family composition), and cultural beliefs (e.g., stigma related to mental illness) into the EBI to enhance cultural sensitivity and facilitate desired outcomes (Kreuter et al., 2003). Decisions regarding which level of adaptation to undertake in different circumstances should be driven by the available resources (e.g., cost, expertise) and by relevant, available data (Domenech Rodríguez & Bernal, 2012).

In Alberta, Canada, surface and deep adaptations were integrated in the cultural adaptation of the Life Skills Training (LST) program for Aboriginal children and youth (Baydala et al., 2009). The LST program, which is a school-based drug and alcohol prevention EBI, was adapted and delivered to grade 3 students at a First Nations school. An adaptation committee was established at the outset of the adaptation process and included community members, school personnel, and tribal Elders. Surface adaptations included translation of program content into Isga, the ancestral language of the people of the Alexis Nakota Sioux Nation. Deep adaptations included the integration of traditional ceremonies and storytelling into the EBI. Module length was increased from 1 hour (as recommended in the original LST program) to 2 hours so that cultural activities and ceremonies relevant to the content of the module could be incorporated during the second hour. Baydala et al. (2009) highlight various lessons learned from this adaptation process. The most prominent lesson was the unexpected complexity and amount of time required to complete the adaptation process. The authors also note that additional funding to hire technical support for the project would have alleviated some of the burden on community members. Nonetheless, the authors emphasize the advantages of culturally adapted EBIs, particularly in the case of deep adaptations where values, beliefs, and the cultural context of the population are intricately woven into EBI adaptation. These advantages included improved engagement, since participants related more closely to the EBI content, and increased ownership of and investment in the EBI by the community.

Setting

Other reasons that may prompt consideration of EBI adaptation include factors such as setting constraints or the knowledge, needs, and preferences of providers. In their review,

TABLE 4.2 Common Goals and Reasons for EBI Adaptation

REASON(S) FOR EBI ADAPTATION	GOAL(S) FOR EBI ADAPTATION	EXAMPLE(S)
New target population	Improve EBI acceptability	■ EBI originally developed for adolescent girls; adapt for women 50+ years old
Cultural adaptation	Increase availability, acceptability, and relevance of EBI for historically underrepresented population	■ Surface adaptation: Language translation of EBI material
	Improve patient engagement and effectiveness of an EBI	■ Deep adaptation: Integration of explanatory models of illness into the EBI
Setting constraints	Improve access	■ Limited staff available to deliver EBI; adapt EBI from individual to group format

Escoffery and colleagues (2018) found that over 60% of the EBIs reviewed included changes to the delivery of the original EBI, due to setting constraints and preferences of providers and consumers. As an example, a clinic may need to deliver an EBI with eight sessions in only four sessions due to limited funding and personnel availability. Consequently, the adaptation required includes reducing the number of in-person sessions and converting some sessions to virtual sessions (Table 4.2).

Common Pitfalls in Practice: An Unsystematic Approach to Adaptation

Empirical evidence indicates that EBIs tend to have a positive impact when adaptations are systematic, well-thought out, and aligned with core functions. EBIs are associated with negative outcomes when adaptations are made reactively and/or without a clear goal in mind (e.g., unsystematically; Moore et al., 2013). Proactive adaptations occur through a process that identifies ways to maximize fit and implementation success, while maintaining core functions of the EBI whenever possible. While adaptations are ideally planned at the beginning of the implementation effort, it is also possible that adaptations can be made proactively during the implementation process itself, when a new potential barrier to fit arises. An example of the latter situation occurred during the COVID-19 pandemic with the wide-spread urgent and rapid transition to EBI delivery via telehealth. When agencies began to anticipate that there would be a period of time during which all care would be delivered virtually, they began to seek training for their staff, order equipment, and develop risk management protocols to facilitate a transition to telehealth (Youn et al., 2020). Even though change occurs during implementation, the process by which it occurs is what distinguishes proactive and reactive adaptation.

In contrast, reactive modifications are changes that occur in an improvised and less systematic manner in response to unanticipated challenges during the implementation process. Modifications may be made by individual practitioners rather than decided upon using a careful, team-based process. Since the changes are improvised, they may be more likely to be fidelity inconsistent. Reactive modifications can lead to fidelity drift

(*continued*)

from the EBI when providers revert to EBIs they feel more comfortable with, or they feel unsure about how to adapt in the moment to address emergent challenges in session.

However, because change is the norm in many settings and not every challenge can be anticipated, reactive modifications are not always avoidable. Providers may improvise in order to meet the needs of an individual they serve, or significant changes may be necessary before a more careful adaptation process can occur. With careful consideration and a clear understanding of the EBI, even when modifications are reactive, EBIs can be tailored in ways that maintain treatment fidelity as well as addresses client needs or contextual constraints. The proactive and intentional application of adaptation process frameworks can mitigate the potential harm of improvised changes and guide systematic approaches to making adaptations.

THE VALUE OF ADAPTATION PROCESS FRAMEWORKS

Adaptation process frameworks, which delineate step-by-step instructions for the full lifecycle of the adaptation process, can help facilitate a thoughtful, thorough, and systematic approach to adaptation. Below we review: (a) consolidated steps from a review of public health EBI adaptations (Escoffery et al., 2019), (b) the Iterative Decision-Making for Evaluation of Adaptations (IDEA; Miller et al., 2020), and (c) the Model for Adaptation Design and Impact (MADI; Kirk et al., 2020). While there are other EBI adaptation frameworks, we focus on these three because they are based on recent literature, comprehensive in scope, and applicable to a range of EBIs.

In a comprehensive review of adaptation frameworks and models for public health EBIs, Escoffery et al. (2019) identified 11 steps that were commonly applied in EBI adaptation. The steps are: (a) assess community or population of interest; (b) understand the original EBI; (c) select an EBI; (d) consult with experts; (e) consult with stakeholders; (f) decide what needs adaptation; (g) adapt the original program; (h) train staff; (i) test the adapted materials; (j) implement; and (k) evaluate.

IDEA is a decision-making framework that is intended to provide guidance in decisions regarding whether to adapt and how to evaluate if the goals of the adaptation were achieved (Miller et al., 2020). It assumes that stakeholders have identified an EBI and are determining whether and how to adapt it for a given setting. It is designed to be iterative and reflective of the nonlinear and dynamic contexts within which implementation occurs. IDEA emphasizes the importance of considering the range of stakeholders who may be impacted by the EBI adaptation during the decision-making process. As seen in the steps that follow which summarize IDEA, it has utility for selecting, tracking, documenting, and evaluating EBI adaptations in healthcare (2020). The IDEA process steps are:

1. determining whether an adaptation to the EBI is required based on initial data, theory, or stakeholder input;
2. considering whether fidelity-consistent (i.e., preserve core functions) or fidelity-inconsistent (i.e., adapt or eliminate core functions) adaptations are required. Decisions should be based on existing literature, evaluation data, and stakeholder input;
3. careful data collection, particularly in situations where fidelity-inconsistent adaptations are made, to inform decisions about alternative adaptations or strategies;
4. considering whether there is sufficient time for a thorough pilot study. If so, strongly consider conducting a pilot study. If not, plan for thorough evaluation throughout the rollout of the (adapted) EBI;

5. based on how "success" is defined at the outset, determining if success of the EBI implementation was achieved; and
6. if the EBI does not achieve expected results based on prior research evidence, deciding: (a) whether further data are needed to understand the reasons for reduced effectiveness in the new population/context, and (b) whether stakeholders are willing to continue the implementation of the "lower voltage" EBI.

MADI highlights possible inter-relationships of how adaptations influence intended and unintended outcomes throughout the adaptation process, emphasizing how a single adaptation may impact multiple outcomes in both expected and unexpected ways (Kirk et al., 2020). For example, the goal of increasing feasibility of EBI delivery may inadvertently result in decreased fidelity. MADI is useful for considering the range of intended and unintended implementation or EBI outcomes that can result from adaptation. It is also valuable for determining which outcomes you may need to monitor (Kirk et al., 2020). For a useful guide, see MADIguide.org.

Combining the work of Escoffery et al. (2019), IDEA, and MADI, Table 4.3 summarizes key steps for EBI adaptation. Certain steps might be skipped or combined for some projects. As illustrated in the case study, some steps, such as consultation with experts or stakeholders, may be repeated as needed throughout the process. It is important to note the integration of an equity lens throughout each step to thoughtfully consider the unique needs of vulnerable communities and settings as they relate to EBI access. Relatedly, it is imperative to consider EBI reach from the very beginning, particularly for historically underrepresented or underserved groups. The sections that follow provide further elaboration on the key adaptation steps in Table 4.3.

TABLE 4.3 Key Adaptation Steps and Descriptions

Ensure to integrate an equity lens into the adaptation process

STEP NAME	STEP DESCRIPTION
1. Conduct a needs assessment	Identify reasons and goals for EBI adaptation: ■ Identify any factors or barriers that may impede progress toward the intended outcome(s) ■ Clearly articulate goals for EBI adaptation based on the preceding point Assess community (e.g., target population, target organization): ■ Identify behavioral determinants and risk behaviors of the new target population using focus groups, interviews, needs assessments, and logic models ■ Assess organizational capacity to implement the EBI
2. Consult with experts	Consult content experts, including original EBI protocol developers, as needed and incorporate expert advice into the program
3. Consult with stakeholders and review assessment data to determine the most appropriate and effective EBI	Seek input from advisory boards and community planning groups where EBI implementation takes place Identify stakeholder partners who can champion program adoption in a new setting and ensure program fidelity Continuously consult with key stakeholders throughout the implementation process

(continued)

TABLE 4.3 Key Adaptation Steps and Descriptions (*continued*)

Ensure to integrate an equity lens into the adaptation process

STEP NAME	STEP DESCRIPTION
4. Decide what needs adapting	Decide whether to adapt or implement the original EBI Demonstrate/provide examples of the selected EBI using new target population and other stakeholders to generate adaptations Determine how original and new target population/ setting differ in terms of risk and protective factors Identify areas where EBI needs to be adapted and include possible changes in intervention structure, content, provider, or delivery methods Retain fidelity to core functions
5. Adapt the original EBI	Develop an adaptation plan Adapt the original intervention contents through collaborative efforts Core functions responsible for change should not be modified
6. Train staff	Select and train staff to ensure quality implementation
7. Pilot and test the adapted materials	Pretest adapted materials with stakeholder group Pilot test adapted EBI in new target population Assess for any unintended outcomes ("ripple effects"); make further adaptations as necessary
8. Evaluate	Document and evaluate the adaptation process and target outcomes as the adapted EBI is implemented Write evaluation questions; choose indicators, measures, and the evaluation design; plan data collection, analysis, and reporting
9. Review results from stakeholders and determine next steps (e.g., further adaptation, discontinuation)	Conduct final interviews, focus groups, and debriefing sessions with stakeholders to understand the EBI adaptation experience from various perspectives Assess for any unintended outcomes; make further adaptations as necessary
10. Implement and continue to evaluate adapted intervention (if warranted, based on Step 9)	Revise implementation plan based on results generated in previous steps Identify and refine outcomes to evaluate decision points for further adaptation, selection of a new EBI, or discontinuation Refine evaluation strategy Execute adapted EBI

HOW DO I KNOW IF I NEED TO ADAPT AN EVIDENCE-BASED INTERVENTION?: CONDUCTING A NEEDS ASSESSMENT

Some adaptation frameworks (Escoffery et al., 2018) discuss the selection of an EBI that fits with the population and setting, emphasizing careful collaboration with stakeholders and a clear understanding of the potential EBIs, their evidence base, and their relevance to the population and setting. However, even after identifying the most appropriate EBI available, there still may be a need for adaptation to improve fit. When assessing EBI fit, it is critical to consult with stakeholders to identify where there may be gaps between the originally developed EBI and the target population and setting (Escoffery et al., 2018; Stirman et al., 2019). Stakeholders may include the individuals who will deliver the EBI; the intended EBI recipients (and sometimes their support systems); administrators and leaders who will need to allocate funding, staffing, time, and resources to support EBI implementation; and potentially thought leaders from the community and organization that will provide the EBI (Petkovic et al., 2020). It may also be important to assess factors that may impact engagement, such as health literacy as well as stigma and attitudes toward seeking treatment. Not only can stakeholders suggest potential barriers and areas for refinement, but they can also identify the key priorities and outcomes that should be optimized throughout the adaptation process (Miller et al., 2020). In many cases, the clinical outcome may not be the only, or even the most important, consideration. For example, in some settings, stakeholders may feel strongly that the EBI needs to be adapted to improve acceptability, satisfaction, or engagement. In other settings, the priority may be improving the feasibility of providing the EBI, such as when staffing shortages preclude individual-level EBI delivery or in settings where much of the population would have difficulty traveling to a clinic.

While assessing fit can happen informally by speaking with stakeholders or people with expertise in providing or implementing the EBI, the use of a formal data-gathering process allows for a more systematic evaluation of fit. Reviewing literature to learn whether the EBI has been provided or tested with similar populations or in similar settings may be part of the initial process of selecting an EBI, or it may occur when fit is being more carefully assessed. Academic partnerships are one way to engage with individuals who could assist with the fit assessment and provide recommendations for adaptations, based on research and evaluation (Morgan et al., 2019). They may inform recommendations based on the research literature or by helping gather relevant information. Whether gathered by individuals outside or within your organization, qualitative (e.g., interviews, focus groups), quantitative (e.g., surveys, pilot, or program evaluation data), or mixed methods (i.e., a combination of qualitative and quantitative methods) can be used to assess fit and to determine potential reasons for adaptation. If you gather your own data, it is imperative to provide stakeholders with sufficient information and sample materials about the EBI to allow for in-depth feedback and assessment of perceptions of the EBI. Stakeholders should have as complete an understanding as possible of what typically happens in the EBI, so they can make informed opinions about whether the EBI could be feasible and acceptable for the population and setting. Stakeholders can additionally offer opinions on how the EBI could be changed to maximize feasibility, acceptability, satisfaction, and engagement. Depending on its format, EBI information can be shared through detailed presentations, examples of the EBI in action (e.g., videos or role plays), and a review of the manuals and materials.

A quantitative approach may entail providing information about the EBI or even providing an opportunity to observe or experience the EBI, followed by surveys such as the Acceptability of Intervention Measure (AIM; Weiner et al., 2017), Intervention Appropriateness Measure (IAM), Feasibility of Intervention Measure (FIM; Weiner et al., 2017) and the Perceived Characteristics of the Intervention Scale (PCIS; Cook et al., 2015). These brief surveys measure stakeholder perceptions of feasibility, appropriateness, and acceptability. The AIM, IAM, and FIM can be administered to a broad group of stakeholders and are intended to be brief, face-valid measures of EBI acceptability, whether the EBI seems appropriate for a particular population or setting, and whether it is likely that the EBI can be successfully carried out as designed. The PCIS has been administered to clinicians but is based on Rogers's (1962) landmark Diffusion of Innovations framework, which emphasizes the influence of intervention characteristics on adoption and implementation. These characteristics include whether the intervention (a) is compatible with the population or setting, (b) seems too complex, (c) can be easily tested and de-implemented if it does not fit or work, (d) is safe for a population, and (e) is perceived to be better than alternatives or the current way of doing things. Surveys can be efficient and provide important clues about the extent to which adaptation may be needed and what goals need to be accomplished through adaptations. However, used alone, surveys might not provide sufficient detail to determine exactly how to adapt. If a large number of stakeholders complete surveys, it is typically not feasible to interview all participants to get a nuanced understanding of their survey responses. As such, it can be helpful to add a free response text box that allows stakeholders to elaborate on their ratings and make suggestions where relevant.

A qualitative approach can complement quantitative data by providing a richer understanding of the responses from the surveys, or it can be used independently. When complementing quantitative data, a subset of survey participants can be interviewed for a more in-depth understanding of perceptions of fit and suggested changes. With or without quantitative data, stakeholder interviews or focus groups can allow for a rich understanding of aspects of the setting, provider perceptions of the EBI and its fit, the needs and opinions of the individuals who are receiving the EBI, and perspectives of administrators who are in positions to support and reinforce the use of EBIs. Interview guides can be developed that are semi-structured and based on a framework that explores factors that influence implementation success. Interview questions can assess factors at different levels (e.g., organization or community, individual provider, and recipient) that may need to be addressed through adaptation. To encourage frank discussion, it is important that the stakeholders view the interviewer as objective, credible, and approachable.

Findings from qualitative and/or quantitative assessments can be summarized and discussed with an advisory board or implementation team. Individuals with expertise in the EBI can review the summary and offer information and ideas about how the EBI can be adapted to address the unique constraints identified during the needs assessment. These suggestions can be reviewed with the individuals who will be providing, supporting, and receiving the EBI. In this way, an adapted EBI can be co-created, which has the added benefit of increasing stakeholder buy-in and increased likelihood of successful and sustained EBI implementation. Adaptation and assessment of fit may need to occur iteratively. In fact, current frameworks and suggested processes for adaptation (e.g., Lyon et al., 2020) emphasize stakeholder engagement, iterative adaptation, and continual assessment and review of the impact of the adaptation.

COMMON PITFALLS IN PRACTICE: ASSUMPTIONS ABOUT ADAPTATION NEEDS

Adaptations can be resource intensive and may not improve desired outcomes over standard EBIs delivered with fidelity (Stirman et al., 2017). Rather than assuming an EBI may need to be adapted, it is wise to consider existing data and stakeholder input regarding whether adaptation will be needed to increase engagement or relevance of treatment content (Lau, 2006). Reviewing empirical evidence is a good first step. If data or theory is lacking for your population of interest, and stakeholder input is not feasible, it is suggested to pilot the EBI without adaptation with a small segment of the population. Results from the pilot can inform whether adaptations are needed before broader EBI implementation (Miller et al., 2020).

CASE STUDY 4.1B CONDUCTING A NEEDS ASSESSMENT IN KURDISTAN WITH PEOPLE SURVIVING TORTURE AND CHEMICAL ATTACKS

STEP 1: IDENTIFY REASONS AND GOALS FOR EVIDENCE-BASED INTERVENTION ADAPTATION

Common barriers to implementing mental health EBIs in less-resourced countries include the limited number of EBIs developed with the target population in mind (most mental health EBIs have been developed and tested in high-resourced countries) as well as a lack of specialist mental health providers available to deliver the EBI (Patel et al., 2010). Accordingly, the goal of Kaysen et al. (2013) was to adapt an intervention to be culturally appropriate for the local Kurdish population and feasible for implementation by community mental health workers.

STEP 2: ASSESS COMMUNITY

In 2008, researchers from Johns Hopkins University completed a qualitative study with torture and chemical attack survivors in Kurdistan. Participants described symptoms that were highly consistent with Western conceptualizations of PTSD, depression, generalized anxiety disorder, as well as complicated bereavement. Additionally, participants described psychosocial problems, such as challenging relationships with family members and ostracism from the wider Kurdish society.

STEP 3: CONSULTATION WITH EXPERTS AND STAKEHOLDERS

Several stakeholders were involved in the adaptation process, including the local nongovernmental organization (Heartland Alliance), local Kurdish mental health-care providers, community mental health workers (i.e., study therapists), the local clinical supervisor, and the Johns Hopkins research team. Based on the results of the qualitative study, the research team sought to identify an EBI to address the prominent issues described by torture and chemical attack survivors. To do so, the research team met with torture and trauma treatment experts and conducted a literature review. The parameters for EBI selection included identifying EBIs that were informed by scientific evidence and could be feasible for implementation in a low-resourced setting. The ultimate decision to select CPT was based on the following rationale: (a) strong evidence base for CPT; (b) thorough manual for training purposes, including training of those with limited clinical expertise; and (c) CPT appeared well-suited for addressing the struggles participants highlighted in the qualitative study.

COMMON PITFALLS IN PRACTICE: NOT ENGAGING ALL NEEDED STAKEHOLDERS

If key stakeholders are excluded during the EBI selection and adaptation process, the EBI can face several risks to success. Implementers may not be aware of important adaptation considerations (e.g., adoption barriers, cultural nuances). Additionally, stakeholders will have varying perspectives on potential unintended consequences based on their unique experiences (e.g., as experts, consumers, community members). Most importantly, without key stakeholders and champions at the table from the beginning, the EBI is unlikely to be sustainable. Proactive collaboration and the integration of input from stakeholders at varying levels are crucial for successful EBI adaptation and long-term sustainability.

DECIDING WHAT NEEDS ADAPTING: THE IMPORTANCE OF CORE FUNCTIONS

It is important to consider the core functions of an EBI prior to making any changes. Recently there has been an emphasis on the importance of preserving the intended function of a core treatment element, even if its delivery looks different (i.e., has a different *form*). In other words, it is more important that an EBI element is serving its core purpose (i.e., function) than whether it looks the same as it did originally. For example, when culturally adapting a diabetes self-management program for the American Samoa population, patients were not directed to professionally led diabetes educational resources as in the original intervention. Instead, community health workers were trained to provide psychoeducation on diabetes during home visits using flipcharts. The adapted form of resources was modified; however, it still achieved the same goal of supporting access to information on diabetes self-care (DePue et al., 2010).

Adaptations that preserve the EBI's core functions are said to be *fidelity-consistent adaptations.* In contrast, *fidelity-inconsistent adaptations* do not preserve the aspects of a treatment believed to drive the treatment effects. Research literature supports the importance of fidelity-consistent adaptations to facilitate positive EBI outcomes (e.g., symptom reduction, decrease in risk behaviors, increase in healthcare utilization; Castro et al., 2004; Escoffery et al., 2019; Moore et al., 2013).

ADAPT THE ORIGINAL EVIDENCE-BASED INTERVENTION: HOW TO DETERMINE EVIDENCE-BASED INTERVENTION CORE FUNCTIONS

Ideally, EBI core functions are identified through the empirical research literature. There has been some research to identify core functions that cut across different types of psychosocial EBIs, diagnoses, or settings (Kennedy & Barlow, 2018; Martin et al., 2018). However, this research is in its infancy and, more broadly, empirical research on specific EBI core functions is limited. When trying to determine core functions of an EBI, you can consult the research literature to see what is known about your specific EBI of interest and/or you can consult with the EBI developers, trainers, and other experts in the EBI to provide guidance on what is known about the treatment's core functions. It is important to work with a team of experts throughout the process of identifying EBI core functions.

If time allows, and there is not sufficient empirical research, you can gather your own data on the EBI's core functions. This type of data can be gathered with approaches like usability testing. Usually done in partnership with EBI experts, this "trial and learning" approach uses a systematic, cyclical process in which small changes are iteratively tested, allowing for the identification of the active ingredients of an EBI (see Blase & Fixsen, 2013). Other options include testing an adaptation with a series of cases or alternating use of the adapted and non-adapted form (e.g., removing one element at a time), collecting data along the way to determine whether the adaptation is having the desired impact. If the adapted form appears to yield less positive outcomes, it may be an indication that the element that was removed is in fact an active ingredient.

When empirical research is inconclusive or unavailable, the next option is to use the theory from which the treatment was developed to help guide your decisions regarding core functions (Dusenbury et al., 2003; Fixsen et al., 2005). This can be done by assessing what is known about the EBI's theory of change (i.e., What mechanisms are proposed to be responsible for the treatment's effectiveness? How does the EBI work?). If there is no research or theory to guide you, you can pull from your practical experience and consider what you have observed about how and why the EBI seems to work when using it with the target population. This should only be undertaken if there is no theory or research to guide adaptation and should be followed up with pilot testing of proposed modifications.

It is important to keep a couple of things in mind when determining if/how to adapt core functions of an EBI. The decision is often based on an assessment of the cost/benefit ratio. For example, it may be necessary to abbreviate an EBI due to factors such as length of stay in a treatment program or limits to reimbursement. In such cases, it may be that a less potent form of an essential EBI element or even removal of a core function may be an acceptable risk, if the potential benefit is more important (e.g., increased access to or reach of the EBI, increased patient engagement in the EBI). Second, it is also important to consider if the adaptation may have an unexpected or undesirable outcome (Kirk et al., 2020). For instance, a proposed adaptation may increase certain benefits (e.g., training all providers in a clinic to provide an EBI increase immediate access to treatment) but may compromise another outcome (e.g., less time to provide care during training increases wait time for services). Sometimes the possible negative impact of an adaptation can be anticipated and planned for to minimize its impact. Kirk and colleagues (2020) suggest that implementation strategies may be used to offset these negative impacts. For example, if an adaptation that can reduce cost may also reduce acceptability, an implementation strategy to increase buy-in could mitigate this potential unintended consequence.

CASE STUDY 4.1C ADAPTATION AND IMPLEMENTATION OF COGNITIVE PROCESSING THERAPY FOR POSTTRAUMATIC STRESS DISORDER IN KURDISTAN

Once CPT was selected, the EBI was adapted to be culturally appropriate and feasible for implementation by community mental health workers. While the essential components of CPT remained the same, training material was adapted to the local culture (Bolton et al., 2014). The adaptation of the training materials was iterative, involved several partners, and was conducted prior to implementing CPT in Kurdistan. First, U.S. trainers and trauma experts reviewed existing CPT training materials and the manual to simplify language and eliminate jargon and American idioms. The revised and simplified materials were reviewed by other members of the Johns Hopkins research team experienced in adapting CPT in low-resourced contexts. The final simplified materials were translated into Kurdish by professional translators based in Kurdistan. Translated materials were reviewed by collaborators and mental healthcare providers in Kurdistan to ensure clarity of content and cultural appropriateness.

Staff were trained in person in Sulaymaniyah, Kurdistan. The 8-day training was conducted in English with translation to Kurdish by a local, professional translator. Trainees included 11 community mental health workers, several local mental health providers, and their local supervisor. The community mental health workers were previously trained as physician's assistants or nurse equivalents. Training content was focused on theory (as relevant to the implementation of the EBI), the structure of the EBI within and between sessions, and step-by-step instruction of how to conduct each of the 12 sessions of CPT, with an emphasis on homework completion. Logistical considerations were discussed during training, such as managing barriers to homework completion and reluctance to attend 12 sessions.

Trainees provided daily feedback to trainers on: (a) clarity of written materials; (b) recommendations to improve cultural fit; (c) recommendations to increase accessibility of written materials for those with low to no levels of literacy; and (d) practical

(continued)

suggestions to limit barriers to implementation in low-resource settings. Feedback was sought daily via group discussion, and daily via an anonymous survey. Before launching the trial, the adapted version of CPT was piloted by the community mental health workers and the clinical supervisor. This step resulted in additional feedback and minor changes to the training materials.

REPORTING, RESEARCH, AND EVALUATION

An important part of the EBI adaptation process is to document and evaluate the impact of the adapted EBI to identify what works in the treatment setting or community. An important step in this process is tracking the adaptations made to the EBI. While planning adaptations makes it somewhat easier to document the changes that are made, some modifications will be made outside the formal adaptation process in response to constraints or challenges that arise in real time. Regardless of the timing of the modifications, clearly specifying what changes were made as well as when, how, and why, allows for a better understanding of the types of changes that may need to be made to improve outcomes or to address constraints or challenges that arise.

THE FRAMEWORK FOR REPORTING ADAPTATIONS AND MODIFICATIONS-EXPANDED (FRAME)

The Framework for Reporting Adaptations and Modifications—Expanded (FRAME) can be considered a comprehensive evaluation framework that facilitates a way to catalog the process of adaptation (Stirman et al., 2019). The following eight aspects in FRAME can be used to describe the nature and types of EBI adaptations: (a) when in the implementation process the adaptation was made (e.g., timing of modification); (b) the extent to which the adaptation was planned/proactive or unplanned/reactive; (c) which stakeholders were involved in the decision to adapt and how to adapt the EBI; (d) what components were modified; (e) the level of delivery at which modifications were made (e.g., individual, organization, community); (f) the type or nature of content-level material; (g) whether adaptations were fidelity-consistent; and (h) the reasons for adaptation, including the goal of the modification and relevant contextual factors that informed the decision.

FRAME (or another framework) can be used to ensure common language and understanding across programs and EBIs regarding the types of adaptations that occur. This understanding can be shared with others who are working on similar implementation efforts and can facilitate an understanding of the types of changes that enhance important outcomes such as feasibility, satisfaction, engagement, or clinical change. Tracking modifications and adaptations can also provide a better sense of why suboptimal outcomes occur. For example, if program evaluation suggests outcomes that are not as strong as those in studies of the original EBI protocol, having a clear sense of what changes were made can shed light on EBI elements that might be important to preserve.

There are a few different strategies for documenting adaptations that vary in their intensity and burden on those who are implementing and documenting. Observation by an outside party who identifies and tracks adaptations using FRAME is perhaps the most objective and detailed approach. However, this strategy involves time and expenses that are rarely available outside of a funded research study. At the same time, there may be approaches where similar programs could observe one another and track factors such as fidelity and adaptation. This technique could facilitate discussion and learning across sites and programs. A codebook is available that operationalizes the different elements of

FRAME (https://med.stanford.edu/fastlab/research/adaptation.html) but decision rules that are specific to the program or EBI would need to be made in consultation with individuals who have a strong knowledge of the EBI. The same website also includes samples of the different methods of tracking adaptation.

Tracking self-reported adaptations may be more feasible. The diagram of FRAME (on the website listed previously) can be used to identify the adaptations or modifications that occur at each encounter or at other intervals, depending on the degree of specificity required to meet the tracking goals. Checklists of content adaptations can also be used by individual providers to track what they do in encounters with the individuals that they serve. Other times, when less precision is needed, adaptations can be tracked and described through interviews or team consensus. Periodically, an interviewer or team lead can work with team members or individual providers to identify and summarize adaptations that have occurred over a specific period of time. Depending on the frequency with which interviews occur, recall and precision may be lower. In a recent study, Johnson and colleagues (2020) found that annual interviews about adaptations resulted in lower agreement with observers than checklists completed after every session. Providers may also be reluctant to report certain types of adaptations if they are perceived as lowering the fidelity of the EBI. However, interviews also allow providers to contextualize their decisions to adapt and to provide a richer description of the goals and rationale.

Thus, to ensure the most accurate sense of which adaptations occurred when, reporting should occur in a context in which the providers are comfortable reporting what changes they have made. It is also recommended that documentation occurs as close as possible to the time the adaptation occurred to increase the likelihood of accuracy. For EBIs that occur across multiple encounters, not all adaptations to the protocol will be detected from observing or reporting on a single encounter. For example, spreading elements across multiple sessions, repeating elements, or changing the length of the protocol will not be detected from observing or reporting on a single encounter. Table 4.4 summarizes advantages and disadvantages of different reporting strategies.

TABLE 4.4 Approaches for Tracking and Documenting Adaptations

REPORTING STRATEGY	PROS	CONS	BEST FOR
Observation	May be most accurate, especially if observation is frequent and objective	Time and personnel intensive; requires trained observer	When precision is needed to understand adaptation at the level of the encounter; when sufficient time and resources exist
Self-report	Relatively fast; can be integrated into documentation for more frequent assessment	Requires provider time and sufficient understanding of protocol to accurately report adaptations	When session or encounter-level reporting is desired and observation is not feasible
Interview	Occurs less frequently; interviewer completes documentation; appropriate when a general summary of adaptations is needed	May be less accurate due to problems with recall; providers may not acknowledge all adaptations they make; requires a more substantial block of provider time	When there is a general summary of adaptations that occur over a specific period of time and a richer description of how and why the adaptations were made is desired

COMMON PITFALLS IN PRACTICE: UNSYSTEMATIC DOCUMENTATION AND TRACKING OF THE IMPACT OF THE ADAPTATION

When EBI adaptations are documented in an ad hoc manner (or not documented at all), it is challenging to understand what led to the EBI outcomes. If an EBI is successful in enhancing outcomes and adaptations are not tracked, it is not possible to learn the different ways that the EBI can be adapted or "flexed" while maintaining positive outcomes. Similarly, if there are suboptimal outcomes following the EBI adaptation, it is difficult, if not impossible, to identify which changes may have been associated with reductions in effectiveness when ad hoc or insufficient documentation occurs. Tracking EBI modifications in a systematic way can inform a clearer understanding of what processes (i.e., core functions) resulted in what outcomes and why. Additionally, the systematic approach of documentation facilitates the use of a common language across programs and EBIs. As discussed, FRAME provides a useful and systematic approach to describe and characterize the process and forms of adaptation that occurred during implementation (Stirman et al., 2019).

CASE STUDY 4.1D IMPLEMENTATION OF COGNITIVE PROCESSING THERAPY FOR PTSD IN KURDISTAN AND CONTINUED REPORTING AND EVALUATION

As noted earlier, CPT was adapted as part of a randomized controlled trial and was compared to a waitlist control condition (Bolton et al., 2014). One hundred one participants participated in the CPT arm of the study. As discussed, feedback from therapists and the local clinical supervisor were continuously sought throughout the trial. Revisions were made to the protocol as needed. Evaluation included assessing process and outcome data. A debriefing meeting was held by the study team with the community mental health workers and clinical supervisor at the end of the trial to solicit feedback about the overall experience. A final set of materials was prepared for the community mental health workers and clinical supervisor as reference material to support their ongoing provision of therapy. Trial results suggested moderate to strong impacts on the outcomes of depression, dysfunction, PTSD, anxiety, and traumatic grief symptoms (Bolton et al., 2014).

SUMMARY

In this chapter, we reviewed key considerations when adapting EBIs, including the use of an equity lens throughout the adaptation process. We provided common reasons and goals for EBI adaptation. We also described the importance of a systematic approach to adaptation that retains fidelity to an EBI's core functions and the utility in using adaptation process frameworks. These frameworks were synthesized into a summary table of the key steps involved in the adaptation of EBIs for ease of reference in implementation practice. The chapter also included methods to systematically document the process and outcomes of EBI adaptations. Throughout the chapter, conceptual information was supplemented with practical examples of EBI adaptations across a variety of contexts, including the adaptation of CPT in a global mental health setting.

KEY POINTS FOR PRACTICE

1. For EBIs that have not been tested on traditionally understudied and underserved populations, adaptation can be an effective tool to improve outcomes when approached in a thoughtful and systematic manner.
2. When considering EBI adaptation, it is important to preserve the parts of the EBI that make it effective (i.e., its core functions).
3. There are a lot of conceptual frameworks and other resources available to help you adapt EBIs.
4. It is important to include key stakeholders in the adaptation process.

COMMON PITFALLS IN PRACTICE

1. Making assumptions about whether EBI adaptation is needed without a careful needs assessment.
2. Not retaining core functions during EBI adaptation.
3. Not tracking the EBI adaptation process and outcomes to understand if EBI adaptation has the desired effect.

DISCUSSION QUESTIONS

1. What factors tell you that you may need to adapt the EBI you are working with? If you are not sure, what approach will you take to determine whether you need to adapt?
2. What is the utility of adaptation process frameworks?
3. What are key considerations for adapting the EBIs you are working with, in the context where you are working?
4. What strategies for assessing adaptations and their outcomes are most likely to be feasible and helpful in the setting where you work?
5. What are potential trade-offs to adaptations in the setting where you work?

ACKNOWLEDGMENTS

This work was completed with support from the Veterans Health Administration. The views expressed in this article are those of the authors and do not necessarily reflect the position or policy of the Department of Veterans Affairs, the United States government, Stanford University, or other affiliates.

REFERENCES

American Psychological Association. (2017). *Clinical practice guidelines for the treatment of Posttraumatic Stress Disorder (PTSD) in adults*. https://www.apa.org/ptsd-guideline/ptsd.pdf

Baumann, A. A., & Cabassa, L. J. (2020). Reframing implementation science to address inequities in healthcare delivery. *BMC Health Services Research, 20*(1), 190. https://doi.org/10.1186/s12913-020-4975-3

Baumann, A. A., Cabassa, L. J., & Wiltsey-Stirman, S. (2017). Adaptation in implementation and dissemination science. In G. A. Colditz, E. K. Proctor, & R. C. Brownson (Eds.), *Dissemination and implementation research in health: Translating science to practice* (pp. 285–300). Oxford University Press. https://play.google.com/store/books/details?id=ycM9DwAAQBAJ

Baydala, L. T., Sewlal, B., Rasmussen, C., Alexis, K., Fletcher, F., Letendre, L., Odishaw, J., Kennedy, M., & Kootenay, B. (2009). A culturally adapted drug and alcohol abuse prevention program for aboriginal children and youth. *Progress in Community Health Partnerships: Research, Education, and Action, 3*(1), 37–46. https://doi.org/10.1353/cpr.0.0054

Bernal, G., Jiménez-Chafey, M. I., & Domenech Rodríguez, M. M. (2009). Cultural adaptation of treatments: A resource for considering culture in evidence-based practice. *Professional Psychology, Research and Practice, 40*(4), 361–368. https://doi.org/10.1037/a0016401

Blase, K., & Fixsen, D. (2013). *Core intervention components: Identifying and operationalizing what makes programs work.* US Department of Health & Human Services: Office of the Assistant Secretary for Planning and Evaluation. https://aspe.hhs.gov/report/core-intervention-components-identifying-and-operationalizing-what-makes-programs-work

Bolton, P., Bass, J. K., Zangana, G. A. S., Kamal, T., Murray, S. M., Kaysen, D., Lejuez, C. W., Lindgren, K., Pagoto, S., Murray, L. K., Van Wyk, S. S., Ahmed, A. M. A., Amin, N. M. M., & Rosenblum, M. (2014). A randomized controlled trial of mental health interventions for survivors of systematic violence in Kurdistan, Northern Iraq. *BMC Psychiatry, 14*, 360. https://doi.org/10.1186/s12888-014-0360-2

Cabassa, L. J., & Baumann, A. A. (2013). A two-way street: Bridging implementation science and cultural adaptations of mental health treatments. *Implementation Science, 8*, 90. https://doi.org/10.1186/1748-5908-8-90

Castro, F. G., Barrera, M., & Martinez, C. R. (2004). The cultural adaptation of prevention interventions: Resolving tensions between fidelity and fit. *Prevention Science: The Official Journal of the Society for Prevention Research, 5*(1), 41–45. https://doi.org/10.1023/b:prev.0000013980.12412.cd

Chard, K. M. (2005). An evaluation of cognitive processing therapy for the treatment of posttraumatic stress disorder related to childhood sexual abuse. *Journal of Consulting and Clinical Psychology, 73*(5), 965–971. https://doi.org/10.1037/0022-006X.73.5.965

Cook, J. M., Thompson, R., & Schnurr, P. P. (2015). Perceived Characteristics of Intervention Scale: Development and psychometric properties. *Assessment, 22*(6), 704–714. https://doi.org/10.1177/1073191114561254

Cornelius, J. B., Moneyham, L., & LeGrand, S. (2008). Adaptation of an HIV prevention curriculum for use with older African American women. *The Journal of the Association of Nurses in AIDS Care: JANAC, 19*(1), 16–27. https://doi.org/10.1016/j.jana.2007.10.001

Creed, T., Valentin, C., Affricot, E., Eustace, E., Shetler Fast, R., Bedard-Gilligan, M., Coleman, S., Forbush, L., Corneil Pierre, U., Fils-Aime, R., Dubuisson, W., Therosme, T., Arelus, D., Robespierre, E., Houde, A., Kelly, K., & Raviola, G. (2019). Adaptation and sustainability of an evidence-based practice for PTSD in Haiti. In *ABCT 53nd annual convention.* https://www.eventscribe.com/2019/ABCT/fsPopup.asp?efp=QkRXSktSV1A4NjU5&PresentationID=603462&rnd=0.3441761&mode=presinfo

DePue, J. D., Rosen, R. K., Batts-Turner, M., Bereolos, N., House, M., Held, R. F., Nu'usolia, O., Tuitele, J., Goldstein, M. G., & McGarvey, S. T. (2010). Cultural translation of interventions: Diabetes care in American Samoa. *American Journal of Public Health, 100*(11), 2085–2093. https://doi.org/10.2105/ajph.2009.170134

Domenech Rodríguez, M. M., & Bernal, G. (2012). Frameworks, models, and guidelines for cultural adaptation. In G. Bernal (Ed.), *Cultural adaptations: Tools for evidence-based practice with diverse populations* (Vol. 307, pp. 23–44). American Psychological Association. https://doi.org/10.1037/13752-002

Dusenbury, L., Brannigan, R., Falco, M., & Hansen, W. B. (2003). A review of research on fidelity of implementation: Implications for drug abuse prevention in school settings. *Health Education Research, 18*(2), 237–256. https://doi.org/10.1093/her/18.2.237

Escoffery, C., Lebow-Skelley, E., Haardoerfer, R., Boing, E., Udelson, H., Wood, R., Hartman, M., Fernandez, M. E., & Mullen, P. D. (2018). A systematic review of adaptations of evidence-based public health interventions globally. *Implementation Science, 13*(1), 125. https://doi.org/10.1186/s13012-018-0815-9

Escoffery, C., Lebow-Skelley, E., Udelson, H., Böing, E. A., Wood, R., Fernandez, M. E., & Mullen, P. D. (2019). A scoping study of frameworks for adapting public health evidence-based interventions. *Translational Behavioral Medicine, 9*(1), 1–10. https://doi.org/10.1093/tbm/ibx067

Farmer, C. C., Mitchell, K. S., Parker-Guilbert, K., & Galovski, T. E. (2017). Fidelity to the Cognitive Processing Therapy protocol: Evaluation of critical elements. *Behavior Therapy, 48*, 195–206. https://doi.org/10.1016/j.beth.2016.02.009

Fasula, A. M., Fogel, C. I., Gelaude, D., Carry, M., Gaiter, J., & Parker, S. (2013). Project power: Adapting an evidence-based HIV/STI prevention intervention for incarcerated women. *AIDS Education and Prevention: Official Publication of the International Society for AIDS Education, 25*(3), 203–215. https://doi.org/10.1521/aeap.2013.25.3.203

Fixsen, D. L., Naoom, S. F., Blase, K. A., Friedman, R. M., Wallace, F., Burns, B., Carter, W., Paulson, R., Schoenwald, S., & Barwick, M. (2005). *Implementation research: A synthesis of the literature.* National Implementation Research Network, University of South Florida.

Gearing, R. E., El-Bassel, N., Ghesquiere, A., Baldwin, S., Gillies, J., & Ngeow, E. (2011). Major ingredients of fidelity: A review and scientific guide to improving quality of intervention research implementation. *Clinical Psychology Review, 31*(1), 79–88. https://doi.org/10.1016/j.cpr.2010.09.007

International Society for Traumatic Stress Studies. (2018). *Posttraumatic stress disorder prevention and treatment guidelines methodology and recommendations*. https://istss.org/getattachment/Treating-Trauma/New-ISTSS-Prevention-and-Treatment-Guidelines/ISTSS_PreventionTreatmentGuidelines_FNL.pdf.aspx

Johnson, C., Lane, J., Sijercic, I., Shields, N., Gutner, C. A., Creed, T., Marques, L., Monson, C. M. M., & Stirman, S. W. (2020). Agreement between observer- and self-reported adaptations to cognitive behavioral therapies for PTSD, depression and anxiety. In *Symposium 15: Adaptations to improve access and quality of evidence-based treatments: Processes for selecting, reporting, and evaluating*. Association for Behavioral and Cognitive Therapies Annual Convention, Virtual.

Kaysen, D., Lindgren, K., Zangana, G. A. S., Murray, L., Bass, J., & Bolton, P. (2013). Adaptation of cognitive processing therapy for treatment of torture victims: Experience in Kurdistan, Iraq. *Psychological Trauma: Theory, Research, Practice and Policy*, *5*(2), 184–192. https://doi.org/10.1037/a0026053

Kennedy, K. A., & Barlow, D. H. (2018). The unified protocol for transdiagnostic treatment of emotional disorders: An introduction. In Barlow, D. H., & Farchione, T. (Eds.), *Applications of the unified protocol for transdiagnostic treatment of emotional disorders* (pp. 1–16). Oxford University Press.

Kirk, M. A., Moore, J. E., Wiltsey Stirman, S., & Birken, S. A. (2020). Towards a comprehensive model for understanding adaptations' impact: The model for adaptation design and impact (MADI). *Implementation Science*, *15*(1), 56. https://doi.org/10.1186/s13012-020-01021-y

Kreuter, M. W., Lukwago, S. N., Bucholtz, R. D. D. C., Clark, E. M., & Sanders-Thompson, V. (2003). Achieving cultural appropriateness in health promotion programs: Targeted and tailored approaches. *Health Education & Behavior: The Official Publication of the Society for Public Health Education*, *30*(2), 133–146. https://doi.org/10.1177/1090198102251021

La Bash, H., Galovski, T., & Stirman, S. W. (2019). Adapting evidence-based psychotherapies while maintaining fidelity. *Current Treatment Options in Psychiatry*, *6*(3), 198–209. https://doi.org/10.1007/s40501-019-00177-9

Lau, A. S. (2006). Making the case for selective and directed cultural adaptations of evidence-based treatments: Examples from parent training. *Clinical Psychology: A Publication of the Division of Clinical Psychology of the American Psychological Association*, *13*(4), 295–310. https://doi.org/10.1111/j.1468-2850.2006.00042.x

Lyon, A. R., Brewer, S. K., & Areán, P. A. (2020). Leveraging human-centered design to implement modern psychological science: Return on an early investment. *The American Psychologist*, *75*(8), 1067–1079. https://doi.org/10.1037/amp0000652

Marsella, A. J. (1988). Cross-cultural research on severe mental disorders: Issues and findings. *Acta Psychiatrica Scandinavia Supplementum*, *344*, 7–22. https://doi.org/10.1111/j.1600-0447.1988.tb08998.x

Marsiglia, F. F., & Booth, J. M. (2015). Cultural adaptation of interventions in real practice settings. *Research on Social Work Practice*, *25*(4), 423–432. https://doi.org/10.1177/1049731514535989

Martin, P., Murray, L. K., Darnell, D., & Dorsey, S. (2018). Transdiagnostic treatment approaches for greater public health impact: Implementing principles of evidence-based mental health interventions. *Clinical Psychology: Science and Practice*, *25*(4), e12270. https://doi.org/10.1111/cpsp.12270

Miller, C. J., Wiltsey-Stirman, S., & Baumann, A. A. (2020). Iterative Decision-making for Evaluation of Adaptations (IDEA): A decision tree for balancing adaptation, fidelity, and intervention impact. *Journal of Community Psychology*, *48*(4), 1163–1177. https://doi.org/10.1002/jcop.22279

Monson, C. M., Schnurr, P. P., Resick, P. A., Friedman, M. J., Young-Xu, Y., & Stevens, S. P. (2006). Cognitive processing therapy for veterans with military-related posttraumatic stress disorder. *Journal of Consulting and Clinical Psychology*, *74*(5), 898–907. https://doi.org/10.1037/0022-006X.74.5.898

Moore, J. E., Bumbarger, B. K., & Cooper, B. R. (2013). Examining adaptations of evidence-based programs in natural contexts. *The Journal of Primary Prevention*, *34*(3), 147–161. https://doi.org/10.1007/s10935-013-0303-6

Morgan, D., Kosteniuk, J., Seitz, D., O'Connell, M. E., Kirk, A., Stewart, N. J., Holroyd-Leduc, J., Daku, J., Hack, T., Hoium, F., Kennett-Russill, D., & Sauter, K. (2019). A five-step approach for developing and implementing a Rural Primary Health Care Model for Dementia: A community–academic partnership. *Primary Health Care Research & Development*, *20*. https://doi.org/10.1017/S1463423618000968

Patel, V., Maj, M., Flisher, A. J., De Silva, M. J., Koschorke, M., Prince, M., & WPA Zonal and Member Society Representatives. (2010). Reducing the treatment gap for mental disorders: A WPA survey. *World Psychiatry: Official Journal of the World Psychiatric Association* , *9*(3), 169–176. https://doi.org/10.1002/j.2051-5545.2010.tb00305.x

Pearson, C. R., Smartlowit-Briggs, L., Belcourt, A., Bedard-Gilligan, M., & Kaysen, D. (2019). Building a tribal–academic partnership to address PTSD, substance misuse, and HIV among American Indian women. *Health Promotion Practice*, *20*(1), 48–56. https://doi.org/10.1177/1524839918762122

Petkovic, J., Riddle, A., Akl, E. A., Khabsa, J., Lytvyn, L., Atwere, P., Campbell, P., Chalkidou, K., Chang, S. M., Crowe, S., Dans, L., Jardali, F. E., Ghersi, D., Graham, I. D., Grant, S., Greer-Smith, R., Guise, J.-M., Hazlewood, G., Jull, J., . . . Tugwell, P. (2020). Protocol for the development of guidance for stakeholder engagement in health and healthcare guideline development and implementation. *Systematic Reviews*, *9*(1), 21. https://doi.org/10.1186/s13643-020-1272-5

Proctor, E. K., Landsverk, J., Aarons, G., Chambers, D., Glisson, C., & Mittman, B. (2009). Implementation research in mental health services: An emerging science with conceptual, methodological, and training challenges. *Administration and Policy in Mental Health, 36*(1), 24–34. https://doi.org/10.1007/s10488-008-0197-4

Rabin, B. A., Brownson, R. C., Haire-Joshu, D., Kreuter, M. W., & Weaver, N. L. (2008). A glossary for dissemination and implementation research in health. *Journal of Public Health Management and Practice: JPHMP, 14*(2), 117–123. https://doi.org/10.1097/01.PHH.0000311888.06252.bb

Reback, C. J., Veniegas, R., & Shoptaw, S. (2014). Getting Off: Development of a model program for gay and bisexual male methamphetamine users. *Journal of Homosexuality, 61*(4), 540–553. https://doi.org/10.1080/00918369.2014.865459

Resick, P. A., Galovski, T. E., Uhlmansiek, M. O., Scher, C. D., Clum, G. A., & Young-Xu, Y. (2008). A randomized clinical trial to dismantle components of cognitive processing therapy for posttraumatic stress disorder in female victims of interpersonal violence. *Journal of Consulting and Clinical Psychology, 76*(2), 243–258. https://doi.org/10.1037/0022-006X.76.2.243

Resick, P. A., Monson, C. M., & Chard, K. M. (2008). Cognitive Processing Therapy Veteran/Military Version: Therapist's manual. In *PsycEXTRA dataset*. https://doi.org/10.1037/e514742018-001

Resnicow, K., Baranowski, T., Ahluwalia, J. S., & Braithwaite, R. L. (1999). Cultural sensitivity in public health: Defined and demystified. *Ethnicity & Disease, 9*(1), 10–21. https://www.ncbi.nlm.nih.gov/pubmed/10355471

Rogers, E. M. (1962). *Diffusion of innovations (First printing)*. The Free Press of Glencoe.

Rogg, I., & Rimscha, H. (2007). The Kurds as parties to and victims of conflicts in Iraq. *International Review of the Red Cross, 89*(868), 823–842. https://doi.org/10.1017/s1816383108000143

Roscoe, J. N., Shapiro, V. B., Whitaker, K., & Kim, B. K. E. (2019). Classifying changes to preventive interventions: Applying adaptation taxonomies. *The Journal of Primary Prevention, 40*(1), 89–109. https://doi.org/10.1007/s10935-018-00531-2

Santiago, C. D., & Miranda, J. (2014). Progress in improving mental health services for racial-ethnic minority groups: A ten-year perspective. *Psychiatric Services, 65*(2), 180–185. https://doi.org/10.1176/appi.ps.201200517

Schoenwald, S. K., Garland, A. F., Chapman, J. E., Frazier, S. L., Sheidow, A. J., & Southam-Gerow, M. A. (2011). Toward the effective and efficient measurement of implementation fidelity. *Administration and Policy in Mental Health, 38*(1), 32–43. https://doi.org/10.1007/s10488-010-0321-0

Schulz, P. M., Resick, P. A., Huber, L. C., & Griffin, M. G. (2006). The effectiveness of cognitive processing therapy for PTSD with refugees in a community setting. *Cognitive and Behavioral Practice, 13*(4), 322–331. https://doi.org/10.1016/j.cbpra.2006.04.011

Stirman, S. W., Baumann, A. A., & Miller, C. J. (2019). The FRAME: An expanded framework for reporting adaptations and modifications to evidence-based interventions. *Implementation Science, 14*(1), 58. https://doi.org/10.1186/s13012-019-0898-y

Stirman, S. W., Gamarra, J. M., Bartlett, B. A., Calloway, A., & Gutner, C. A. (2017). Empirical examinations of modifications and adaptations to evidence-based psychotherapies: Methodologies, impact, and future directions. *Clinical Psychology: Science and Practice, 24*(4), 396–420.

Stirman, S. W., Miller, C. J., Toder, K., & Calloway, A. (2013). Development of a framework and coding system for modifications and adaptations of evidence-based interventions. *Implementation Science, 8*(1), 1–12. https://doi.org/10.1186/1748-5908-8-65

Weiner, B. J., Lewis, C. C., Stanick, C., Powell, B. J., Dorsey, C. N., Clary, A. S., Boynton, M. H., & Halko, H. (2017). Psychometric assessment of three newly developed implementation outcome measures. *Implementation Science, 12*(1), 108. https://doi.org/10.1186/s13012-017-0635-3

Youn, S. J., Creed, T. A., Wiltsey-Stirman, S., & Marques, L. (2020, May 20). *Hidden inequalities: COVID-19's impact on our mental health workforce*. Anxiety & Depression Association of America. https://adaa.org/learn-from-us/from-the-experts/blog-posts/professional/hidden-inequalities-covid-19s-impact-our

5

Understanding Barriers and Facilitators for Implementation Across Settings

Maria E. Fernandez, Laura Damschroder, and Bijal Balasubramanian

Learning Objectives

By the end of this chapter, readers will be able to:

- Explain how various contextual factors, referred to as barriers and facilitators, can influence implementation success
- Describe a process for using existing implementation science knowledge, frameworks, and contextual data to identify barriers and facilitators to implementation
- Recognize how constructs from theories, models, and frameworks can help inform the identification of barriers and facilitators to implementation
- Explain how to assess the importance of barriers and facilitators to implementation and how to prioritize the targeting of those most able to improve implementation.

CASE STUDY 5.1A IMPLEMENTATION OF THE TELEPHONE LIFESTYLE COACHING PROGRAM (Damschroder et al., 2017)

The U.S. Veterans Health Administration (VHA) recently conducted a large 2-year pilot to implement an evidence-based program called Telephone Lifestyle Coaching (TLC) with 25 medical centers across the country (Dale et al., 2008; Donnelly et al., 2013; Gold et al., 2000; McKay et al., 2005; Perri et al., 2008; Stead et al., 2013; U.S. Preventive Services Task Force [PSTF], 2003). TLC provided telephone-based coaching to help patients enact healthier behaviors (e.g., healthy weight, smoking cessation). Medical centers had to identify patients who would benefit from TLC and then refer them to a centralized coaching center. When the referral was received a coach called the patient, oriented them to the program, then provided up to nine coaching sessions over a span of 6 months.

By the end of 19 months, 9,357 patients had been referred to TLC, and significant variation in rate of referral was observed across the 25 medical centers. The center with the highest rate of referrals had seven times more referrals than the center with the lowest rate of referrals (Figure 5.1). The guiding question was: What were the factors that contributed to such large differences in referral rates?

To better understand what happened and identify the barriers and facilitators that influenced the wide variation in implementation of TLC across medical centers, a team of researchers partnered with policy leaders in the VHA to evaluate the experiences of medical center clinicians and staff who participated in the pilot (Damschroder et al., 2016). Respondents cited numerous challenges about program delivery (not about the content of the program), including barriers and facilitators associated with each medical center. The evaluation team noted that medical center context was likely largely responsible for the differences observed. They used implementation science frameworks and methods to better understand how contextual factors translated to variable implementation success.

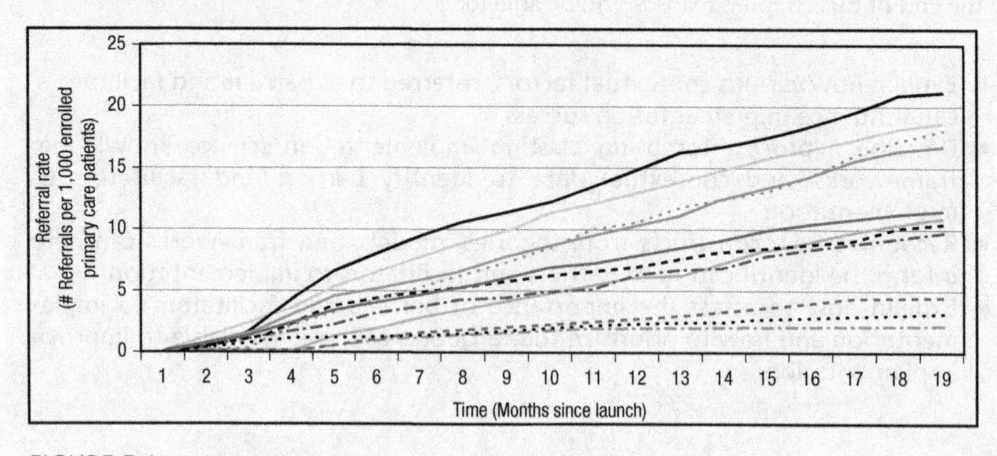

FIGURE 5.1 Variable referral rates from the TLC implementation study.

INTRODUCTION

The purpose of implementation science is to better understand how innovations get implemented in the field and to intervene to improve implementation. More effective implementation will result in better outcomes. In healthcare, successful implementation can increase equitable access to diagnostic testing and care, speed recovery, improve long-term management of chronic diseases, increase life expectancy, and improve quality of life. When a new program, policy, or practice is developed (whether by a researcher, healthcare provider, public health practitioner, an educator or other individual/organization) *everyone* wants to know if it is effective. Once a program is considered effective ("evidence-based") then it can be replicated and the whole world can benefit, right? Not quite. There are many reasons why an evidence-based intervention (EBI) may fail even if that intervention achieved astounding results previously. In the example given in the Case Study, even though the TLC program that was being implemented enjoyed a very strong evidence base for the outcomes that the medical centers were aiming to achieve (Dale et al., 2008; Donnelly et al., 2013; Gold et al., 2000; McKay et al., 2005; Perri et al., 2008; Stead et al., 2013; PSTF, 2003), unanticipated implementation barriers had a disruptive effect.

Despite the best efforts of practitioners, even innovations proven to be highly effective in certain settings are often not broadly adopted or implemented as they were intended to be. To address the root causes of this "implementation gap," it is important to first understand how and why an implementation effort succeeded or failed, and how that understanding can be leveraged to improve future implementation efforts.

Whether or not an implementation effort succeeds or fails is affected by amorphous factors, often referred to as **context**, such as the culture and history of the implementing organization, characteristics of the individuals involved in the implementation effort, leadership, or local policies and regulations. Different disciplines use different lenses through which to conceptualize context. For example, experts in organizational development may focus on the clinic culture, team functioning, or leadership structures (Birken et al., 2017; Foster et al., 2007). Health promotion experts viewing a problem from an ecological perspective may focus on various levels (provider, organizational, policy) and the "actors" within those levels that need to enact adoption and implementation behaviors. Still other researchers may use a lens based on theories of complexity that focus more on *interactions* rather than discrete individual actions or agents (Plsek & Wilson, 2001)

Context is a complex concept with definitions often varying by discipline. Given this variability, how do we account for the right contextual factors *in practice* to improve the likelihood of successful implementation of an innovation which is already proven to be effective in other contexts? How can the innovation be better understood? How can implementation science help with this challenge? The aim of this chapter is to answer these questions. In the following, we describe a process for identifying the various factors that can influence implementation. We explain how implementation science theories, models, and frameworks can help guide the identification of contextual barriers and facilitators, and how to apply common methods for assessing and prioritizing them.

DEFINING CONTEXT

Whether an innovation is new or has been sub-optimally used, to improve the implementation of any EBI (e.g., a practice, program, a policy) we must understand the innovation itself, its intended use, and the factors that impact the extent to which it is used in the real world (the focus of this chapter). In implementation science the various factors influencing implementation are often referred to as **barriers and facilitators**, which refer to those things that make it harder or easier to get something implemented. A barrier could also include things that were not in place that should have been (e.g., leadership support) that made it difficult for successful implementation. Another term that is often used is **implementation determinant**, because these factors *determine* whether and/or how well an innovation gets implemented. Whether these factors are referred to as barriers and facilitators or determinants, they can be encompassed by the global term: *context*.

Although there is general consensus about the importance of contextual influences on implementation, practically, the field of implementation science has not yet adopted a consistent definition of context (McDonald, 2013). It has been described broadly, as "a multi-dimensional construct…anything that cannot be described as an intervention or an outcome" (Gagliardi et al., 2014; McDonald, 2013). Others define context as a construct with multilevel determinants that either were pre-existing, come up during implementation (emergent), or change throughout the implementation process (dynamic). These various definitions underscore the notion that context is broad, constantly changing, interactive, and complex (Butler et al., 2017; Rogers et al., 2020) and should be considered at more than one level. For practical purposes we define **context** as the factors that influence the implementation of an evidence-based innovation.

When determining which contextual factors will or did influence implementation, it is useful to keep in mind the following: (a) Context is multilevel, (b) contextual factors can serve as barriers or facilitators to implementation, (c) context can change over time, and (d) some contextual factors are modifiable while others are not. Understanding these four core principles can help implementers identify relevant contextual factors impacting or likely to impact their implementation effort, evaluate how important they are, and decide which may be targets for intervening to improve implementation outcomes.

Why and When Should We Consider Context?

The context in which interventions or innovations are implemented influences implementation. Interventions effective in one context can fail in another context, particularly when the role of specific contextual factors in previous implementation efforts is not well understood. In fact, the success of many EBIs in improving healthcare have not been replicated (Porter, 2010) because of context-specific variations. Examining contextual influences on implementation can help explain the "how and why" of intervention effectiveness and impact. Assessing and reporting contextual factors that influence implementation is not only important for improving specific implementation efforts, but also for contributing to the knowledge that can be applied to other settings, thus enhancing intervention impact (Stange & Glasgow, 2013).

When implementation context is examined retrospectively, we might seek to understand the contextual factors influencing implementation by looking back at an implementation effort that did not turn out as well as planned. In doing so we try to determine what went wrong, and what we can do to improve future efforts. Prospectively, we seek to understand the contextual factors that may represent barriers or facilitators of implementing a planned EBI so that we can be prepared to deal with the barriers and/or capitalize on or leverage the facilitators. Indeed, the concept of organizational readiness for implementation (described later in the chapter) is based on this idea. Understanding contextual barriers and facilitators can also inform the development or selection of strategies to increase adoption, use, and/or maintenance of the innovation.

CORE PROCESSES FOR IDENTIFYING BARRIERS AND FACILITATORS OF IMPLEMENTATION

Given the multicomponent and multilevel nature of implementation context, how can a practitioner identify important barriers and facilitators that could be influencing implementation? First, we must consider the potential contextual factors, then gather evidence (using existing experience, literature, theories and frameworks, and new data) about which of these are related to implementation in the specific setting, and then prioritize among the several factors that should be addressed.

It is not uncommon for people involved in implementation efforts to brainstorm factors they believe could influence implementation and to think about solutions (implementation strategies) that might address them. However, they may not consistently use the most recent available information and/or established tools that can help them identify critical factors. Some of the best resources available include the published literature about implementation barriers and facilitators for the innovation of interest (or a similar one), implementation science theories and frameworks that help sort through what might influence implementation, and newly collected data from people and sites that have been (or will be) involved in implementation. Even when implementers do review literature and theories, and collect additional research data, it is still not always clear exactly how and when the information should be used to understand and address barriers and facilitators (Buunk & Van Vugt, 2013; Ruiter et al., 2013). In the following, we describe a series of steps (or processes) for identifying barriers and facilitators to implementation.

Core processes are a set of helpful actions or tools that can provide a systematic way to answer questions raised while exploring potential barriers and facilitators to implementation. Using core processes can make it less likely to miss factors that are important and can help prioritize which should be addressed. The processes in the following are a modified version of those used in Intervention Mapping (Bartholomew-Eldredge et al., 2016; Fernandez et al., 2019) and Implementation Mapping (Fernandez et al., 2019). (See the following and further described by Ruiter and Crutzen, 2020.) These core processes also align well with Stange and Glasgow's framework (2013) for guiding the assessment of context. The remainder of this chapter is organized into four core processes, presented along with examples:

1. *Brainstorm* potential barriers and facilitators (based on experience, past needs assessments, and published literature)
2. *Use theories and frameworks*
3. *Collect new data*
4. *Prioritize* the most important and changeable factors

There has been increasing recognition recently of the importance of ensuring that practitioners, other stakeholders, and communities are engaged in implementation research and practice (Blachman-Demner et al., 2017; Pinto et al., 2021). Community and stakeholder engagement in any implementation effort (whether research or not) is critical, and should be integrated with the core processes described in the following. Input from stakeholders, including practitioners, patients, community members, decision-makers, and implementers, can help create a shared vision for the implementation effort, ensure that it will meet needs, build support for the implementation effort, and increase the likelihood that the EBI or other innovation will be sustained over time. Community and stakeholder engagement should occur at an early stage and continue through the evaluation of the effort.

In a review of dissemination and implementation (D&I) models to identify community-specific engagement constructs, Pinto (Norris et al., 2017) and colleagues noted that models reflected the following constructs: communication, partnership exchange, community capacity building, leadership, and collaboration. The authors suggest that implementation practitioners can help ensure that researchers select D&I models more likely to improve community involvement. A qualitative study described how stakeholders in a large healthcare system defined engagement (Norris et al., 2017). Some of the key points were that stakeholders should be involved in decision-making with engagement, meaning that a process of shared decision-making with input of those most impacted is what would lead to buy-in and commitment. Stakeholders also noted that engagement is a two-way interaction beginning early in the implementation effort with an emphasis on respectful exchanges where stakeholders would feel understood. There are many resources for ensuring that community engagement is an integral part of understanding barriers and facilitators to implementation. Glandon and colleagues (2017) provide a compilation of the *10 Best Resources for Community Engagement and Implementation Research*. Practice-based efforts that are not research focused can also benefit greatly from these resources to ensure that community and stakeholder perspectives are central in any effort to identify barriers and facilitators to implementation.

CORE PROCESS 1: BRAINSTORM POTENTIAL BARRIERS AND FACILITATORS USING EXPERIENCE, EVIDENCE, AND ENGAGEMENT

Following a deliberate process will help ensure that implementation planners arrive at a comprehensive list of barriers and facilitators most likely to influence implementation. Core process 1, *brainstorm*, emphasizes relying on both the experience of the planning team and other relevant stakeholders, as well as the literature. While practitioners may not have a broad wealth of implementation research-related knowledge pertaining to a given intervention or already know the best implementation strategies to deliver it, they do possess valuable hands-on experience. This rich experience is not always captured or easily extracted from available literature. In many cases, the hands-on experience of the practitioners involved aligns well with published evidence. In other cases, non-alignment sheds light on unexplored factors or reveals ones that may have been important in another setting but not the current one. In either case, discussion about how barriers and facilitators may be the same or different in a particular setting as compared to what others have found (documented in reports or in the published literature) can be useful for decision-making about what needs to be addressed.

For example, during a brainstorming session an implementation planning team may all feel strongly that a barrier to implementation in the past has been an organization's reliance on email for communicating important knowledge to healthcare workers about new practice changes or innovations. The planning team's perception of email communication as a barrier may not align with a literature review that indicates that email communication has been used effectively for imparting important knowledge about implementation of an intervention in other studied settings. It is important to remember that this literature review finding may or may not directly translate to the setting/ organization in question, even if superficially the settings seem similar. In this case planners should reconsider whether email communication is truly a barrier to effective implementation in their context, and if past issues with email communication still exist. They may conclude that the important point that both the literature and their team agree on is that communication about prioritizing the innovation is what is important. They can then decide on whether they want to improve their email communication or find another channel. Checking experiential observations versus the published evidence provides planners with a new vantage point from which they can reiterate their initial conclusions, if necessary.

It is important for planning teams to recognize that neither practitioner experiences nor published evidence are innately "right." These sources of information are simply tools that can be used to create a more insightful implementation plan. Cross-checking group brainstorming of barriers and facilitators with the literature may provide a clear indication that the group's conclusions missed key factors or were unrealistic. Alternatively, stakeholders within a given organization know that setting better than anyone and may at times find that the existing published evidence does not map well to their organization. In certain instances, it is acceptable for planners to discount published evidence based their own intuition or hands-on experiences. Similarly, a lack of evidence supporting group conclusions should not automatically discount the conclusion reached based on real-world experience. To more fully understand barriers and facilitators able to influence implementation in a specific context, both real-world experiences and published evidence should be considered. Acknowledging the importance of both will result in an implementation plan that is more likely to achieve the desired outcomes.

CORE PROCESS 2: USING THEORIES, MODELS, AND FRAMEWORKS TO IDENTIFY BARRIERS AND FACILITATORS TO IMPLEMENTATION

In trying to identify potential contextual factors that influence implementation we may wonder which are most likely and which matter most. Considering the range of potential factors is important because unless we are open to the possibilities of what could influence implementation, we run the risk of making assumptions based on our hunches or missing something important. The challenge, however, is that we don't know what we don't know. Using theories, models, and frameworks can help. In this section, we provide examples of implementation science theories, models, and frameworks that have been used to better understand the potential barriers and facilitators influencing implementation success and failure. Use of such frameworks can have an important bearing on the success of the planned implementation of the intervention.

With the array of implementation science theories, models, and frameworks available, practitioners often ask: How do I know what theory or framework to use? The answer, unfortunately, is often that it depends on what you need it for. Nilsen described a useful categorization of implementation science models dividing them into **process models** that describe the steps or phases in translating research to practice, **evaluation models** that provide guidance about the implementation outcomes, and **determinant models** that help understand or describe the factors (barriers and facilitators) influencing implementation (Nilsen, 2015). A helpful resource to guide choosing a framework is the Theory Comparison and Selection Tool (T-CaST; technical assistance website: https://impsci.tracs.unc.edu/tcast/) developed by Birken and colleagues (2018). They list practical considerations including how usable, how testable, how applicable, and how acceptable the framework is for you and other key people you work with.

For this chapter, which is focused on understanding the factors (or determinants) influencing implementation, a closer look at *determinant models* is warranted. Within this class of models, prime differentiators include:

- Comprehensiveness: Some models have more constructs than others
- Levels: Some models focus on many levels (i.e., community, organization, individual)
- Contexts of application: Some models are more relevant in healthcare, others in schools, others in community settings

When considering which specific determinants model to employ, implementers should take these attributes into account. It is not necessary to limit the selection to only one model or framework. One model may be more helpful for understanding potential personal barriers that may exist within individuals in organizations (e.g., knowledge, skills, self-efficacy), while other models may focus on the implementation environment or setting (e.g., implementation climate).

The use of implementation determinants models (and theories and frameworks) can help researchers and practitioners understand barriers and facilitators for three purposes: (a) to understand why things happened, (b) to predict what might happen, and (c) to inform the selection or development of implementation strategies to increase adoption, implementation, and/or maintenance of EBIs. In the Case Study 5.1A, the Consolidated Framework for Implementation Research (CFIR) framework helped understand how contextual factors explained what had occurred during implementation. This information was used to understand why things happened the way they did and why there may have been a difference across health centers, and ultimately to develop strategies to address them such that implementation is improved.

In this section, we briefly describe key implementation science frameworks that can be used to help identify barriers and facilitators to implementation. We also apply one of them (the CFIR) to provide a glimpse into the range of lenses used to understand context. Fundamentally, we use these frameworks to understand how context affects our ability to successfully implement EBIs.

The Social Ecological Model (SEM; Bronfenbrenner, 2009) is a framework that can help illuminate the multiple levels of contextual factors that can influence implementation. Developed by psychologists over 50 years ago and applied commonly in the field of health promotion (McLeroy et al., 1988; Wold & Mittelmark, 2018), the SEM describes the interaction between individual, organizational, community, and societal factors. It shows that individuals (e.g., patients, community members) are influenced by their relationships to family, peers, partners, and other social networks; by community organizations such as churches, schools, and workplaces; by social and cultural norms; and by their broader societal, political, and physical environments. The term ecology refers to the relationships between people (or organisms) and their environments and **ecological models** focus on the interdependence of these environmental levels and individuals.

Ecological models recognize multiple levels of influence on health behaviors, including (Rimer & Glanz, 2005):

- Intrapersonal/individual factors: An individual's traits, including factors that influence behavior such as knowledge, attitudes, and beliefs.
- Interpersonal factors: Relationships and social networks, including interactions with other people, can provide social support or create barriers to implementation.
- Institutional and organizational factors: The organizational rules and policies, formal and informal structures, processes, and organizational culture that could influence implementation.
- Community factors: The formal or informal social norms that exist among individuals or organizations that can enhance, limit, or impede implementation.
- Public policy factors: Local, state, and federal policies and laws that can influence implementation by regulating or supporting practices (e.g., chronic disease detection, control, and management).

A central idea underlying SEM is that individuals (and organizations) do not exist in a vacuum. Instead, everything impacts everything else and changing a system influences both individual and collective behaviors. Various levels of contextual influence, then, could impact implementation. While it may not be possible to determine exactly how factors at various levels interact, affect, and change each other, it is still useful to identify and describe what they are and to know that changing one factor is likely to affect others.

Unlike some other frameworks covered in the following, SEM does not offer specific factors or determinants to consider. Nevertheless, it can be useful in thinking about what barriers and facilitators may exist within each level. For example, to implement a particular innovation (e.g., COVID-19 vaccines), one should consider how interpersonal factors (provider recommendation), organizational factors (clinic leadership prioritization of COVID-19 vaccines), community (access to vaccination), and policy (federal incentives for clinic) can influence implementation.

The SEM has been used to identify potential barriers and facilitators barriers that could predict implementation success or failure thus informing the selection of implementation strategies to address them. A recent study used the SEM to identify facilitators and barriers to implementation of opioid treatment programs in prisons (Komalasari et al., 2021). The study found barriers such as intrapersonal factors (misperceptions), interpersonal barriers (inflexible treatment processes), and social-structural factors (resource constraints), and highlighted the interaction between interpersonal and organizational factors. The strategies that were suggested included: those that addressed multiple levels including education and training for prisoners and staff, the re-assessment of practices and policies relating to the delivery of methadone, and a focus on harm reduction in prisons including the role of families and social support.

The SEM has also been applied to investigate the determinants that influence implementation in low- and middle-income countries (LMICs), allowing for a deep examination of multiple effects and interrelatedness of social factors in a given environment. For example, a study conducted in sub-Saharan Africa used the SEM framework to categorize themes in order to highlight the multi-faceted factors (individual, community, organizational, and policy) that play a significant role in the implementation of a Diabetes Self-Management Education and Support program (Bamuya et al., 2021). The SEM framework provided a solid foundation for investigating personal and environmental factors that determined change, as well as an understanding into how the program could be implemented and embedded within larger type 2 diabetes mellitus services in the region (Bamuya et al., 2021).

Table 5.1 (Rogers et al., 2020) is a non-exhaustive compilation of contextual factors at different levels from a recent systematic review of the literature that can help implementers quickly find relevant categories of barriers and facilitators at different levels. While the factors listed in Table 5.1 are purposefully general, they can be further specified to more clearly represent those factors that influence implementation in a particular setting.

TABLE 5.1 Example Contextual Factors (Rogers et al., 2020) by Level From the Literature

INDIVIDUAL	TEAM	ORGANIZATIONAL	EXTERNAL (REGION)
Perceptions/attitudes	Teamwork	Resources	Economic environment
Autonomy	Team resources	Culture	Health system characteristics
Involvement	Team skills	Climate	Political environment
Socio-economic background	Team relationships	Support	Social environment
Self-efficacy	Team stability	Characteristics	External incentives
Experience	Team morale	Leadership	
Commitment/motivation	Team workload	Trust	

Normalization process theory (NPT) was developed to help explain the social process by which new treatments are implemented, embedded, and fully integrated to ensure that new treatments are routinely used within clinical settings to improve patient outcomes (May et al., 2009). NPT focuses specifically on what people do within organizations. Like other implementation science frameworks, NPT focuses on explaining how collective efforts can lead to change in collective behaviors; working collectively requires understanding relational dynamics of the organization, and who (e.g., doctors, nurses, clerks, leaders) and how people can work together to enact changes needed to ensure routine delivery of a new EBI.

NPT describes four key areas of action that are needed for successful implementation of a new EBI. First, the people involved must engage in sense-making, individually and collectively, to achieve ***cohesion***. This means that people are literally working to make sense of the change by building a shared understanding of how the change differs from usual ways of working, solidifying the purpose behind the change, operationalizing how work routines will be affected, and theorizing its potential value. The second area of action is ***cognitive participation***, which highlights the relational work needed to build and sustain a community of practice dedicated to the change. People involved need to take on key roles to drive or lead implementation efforts, recognize that they need to work with colleagues in new ways, see their participation in the change as a legitimate part of their work, and support the change. Third, ***collective action*** is the operational work necessary to integrate the new practice with established work processes. Collective action is also building accountability and confidence among people involved in the change, establishing roles and responsibilities with necessary skill-building, and tailoring and adapting to fit local contexts. The fourth and final area of action is ***reflexive monitoring***, which is necessary to assess and understand how effective and useful the new treatment is to everyone involved. Monitoring helps to systematize the change, engage in collaborative and individual appraisal, and to reconfigure as needed based on continued reflexive monitoring. NPT provides a guide to help users systematically identify and evaluate barriers and facilitators to successful implementation.

NPT defines and describes potentially influential factors based on theory and affirmed by many empirical studies (May et al., 2009). Each NPT domain can be methodically assessed. Researchers and implementers that use and report on their experiences using language and concepts described by NPT can learn from each other much more readily because they are using a shared language and conceptual framework. Many frameworks, like NPT, have technical assistance websites to help users apply the framework (May et al., 2015). For example, http://normalizationprocess.org/ provides instructions for applying the framework, how results can be used to guide implementation efforts, and provides a 23-question assessment instrument, called NoMAD, that elicits quantitative ratings of the extent to which each of the four domains are in place. There is also a bibliography of articles that all use NPT so users can find other studies that were guided by NPT.

O'Reilly et al. (2017) conducted a review of efforts to implement interdisciplinary teamwork within primary care settings, organizing their findings using NPT's four domains. For *cohesion*, although the idea of multidisciplinary teams made sense to providers, they did not always see the value of sharing responsibility of patient care with other health professionals. Second, for *cognitive participation*, providers were key champions for driving change and yet were also the source of strongest resistance to implementation efforts. Third, for *collective action*, results were mixed but clarity and trust about division of labor across health profession roles was an important facilitator. Fourth, for *reflexive monitoring*, the authors found little evidence of team-based appraisal (O'Reilly et al., 2017). The findings of this review provide a high-level overview from a collection of studies that all used the NPT framework.

NPT can also be used to diagnose or explain why an intervention did not work and help point to better strategies to use in future efforts. **Audit and feedback** is a commonly

TABLE 5.2 List of Strategies to Address Challenges by NPT Domain

NPT DOMAIN	CHALLENGES REVEALED	STRATEGIES TO ADDRESS CHALLENGES
Coherence	None.	
Reflexive monitoring	Doctors questioned credibility which undermined their willingness to engage in reflexive monitoring.	Ensure data matters to recipients Model how data can be used to drive practice changes
Cognitive participation	Lack of technical skills impeded ability to interact with the data.	Prove access to someone to assist with data interpretation Provide training on interpreting practice data
Collective action	Physicians struggled to identify actions they could do based on the data.	Provide opportunity for social interaction Circulate examples of effective actions

Source: From May, C., Rapley, T., Mair, F. S., Treweek, S., Murra, E., Ballini, L., Macfarlane, A. Girling, M., & Finch, T. L. (2015). Normalization process theory on-line users' manual, toolkit and NoMAD instrument. http://www .normalizationprocess.org

used intervention to provide data about clinical processes (e.g., consistency of measuring and documenting blood pressure) and patient outcomes (e.g., rates of uncontrolled blood pressure and cardiovascular disease) to healthcare professionals. Often comparative benchmarks are included so people can see how their performance compares with their peers. Based on data reports, providers can identify gaps in care that need to be improved. For example, data showing low rates of documented blood pressure for patients points to the need to identify solutions to ensure more consistent blood pressure monitoring. Though providers may understand the value of this reporting and the importance of improving clinical processes and outcomes (i.e., high *coherence*), other challenges dampen providers' participation. Guided by NPT, Desveaux et al. conducted qualitative interviews with physicians across five clinics in Canada (Desveaux et al., 2021). The authors found that the credibility of the data source and credibility of the data itself were barriers to *reflexive monitoring* by providers. Second, they found that while providers may see that they were below benchmark, they did not always have the skills needed to interpret what that data meant for their own practice. Providers also struggled to identify solutions or actions they could take that would address that gap to improve performance. Table 5.2 summarizes these findings and lists strategies that can be used to address those challenges in future implementations. This example study demonstrates how NPT can be used to methodically identify challenges that then can inform needed strategies to overcome those challenges.

In summary, NPT can be used to collect quantitative ratings of domains using the NoMAD instrument or to elicit more in-depth information through qualitative interviews. The goal for NPT is to help explain potential (if assessed before implementation) or actual (if assessed after implementation) facilitators and barriers to sustained integration of a new treatment into routine practice.

The Consolidated Framework for Implementation Research (CFIR)

Like NPT, the CFIR (Damschroder et al., 2009) was developed to better understand and communicate complex factors arising from settings within which implementations occur.

The CFIR was developed based on published theories, models, and frameworks, and consolidates from them factors that may influence implementation success. The CFIR identifies determinants (i.e., factors/constructs/influences that may lead to success or failure of implementation efforts), and its constructs capture collective perceptions about local context. For example, the perception of employees about the degree of leadership engagement (a CFIR construct examining the commitment, involvement, and accountability of leaders and managers) in support of planned implementation of an innovation. Understanding manifestation and dynamics of these factors can help point toward which implementation strategies may be needed to navigate or mitigate potential barriers and facilitators (when assessed pre-implementation) or to explain outcomes (when assessed post-implementation). Commonly, individuals who help inform contextual assessment of constructs are referred to as **stakeholders** and may include individuals at many levels of the organization (clinicians, administrators, and leaders) or community setting, along with potential beneficiaries (e.g., patients) of the newly implemented program. Stakeholders are simply all individuals who influence or are influenced by implementation of a new program. Table 5.3 lists constructs across the CFIR's five domains of context.

The first domain within the CFIR, **characteristics of the intervention**, relates to perceptions of the innovation by implementers (e.g., *adaptability, complexity, cost, relative advantage, evidence strength and quality*; see Table 5.3 for a list of all subdomains). For example, perceptions of *evidence strength and quality* of the innovation may influence willingness to implement or deliver the innovation to their patients. If stakeholders uniformly report positive perceptions of the evidence, believing the program will benefit their patients, they will be more receptive to implementing it. In Case Study 5.1A implementation leaders at each medical center underwent training about TLC and the research evidence supporting its use, and were provided with informational brochures, presentation templates, and booklets they could use with their providers to help educate and ensure everyone (especially referring physicians) was aware of the evidence base showing how effective TLC can be for patients (Damschroder et al., 2016).

The second CFIR domain is outer setting, and contains constructs such as *patient needs and resources* (the extent to which the organization understands its patients and the barriers and facilitators patients may experience within their community or home). Outer setting also includes consideration of market forces, or policies including reimbursement regulations, all which can affect implementation outcomes (see Table 5.3 for all subdomains). For example, in Case Study 5.1A, most stakeholders welcomed the TLC program because they believed it would allow their patients to receive coaching within their own home rather than suffer long commutes to a clinic for in-person coaching.

The third domain within the CFIR is **inner setting**, which contains the longest list of constructs. The many aspects of the inner setting reflect the complex array of influences within clinical settings. The constructs found in the inner setting include *structural characteristics, networks and communications, culture, implementation climate*, and *readiness for implementation* (see full listing of subdomains in Table 5.3). Within Case Study 5.1A, *networks and communications* (the nature and quality of webs of social networks and formal and informal communications within an organization) varied widely across the centers and was associated with implementation outcomes. Two of the most successful medical centers had implementation leaders with strong working relationships with the physicians who were the main source of patient referrals to the TLC. Sites with the lowest referral rates did not have these connections nor were they able to work with their physicians to generate referrals. Another factor associated with implementation outcomes was *compatibility* of TLC with other pre-existing programs and processes. Within the highest referral centers, individuals welcomed TLC as a synergistic program to expand their existing programs. In contrast, at the lowest referring centers, TLC was regarded as a competitor to an existing

TABLE 5.3 List of CFIR Constructs With Short Definitions

	TOPIC/DESCRIPTION	SHORT DESCRIPTION
I. Intervention characteristics		
A	Intervention source	Perception of key stakeholders about whether the intervention is externally or internally developed
B	Evidence strength and quality	Stakeholders' perceptions of the quality and validity of evidence supporting the belief that the intervention will have desired outcomes
C	Relative advantage	Stakeholders' perceptions of the advantage of implementing the intervention versus an alternative solution
D	Adaptability	The degree to which an intervention can be adapted, tailored, refined, or reinvented to meet local needs
E	Trialability	The ability to test the intervention on a small scale in the organization (Stead et al., 2013), and to be able to reverse course (undo implementation) if warranted
F	Complexity	Perceived difficulty of implementation, reflected by duration, scope, radicalness, disruptiveness, centrality, and intricacy and number of steps required to implement
G	Design quality and packaging	Perceived excellence in how the intervention is bundled, presented, and assembled
H	Cost	Costs of the intervention and costs associated with implementing that intervention including investment, supply, and opportunity costs
II. Outer setting		
A	Patient needs and resources	The extent to which patient needs, as well as barriers and facilitators to meet those needs, are accurately known and prioritized by the organization
B	Cosmopolitanism	The degree to which an organization is networked with other external organizations
C	Peer pressure	Mimetic or competitive pressure to implement an intervention; typically because most or other key peer or competing organizations have already implemented or are in a bid for a competitive edge
D	External policy and incentives	A broad construct that includes external strategies to spread interventions including policy and regulations (governmental or other central entity), external mandates, recommendations and guidelines, pay-for-performance, collaboratives, and public or benchmark reporting

(*continued*)

TABLE 5.3 List of CFIR Constructs with Short Definitions (*continued*)

	TOPIC/DESCRIPTION	SHORT DESCRIPTION
III. Inner setting		
A	Structural characteristics	The social architecture, age, maturity, and size of an organization
B	Networks and communications	The nature and quality of webs of social networks and the nature and quality of formal and informal communications within an organization
C	Culture	Norms, values, and basic assumptions of a given organization
D	Implementation climate	The absorptive capacity for change, shared receptivity of involved individuals to an intervention and the extent to which use of that intervention will be rewarded, supported, and expected within their organization
1	Tension for change	The degree to which stakeholders perceive the current situation as intolerable or needing change
2	Compatibility	The degree of tangible fit between meaning and values attached to the intervention by involved individuals; how those align with individuals' own norms, values, and perceived risks and needs; and how the intervention fits with existing workflows and systems
3	Relative priority	Individuals' shared perception of the importance of the implementation within the organization
4	Organizational incentives and rewards	Extrinsic incentives such as goal-sharing awards, performance reviews, promotions, and raises in salary and less tangible incentives such as increased stature or respect
5	Goals and feedback	The degree to which goals are clearly communicated, acted upon, and fed back to staff and alignment of that feedback with goals
6	Learning climate	A climate in which (a) leaders express their own fallibility and need for team members' assistance and input; (b) team members feel that they are essential, valued, and knowledgeable partners in the change process; (c) individuals feel psychologically safe to try new methods; and (d) there is sufficient time and space for reflective thinking and evaluation
E	Readiness for implementation	Tangible and immediate indicators of organizational commitment to its decision to implement an intervention

(*continued*)

TABLE 5.3 List of CFIR Constructs with Short Definitions (*continued*)

	TOPIC/DESCRIPTION	SHORT DESCRIPTION
1	Leadership engagement	Commitment, involvement, and accountability of leaders and managers with the implementation
2	Available resources	The level of resources dedicated for implementation and on-going operations including money, training, education, physical space, and time
3	Access to knowledge and information	Ease of access to digestible information and knowledge about the intervention and how to incorporate it into work tasks
IV. Characteristics of individuals		
A	Knowledge and beliefs about the intervention	Individuals' attitudes toward and value placed on the intervention as well as familiarity with facts, truths, and principles related to the intervention
B	Self-efficacy	Individual belief in their own capabilities to execute courses of action to achieve implementation goals
C	Individual stage of change	Characterization of the phase an individual is in, as they progress toward skilled, enthusiastic, and sustained use of the intervention
D	Individual identification with organization	A broad construct related to how individuals perceive the organization and their relationship and degree of commitment with that organization
E	Other personal attributes	A broad construct to include other personal traits such as tolerance of ambiguity, intellectual ability, motivation, values, competence, capacity, and learning style
V. Process		
A	Planning	The degree to which a scheme or method of behavior and tasks for implementing an intervention are developed in advance and the quality of those schemes or methods
B	Engaging	Attracting and involving appropriate individuals in the implementation and use of the intervention through a combined strategy of social marketing, education, role modeling, training, and other similar activities

(*continued*)

TABLE 5.3 List of CFIR Constructs with Short Definitions *(continued)*

	TOPIC/DESCRIPTION	SHORT DESCRIPTION
1	Opinion leaders	Individuals in an organization who have formal or informal influence on the attitudes and beliefs of their colleagues with respect to implementing the intervention
2	Formally appointed internal implementation leaders	Individuals from within the organization who have been formally appointed with responsibility for implementing an intervention as coordinator, project manager, team leader, or other similar role
3	Champions	"Individuals who dedicate themselves to supporting, marketing, and 'driving through' an [implementation]" (p. 182), overcoming indifference or resistance that the intervention may provoke in an organization
4	External change agents	Individuals who are affiliated with an outside entity who formally influence or facilitate intervention decisions in a desirable direction
C	Executing	Carrying out or accomplishing the implementation according to plan
D	Reflecting and evaluating	Quantitative and qualitative feedback about the progress and quality of implementation accompanied with regular personal and team debriefing about progress and experience

Source: Damschroder, L. J., Aron, D. C., Keith, R. E., Kirsh, S. R., Alexander, J. A., & Lowery, J. C. (2009). Fostering implementation of health services research findings into practice: A consolidated framework for advancing implementation science. Implementation Science, 4, 50. https://doi.org/10.1186/1748-5908-4-50

program. Another bottleneck unique to one low referral center was the inability for anyone other than physicians to refer patients.

The fourth CFIR domain is the **characteristics of individuals** who are involved with implementation. The actions of individuals within an organization or community influence implementation and are influenced by characteristics of those individuals such as their *knowledge, attitudes, and beliefs about the intervention, self-efficacy*, their *individual stage of change*, their *individual identification with the organization*, and *other personal attributes*. These characteristics can heavily influence implementation. For example, if a physician does not believe their patients will benefit from a new intervention, they will not refer to the program.

The fifth domain is **process**, which describes the procedure for implementation and contains four constructs: *planning*, *executing* the plan, *engaging* key individuals, and *reflecting and evaluating* progress (see Table 5.3 for a full list of subdomains). These four activities are common best practices identified by many different methods of implementation. The CFIR does not direct implementers on how to address each of these constructs but, rather, posits that failure to do these key things will potentially influence implementation efforts. For example, in Case Study 5.1A, the degree to which individuals succeeded in ***engaging*** key stakeholders was associated with implementation outcomes. At the highest referral centers, the implementation leader reached out to primary care providers using multiple communication channels and repeated messaging to help reinforce the availability of TLC. This did not occur in the less successful centers.

The CFIR can help users systematically explore many of the possible barriers and facilitators across different levels that could influence implementation. Like the NPT, the CFIR can be used to systematically assess context to identify actual, or potential barriers and facilitators by using common language, terms, and definitions for constructs arranged across five domains. In this way, the CFIR provides language by which complex contexts can be articulated. The CFIR technical assistance website (https://cfirguide.org) provides guidance on the application of the framework including how to prioritize constructs within the longer list to a shorter list of high-priority constructs (CFIR Research Team-Center for Clinical Management Research, 2021).

CASE STUDY 5.1B USING THE CFIR TO PLAN TLC IMPLEMENTATION

During the implementation of TLC (as described in Case Study 5.1A), the research team engaged national policy leaders in a series of consensus discussions to identify a shortlist of the CFIR constructs with most potential influence on implementation outcomes. Past on-the-ground experiences with implementing similar programs and early research findings from other similar studies were used to inform the choice of constructs. For example, both research findings and experiences within the VA healthcare system pointed to the significant role of engaged champions including implementation leaders—highly capable, intrinsically motivated individuals can drive toward meeting implementation goals while the absence of these qualities can present enormous challenges for implementation. As a reminder, there was a seven-fold difference in the rate at which patients were referred to TCL within medical centers with the highest versus lowest referral rates. The CFIR was used to methodically guide, identify, and understand barriers and facilitators that might explain why there was such a wide range in success. For example, the role of implementation leader was highly correlated with referral rates: Medical centers with the highest rates of referrals all had more than a single implementation leader who were enthusiastic

(*continued*)

CASE STUDY 5.1B USING THE CFIR TO PLAN TLC IMPLEMENTATION (*continued*)

and highly committed to successful implementation of TLC but most of the medical centers with the lowest rates of referral did not identify an implementation leader or champion (because of vacancies) or had a single individual without enough support. The methodical use of the CFIR helped to reveal this plus six other key barriers (or facilitators) that were significantly correlated with implementation outcomes. The online website (www.CFIRGuide.org) provides detailed descriptions, templates, and tools to aid use of the CFIR. For the TLC implementation evaluation, a master guide for use when interviewing key individuals about their context was created in part by using a tool that allows users to click and select constructs and use this to guide interviews of people involved with implementation (e.g., program coordinators, dietitians, physicians, clinic leaders) at 11 of the 25 medical centers that participated in the pilot. The online codebook was used to guide coding of data elicited from 128 interviews. Next, online guidance describes how to rate interview data using a quantitative scale that indicates barriers (ratings less than zero) versus facilitators (ratings above zero). In the TLC evaluation, these ratings were used to explore correlation of each of the evaluated CFIR constructs with implementation outcomes across the medical centers; seven CFIR constructs were correlated with implementation outcomes within the TLC evaluation. This illustrative study shows how frameworks like the CFIR provide the foundation for conducting systematic, stepwise processes for assessing complex factors related to context.

An example of how the CFIR was used to better understand the implementation planning process can be seen in the technology-delivered asthma care intervention *Breathewell*, rolled out in an integrated care organization (King et al., 2020). The researchers interviewed implementation team members using questions that were adapted from the CFIR Interview Guide Tool. Findings from this study showed that CFIR constructs, such as alignment with the system's organizational *culture* and the perception of *compatibility* of the intervention with workflows and systems, were important considerations. They also found that low confidence that the intervention would be adopted and maintained over time was likely due to low levels of several important CFIR constructs such as *leadership engagement, relative priority*, and *tension for change*. In this study, the authors underscore the usefulness of the CFIR in helping explain why implementation succeeded or failed and assert that when used proactively, the CFIR can be used to identify salient modifiable factors that can and should be used to guide choice of implementation strategies.

The CFIR can also be used to prospectively plan for implementation. For example, English (2013) used the CFIR to help guide development of an intervention to improve pediatric services for children in Kenya, where the authors identified the key role of peer collaborations within hospitals (*networks and communication*) and between hospitals (*peer pressure*; English, 2013). The plan to address this barrier is to develop improvement collaboratives to provide mentorship and support to hospitals and key personnel within hospitals. The collaboratives will help to build broad communities of practice to strengthen a sense of shared identity, expose leaders and implementers to the persuasive force of their peers, and promote shared learning. This is an example of how frameworks such as the CFIR provide a solid foundation from which to assess potential barriers and facilitators of implementation (whether prospectively or retrospectively).

Organizational Readiness: Being Ready—or Not—for Implementation

The relationship between readiness and implementation outcomes is well established and the degree to which an organization can effectively implement an EBI is strongly associated with its *readiness* to do so (Drzensky et al., 2012; Holt & Vardaman, 2013; Scaccia et al., 2015; Weiner et al., 2008). The study of an organization's readiness is strongly associated with the identification of barriers and facilitators. In fact, readiness is considered a facilitator to implementation, while a lack of organizational readiness is considered a barrier (Domlyn & Wandersman, 2019; Drzensky et al., 2012; Holt & Vardaman, 2013; Weiner et al., 2009). It is therefore no surprise that in the field of implementation science, the assessment of readiness has historically been used to identify discrete barriers and facilitators within an organization or setting (Weiner et al., 2020). Understanding the reasons why an organization, community, or other setting is ready, or not, to implement something new is essentially the same as understanding the implementation barriers (reasons why the organization may not be ready) and facilitators (factors that make the organization ready). In CFIR, **readiness** is defined as the "tangible and immediate indicators or organizational commitment to its decision to implement and intervention" and includes sub-constructs of *leadership engagement, available resources,* and *access to knowledge and information* (CFIR Research Team-Center for Clinical Management Research, 2021, p. 4). While many definitions such as the one used in the CFIR consider readiness a necessary precursor for implementation to occur effectively, more recent definitions describe its importance throughout the process of adoption to include implementation and sustainment (Scaccia et al., 2015; Weiner et al., 2008).

Scaccia and Wandersman (2015) describe readiness as being made up of three main parts (abbreviated as $R = MC^2$): **R**eadiness = ***M****otivation* to implement an EBI, *innovation specific* ***C****apacities* needed to deliver the EBI (i.e., the specific knowledge and skills needed to implement a particular EBI), and the *general* ***C****apacities* of an organization needed to support implementation (e.g., adequate staffing, engaged leadership, resources). One implication is that if any of the components is very low, the organization or community may not be ready to implement an EBI and attempts to implement the EBI before the missing element is addressed will likely be unsuccessful. The assumption is that the likelihood of success could be intentionally increased following an assessment of readiness, through attention to building the capacities and motivations for implementation.

The idea is highly intuitive that for organizations or communities to be "ready," there needs to be support, capacity, and motivation. Nevertheless, most practitioners struggle with how to assess readiness and what to do with the information about readiness once they have it. While it is beyond the scope of this chapter to fully describe readiness measures, there are several previously developed and well-established measures that are designed to assess organizational readiness (Scaccia et al., 2015; Wandersman & Scaccia, 2017; Weiner et al., 2008). There are also ready-to-use planning tools available to assist implementation planners with the process of assessing readiness. Two such tools are the *Readiness Thinking Tool* (RTT) and the *Readiness Diagnostic Survey* (RDS). Both tools are designed to assess organizational readiness using the $R = MC^2$ framework and are described under Core Process 3 (collecting new data) in the following.

Implementation teams have largely used readiness assessments to diagnose where organizations (or other implementing settings), may be low on specific elements of readiness. The data can be depicted in heat maps and then used to elicit discussion with stakeholders about what should be prioritized, or for planning appropriate implementation strategies to increase readiness. For example, in a recent article, Domlyn (2021) describes a readiness building process centered around $R = MC^2$ and provide case studies at local, state, and national levels. It is important to understand the level and sources of readiness in your implementation context, as assessment and building of readiness can help practitioners prioritize the most effective actions (Domlyn et al., 2021).

USING THEORIES AND FRAMEWORKS IN LOW- AND MIDDLE-INCOME COUNTRIES

Given that the majority of interactive systems frameworks (ISFs) have been developed in high income countries (HICs), one important question is: When working in LMICs, how relevant and useful are these HIC-centered frameworks at identifying barriers and facilitators? The applicability of such frameworks in LMICs may prove difficult for several reasons, especially when there are key differences in how resources and processes for service delivery are constrained, regulated, and procured. To address this challenge, IS principles and tools such as the CFIR have been adapted, sometimes as an intentional precursor to implementation in a specific region or country. Researchers in India, for example, adapted various ISFs (e.g., the CFIR, *UK Medical Research Council's [MRC] framework for implementing complex interventions*) as part of their process of developing a new intervention design approach appropriate for use in India. The resulting approach not only helped strengthen and support existing delivery systems, but also established new support systems for implementing mental health services which were eventually integrated into the existing system (Ramaswamy et al., 2018).

There is growing use of the CFIR in LMICs as it continues to be adapted to various country and regional contexts—for example, to investigate the acceptability of a health intervention in Zambia (Jones et al., 2018) or to understand the sustainability of a health intervention in Ghana (Gyamfi et al., 2020)]—demonstrating that existing frameworks can be tailored to specific research requirements. The CFIR can be used to facilitate data collection using a deductive method and/or to sort out data collected using an inductive approach during the data analysis stage (Means et al., 2020). As an example, Ezezika et al.'s (2021) review of studies examining barriers and facilitators to implementation of large-scale nutrition interventions in Africa used CFIR to extract data from the studies. The authors noted that using CFIR helped them organize the identification of barriers and facilitators and resulted in the documentation of 16 out of 39 CFIR constructs. Thematic areas included policy and legislation; leadership management; resources mobilization; and cultural context and adaptability.

Another recent review looked at where and how the CFIR had been applied in LMIC contexts. Means and colleagues found that the CFIR was used in 34 studies across 21 countries, and applied to 18 different health topics (Means et al., 2020). The studies used CFIR in various ways, including: to help guide data collection to identify barriers to implementation, to assess the extent to which a program was delivered and the barriers and facilitators that influenced implementation, and to determine what factors influenced implementation retrospectively. Based on a survey conducted with authors, the review found that organizational *culture* (part of the *inner setting* domain) and *engaging* (part of the *process* domain) were the constructs most often cited as compatible with use in global implementation research. *Patient needs and resources* and *individual stages of change* were the two constructs noted as incompatible for the local application of the framework. Of the factors deemed important but absent from the original CFIR included the *influences of the team* on implementation and *characteristics of systems*. This led to a proposed new domain: *characteristics of systems*. This additional domain considers facilitators and barriers at the health systems-level that go beyond those influencing only the implementing organization.

HEALTH EQUITY CONSIDERATIONS

In this chapter, we describe how implementation frameworks, particularly determinants frameworks, can help inform the identification of contextual factors influencing implementation. One limitation to these frameworks is the lack of explicit focus on health equity.

It is unlikely that frameworks lacking a health equity focus can provide important insight into health equity–related determinants. This omission limits the ability of implementation science to create tools that examine health equity determinants for implementation, and further limits the ability to intentionally target implementation determinants that will improve health equity. Health professionals and organizations are becoming increasingly aware of the impacts of systemic racism and social injustice on health. Increasing willingness to critically examine this truth has allowed light to be shed on the continued health inequities experienced by marginalized communities (e.g., healthcare discrimination, inequitable innovation access). Effort to ensure that implementation is equitable is critical, and implementation science has the potential to be a tool or catalyst for increasing health equity. Brownson and colleagues (2021) described several recommendations to improve health equity in implementation science that addresses identified gaps in the evidence base, methods, and measurement and in addressing contextual factors influencing implementation (Brownson et al., 2021). Of these, the most relevant to this chapter include: linking social determinants with health outcomes, using equity-relevant metrics, and integrating equity into implementation models (2021).

The **Health Equity Implementation framework** (HEI framework) incorporates both an implementation science framework (Kilbourne et al., 2006) and a healthcare disparities framework (Harvey & Kitson, 2016) and thus, can be useful for ensuring the consideration of health-equity related barriers and facilitators to implementation (Woodward et al., 2019). A key feature of the HEI framework is its attention to multilevel healthcare disparities factors that influence implementation, and considers factors negatively impacting vulnerable populations caused by social and historical sidelining. The premise is that social influence affects all contextual factors influencing implementation and includes the economies, policies, and sociopolitical forces within which patients, providers, and other recipients are living and attempting to be healthy or provide healthcare (2019). The HEI framework guides the consideration of societal influence as various potential barriers and facilitators are assessed. For example, identifying factors within the clinical encounter that could affect implementation issues such as unconscious or explicit racial bias during a clinical encounter, can help ensure that the strategies developed to improve implementation directly address these concerns. The developers of the HEI framework used it to design interview guides that explored possible causes of healthcare disparities at multiple levels. This led to a greater ability to identify and interpret barriers and facilitators to the implementation challenge they faced when expanding treatment to Black patients (2019). The authors point out that knowledge about specific health equity–related barriers can help inform adaptations to implementation strategies to address barriers that might be specifically relevant for certain groups. They also note that the identification of facilitators to implementation can help identify policies, practices, or procedures that should be maintained.

CORE PROCESS 3: COLLECTING NEW DATA ON BARRIERS AND FACILITATORS

Even after considering the experience of those in a particular context, drawing from available evidence (in the literature or unpublished reports), and considering theories and frameworks, practitioners may want to gather new data (evidence) about what may influence (or be influencing—during an on-going effort) implementations. Assessing barriers and facilitators that occur within the multi-dimensional and multi-level aspects of context requires collecting both quantitative and qualitative data. This can occur at baseline (before implementation begins) and throughout implementation of innovations. The most complete picture is created when findings across multiple methods are integrated. Complementing the breadth of information gathered through quantitative data (such as surveys) with the depth and richness of information from qualitative data (such as interviews and observations) and integrating findings across these data can provide a fuller picture of the contextual factors that might influence implementation success (Fernandez et al., 2018).

Quantitative Data

The collection of quantitative data to measure implementation context commonly includes use of surveys, clinical data from electronic health records, and administrative data routinely collected by organizations like health systems about their operations, reimbursement, and policies. Contextual factors may be assessed by surveying teams, employees, and/or organizations. A key consideration in use of surveys is the availability of valid and reliable measures and instruments.

Some research teams have created open-source repositories of existing instruments and measures, often mapped to implementation frameworks and theories, that may be useful to researchers (https://impsciuw.org/implementation-science/research/measures/; https://dissemination-implementation.org/content/measures.aspx) (Dissemination & Implementation Models in Health Research & Practice, 2021; Washington, 2021). A repository of measures related to CFIR items was created by the Society for Implementation Research Collaboration (SIRC; https://societyforimplementationresearchcollaboration.org/what-is-sirc/). Other available CFIR measures include a measure of the Inner Setting Constructs (Fernandez et al., 2018) and another measure that includes subscales to measure several other constructs within the CFIR (Kegler et al., 2018).

There are several tools to assess organizational readiness. Weiner et al. published a review of measures for organizational readiness and, more recently, a chapter that describes differences in how organizational readiness has been described and measured (Weiner et al., 2008, 2020). One take-away was that much more research is needed to understand how best to measure readiness and use information about it to improve implementation. Nevertheless, there are some readiness assessment tools that have been used by practitioners to assess readiness for implementing an innovation that can provide information about what factors may need to be improved to maximize implementation outcomes. One widely used tool, developed to measure readiness for implementation in clinical settings, is the Organizational Readiness to Change Assessment (ORCA; https://www.nccmt.ca/knowledge-repositories/search/187; Helfrich et al., 2009). The survey consists of 77 items measuring: strength of the evidence for the proposed innovation or change; quality of the organizational context to support the change; and the capacity of the organization to facilitate the change.

The *RTT* (Wandersman Center, 2019) and the *RDS* (Scaccia et al., 2015) are designed to assess organizational readiness using the $R = MC^2$ framework described earlier (see Process 2), both using a 7-point Likert scale. The *RDS* is an online tool which can be completed in 20 to 25 minutes. After responding to the prompts, the planner receives a customized readiness report that they can use to better inform their course of action. The *RTT*, by contrast, can be completed in just 4 to 5 minutes. Unlike the *RDS*, however, this tool does not provide a report. Rather, the expectation is that the planning team will discuss the responses and brainstorm around how to use the information they reflect. The planner is prompted to rate their organization's readiness in three categories: *motivation*, *innovation-specific capacity*, and *general (organizational) capacity*. Questions touch-upon the organization's culture, internal relationships, climate, staff capacity, leadership, and other key metrics.

The Context Assessment for Community Health (COACH) tool is a tool for assessing context specifically designed for use in LMICs. The COACH tool is based on the context dimension of the Promoting Action of Research Implementation in Health Services (PARIHS) framework (Bergström et al., 2015; Kitson et al., 2008). COACH was developed and tested among 690 health workers in Bangladesh, Vietnam, Uganda, South Africa, and Nicaragua. This tool can be more appropriate in LMICs when characterizing the local healthcare context to identify implementation barriers and facilitators, and when tailoring implementation strategies.

Electronic health records and administrative data provide additional sources to measure contextual factors such as patient demographic and insurance mix in a health system or financial performance of an organization. Throughout the identification and collection of quantitative data on contextual factors, it is important to remember that these factors are often correlated and operate interdependently.

Using Checklists to Help Identify Barriers and Facilitators to Implementation

Case Study 5.1B showed how the CFIR can be used to guide context assessment. In the case study, this occurred after the implementation effort; however, it can be done prior to implementing change. In fact, it is often desirable to use checklists and templates multiple times before, during, and after implementation to get a real-time and actionable understanding of how barriers and facilitators influence implementation (Balasubramanian et al., 2017; Shaw et al., 2013).

The field of implementation science is relatively new and much more research is needed in developing new measures for a variety of constructs (such as planning and stakeholder engagement) and adapting existing measures to different populations and settings. Developing measures to assess contextual factors that could be influencing implementation is challenging partly because it can be difficult to translate concepts (or theoretical constructs) into everyday language. Most assessments based on CFIR have used qualitative methods for this reason. However, some quantitative measures of CFIR constructs do exist (CFIR Research Team-Center for Clinical Management Research, 2021; Fernandez et al., 2018). Damschroder and colleagues from the CFIR Research Team in Ann Arbor, Michigan developed *The Barrier Buster Tool* (BBT) as a practical measure to assess context (CFIR Research Team-Center for Clinical Management Research, 2021; Kirk et al., 2016). They conducted a study using a "Think Aloud" technique to develop a short, straightforward survey or checklist based on CFIR. The intent was to develop a tool that could be used by front-line teams in healthcare settings. To help identify the constructs that should be included in the BBT, they included those most frequently listed in published research based on a systematic review of use of the CFIR (Kirk et al., 2016).

The study found that prompts that were specific and referred to a particular implementation effort (rather than abstractly worded questions about general change) were much clearer and made it easier to identify specific barriers and facilitators that were relevant for a particular implementation effort. The resulting tool captures key factors believed to impact implementation efforts and was designed to help teams identify barriers and facilitators at various points throughout the implementation process. Designed to be used before implementation, the BBT can help teams anticipate potential barriers, thus helping them strategize how to overcome, lessen, or avoid them. Teams intending to use the tool may want to tailor it to their specific implementation effort.

CORE PROCESS 4: PRIORITIZING BARRIERS AND FACILITATORS TO BE ADDRESSED

Employing the three core processes we have discussed assists with identifying the many contextual factors that may influence implementation and characterizing them as barriers or facilitators of implementation. Depending on how many there are, organizing and prioritizing barriers and facilitators derived from various sources (theory, evidence, experience, stakeholder engagement) could prove challenging. In the following, we describe how tools from Implementation Mapping can help.

USING IMPLEMENTATION MAPPING TO PUT IT ALL TOGETHER

It can be challenging to sort through the available information about barriers and facilitators, prioritize the most important factors, and then connect the dots between what influences implementation and deciding what to do to improve it. While strategy selection and development is addressed in another chapter, here, we describe how **Implementation Mapping** (IM; Fernandez et al., 2019), a process to help practitioners plan implementation strategies, can also help in organizing and prioritizing information about barriers and facilitators to implementation. Tools within IM that are particularly helpful include a logic model to illustrate causal relationships (which and how various factors affect outcomes), and a table to organize information from various sources and help in prioritization.

Using IM logic models can help the practitioner visualize the expected causal factors influencing implementation success or failure. Logic models are graphic representations of the (hypothesized) causal relationships between determinants (e.g., barriers and facilitators of implementation) and outcomes, and are commonly used for planning and evaluation. They can be extremely useful for engaging stakeholders and teams in collaborative planning (Funnell & Rogers, 2011; Kellogg Foundation, 2004; National Institute of Allergy and Infectious Diseases, 2020). IM logic models show how the determinants of implementation behaviors and the implementation environment (context) influence implementation outcomes, and ultimately, health outcomes. When using these logic models to plan implementation strategies, they also show how the methods used in the implementation strategy are supposed to affect the barriers and facilitators of implementation (sometimes called *strategy mechanisms of action*).

In Figure 5.2, the logic of what influences implementation goes from left to right. Thinking about how to fill in the logic model, however, should go from right to left. First, determine what the expected health outcomes are and *who* must do *what* to implement the innovation such that those outcomes are achieved. Specifying the explicit implementation tasks (or actions) needed helps answer the next question of "*why*" (*why would this implementor do or not do that task?*) leading to the identification of various factors (barriers and facilitators) that can influence implementation. We also might ask: What contextual (external factors) may make implementation harder or easier? These contextual factors can be things that influence the implementation behaviors (skills to implement the innovation), or conditions of the implementation context (resources, culture). Practitioners can develop a logic model of the problem or a logic model of change that fits their implementation context. A logic model of the problem would focus on all barriers to implementation, while a logic model of change would focus on all factors that facilitate implementation. Another option is to include both barriers and facilitators in the same logic model and annotate them (e.g., with a plus or minus) to show whether they help or hinder implementation.

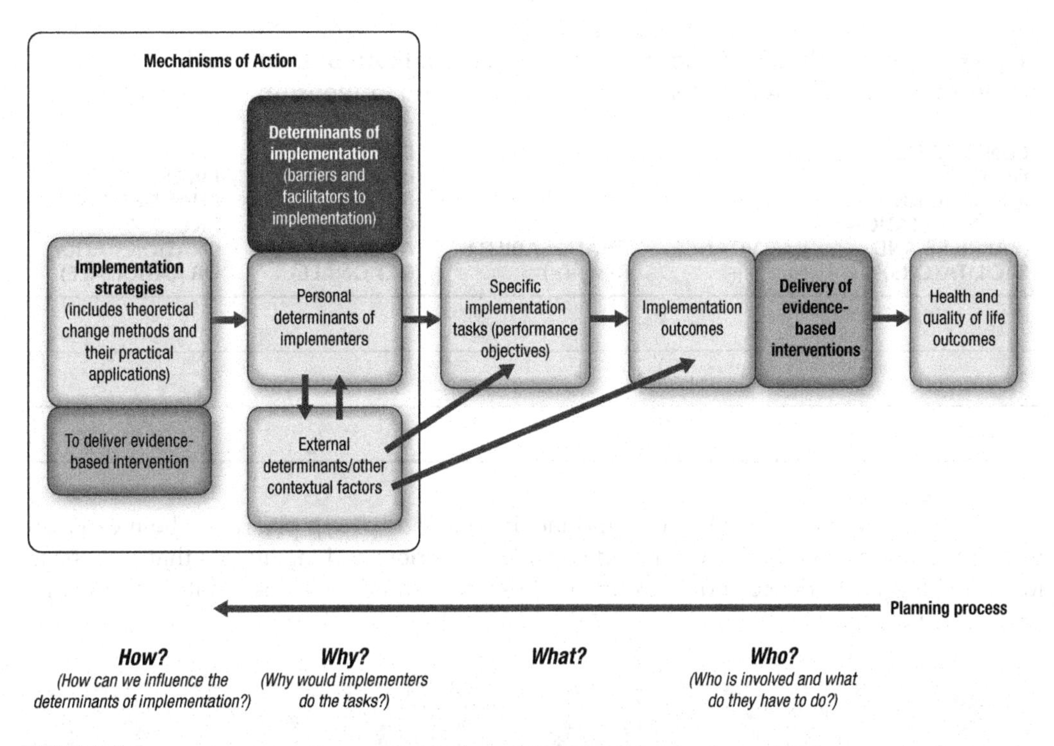

FIGURE 5.2 Implementation Mapping (IM) logic model for identifying barriers and facilitators to implementation
Source: Fernandez, M. E., Ten Hoor, G. A., van Lieshout, S., Rodriguez, S. A., Beidas, R. S., Parcel, G., Ruiter, R. A. C., Markham, C. M., & Kok, G. (2019). Implementation mapping: Using intervention mapping to develop implementation strategies. *Frontiers in Public Health, 7*, 158. https://doi.org/10.3389/fpubh.2019.00158

A PROCESS FOR PRIORITIZING CONTEXTUAL FACTORS

There are several frameworks that have been used for prioritization in healthcare and public health practice. One useful approach, originally developed by Green and Kreuter (1999, 2005, 2022) consists of an evaluation of each factor's importance and changeability. Judging **importance** means determining how likely it is that a particular factor is causally related to implementation. Is this factor (facilitator) necessary for implementation to occur? If this factor (barrier) is present, is there no way implementation will occur optimally? How closely is the factor aligned with or associated with implementation (was it present or absent during successful implementation efforts)? The other criterion that implementation teams may want to consider is **changeability**—the ease or difficulty of changing a factor. This criterion is particularly relevant if you are identifying barriers and facilitators that will be addressed through implementation strategies. Obviously, factors that are relatively easy to change and important are ones that should be prioritized. Additionally, those that may be harder to change but highly important (*implementation climate, leadership engagement*) should also become priorities. Some factors may be easy to change but not deemed particularly important because their presence may not (on their own) translate to optimal implementation (e.g., *knowledge* of an innovation). Nevertheless, these factors may still be considered a priority if they represent a necessary precursor for implementation to occur. Factors that are both less impactful and difficult to change should not be prioritized. We outline a simple table (Table 5.4) in the following that can be used to assess the importance and changeability of various contextual factors. Of course, stakeholders may choose other criteria to consider when prioritizing barriers and facilitators and if they do, they can be easily added to a table like this.

TABLE 5.4 Example of a Table to Organize the Summary of Evidence for Importance and Changeability of Contextual Factors Influencing Implementation

CONTEXTUAL FACTORS INFLUENCING IMPLEMENTATION (BARRIERS AND FACILITATORS)	IMPORTANCE (0, +, ++)	CHANGEABILITY (0, +, ++)	EVIDENCE FOR IMPORTANCE (INCLUDE CITATIONS AND/OR RATIONALE)	EVIDENCE FOR CHANGEABILITY (INCLUDE CITATIONS AND/ OR RATIONALE)

Using tables to organize barriers and facilitators and to help prioritize them can also be helpful. In Case Study 5.2, we include a table of barriers and facilitators that lists those identified from experience and literature, theories and frameworks, new data, and the prioritized list of factors.

CASE STUDY 5.2 EXPLORING BARRIERS AND FACILITATORS OF IMPLEMENTATION OF *SALUD EN MIS MANOS*, A BREAST AND CERVICAL CANCER SCREENING INTERVENTION FOR HISPANIC WOMEN

Despite ample evidence of effectiveness and clearly established guidelines for breast and cervical cancer screening and HPV vaccination, Latinas have disproportionately lower rates of these cancer control behaviors compared to non-Latina Whites. *Salud en Mis Manos* (SEMM) or *Health in My Hands*, is an evidence-based Lay Health Worker (LHW)-delivered screening and vaccination intervention. Adapted from the *Cultivando la Salud* program (Fernandez et al., 2009), the intervention components and delivery strategies are based on effective approaches recommended by the Guide to Community Preventive Services (Attipoe-Dorcoo et al., 2021; Sabatino et al., 2012). Although SEMM had solid evidence of effectiveness for increasing screening and has been implemented successfully in community settings in Texas, it has not been widely adopted or implemented by community health centers. The goal of the SEMM-Dissemination and Implementation Assistance (SEMM-DIA) program was to develop implementation strategies to increase implementation of SEMM in Federally Qualified Health Centers (FQHCs) to achieve broader impact. The team used the four core processes described in this chapter to identify barriers and facilitators to inform the development of strategies to accelerate and improve implementation and sustainment of the program in FQHCs.

The planning team was made up of a multidisciplinary group of researchers, program planners, and community partners. Engagement of community members and stakeholders was a critical part of both the development and adaptation of the program as well as planning its implementation. The team conducted brainstorming sessions focused on creating a broad list of potential contextual factors that could

(*continued*)

CASE STUDY 5.2 EXPLORING BARRIERS AND FACILITATORS OF IMPLEMENTATION OF *SALUD EN MIS MANOS*, A BREAST AND CERVICAL CANCER SCREENING INTERVENTION FOR HISPANIC WOMEN (*continued*)

influence the adoption and implementation of SEMM in clinic settings. During the original development of the SEMM program, there had already been substantial work done to understand factors associated with LHW delivery of the program and the implementation strategies focused on building capacity and motivation of front-line implementors (LHWs) was well developed (e.g., training, fidelity tracking). Therefore, although the team was open to making modifications to those implementation strategies, and certainly to consider new barriers or facilitators given the new implementation context (clinics versus communities), the focus of the brainstorming session was to identify clinic-level contextual factors that could influence adoption and implementation.

The brainstorming sessions generated a list of contextual factors by asking a series of questions to prompt the discussion that followed. Collaborators came to the table with experience working with community health centers, delivering LHW programs, and an understanding of barriers and facilitators to implementation of LHWs programs based on the literature. Discussions started by identifying who may be involved in decision-making related to adoption and implementation of SEMM followed by question prompts such as: *What do clinics need to do to implement SEMM? Who would have to do what? Why would the implementors carry out those tasks? Why wouldn't they?* and *What might make it easier or more challenging to implement SEMM in a community health center?*

Discussions also focused on recognizing the contextual factors in which SEMM would be implemented (e.g., what are some of the most common organizational barriers to implementing a program like SEMM in a community health center?). After brainstorming potential barriers and facilitators, the team made a list of potential answers.

A review of implementation science literature supported the provisional list of factors influencing implementation. The team determined that clinic leadership, the community health worker, and program champion as key program actors who will implement and maintain the SEMM program and the key determinants of implementation. Barriers and facilitators that emerged from the brainstorming sessions were entered into a table (see Table 5.5) and review of literature confirmed that these factors were consistent with ones that had been previously identified in similar implementation efforts. The team then considered constructs from prominent health behavior (Social Cognitive) and implementation science determinants frameworks (CFIR and organizational readiness) that could confirm that identified barriers and facilitators corresponded with constructs in the theories and frameworks. They also identified other constructs that may not have come up in the brainstorming but seemed relevant or had been previously identified as important in similar implementation efforts. These were entered into the second column of Table 5.5.

The planning team recognized a need to obtain first-hand, real-time understanding of implementation factors from members of the community clinics, particularly people who may be involved in the implementation effort. The team conducted

(*continued*)

CASE STUDY 5.2 EXPLORING BARRIERS AND FACILITATORS OF IMPLEMENTATION OF *SALUD EN MIS MANOS*, A BREAST AND CERVICAL CANCER SCREENING INTERVENTION FOR HISPANIC WOMEN *(continued)*

TABLE 5.5 Example Barriers and Facilitators to Implementation of SEMM in Community Health Centers

BRAINSTORMED POTENTIAL BARRIERS AND FACILITATORS (BASED ON EXPERIENCE, PAST NEEDS ASSESSMENTS, AND PUBLISHED LITERATURE)	ADDITIONS OR CONFIRMATION FROM THEORIES, MODELS, AND FRAMEWORKS	FINDINGS FROM NEW DATA (IN-DEPTH INTERVIEWS, SURVEYS)	PRIORITIZED LIST
<u>Barriers:</u> ■ Lack of adequate resources for implementing SEMM and ongoing operations ■ No existing lay health workers ■ Competing priorities (COVID-19) ■ Leadership may not support (and articulate) implementing SEMM ■ Lack of skills and confidence in planning and implementing SEMM	■ Relative advantage ■ Priority ■ Trialability/ability to pilot ■ Program champion ■ Comparability ■ Complexity ■ Staff capacity ■ Specific implementation climate support ■ Commitment ■ Goals and Feedback	■ CHWs are able to wear multiple hats ■ Program champion is critical to the success of the innovation ■ Broad reach of SEMM is important to reach more patients ■ Concerns with needing to further expand CHWs role for program implementation	■ Program champion and CHWs are instrumental for implementation ■ Specific implementation climate support—*for example, staff and leadership supports implementation of SEMM* ■ Facilitating beliefs: ■ SEMM is in sync with organizational values and norms ■ SEMM is an easy-to-implement program (simplicity vs. complexity) ■ SEMM has unique benefits that make it relevant compared to other programs (relative advantage) ■ Priority—for example, implementing SEMM is a priority
<u>Facilitators:</u> ■ Perception that: ■ SEMM is easy to use ■ Implementing SEMM will help achieve quality	■ Learning climate ■ Intra-organizational relationships	■ Collaboration with other organizations, agencies and partners important	■ Trialability/ability to pilot—for example, SEMM has been implemented in similar clinic settings with minimum support and risk

CASE STUDY 5.2 EXPLORING BARRIERS AND FACILITATORS OF IMPLEMENTATION OF *SALUD EN MIS MANOS*, A BREAST AND CERVICAL CANCER SCREENING INTERVENTION FOR HISPANIC WOMEN (*continued*)

TABLE 5.5 Example Barriers and Facilitators to Implementation of SEMM in Community Health Centers (*continued*)

BRAINSTORMED POTENTIAL BARRIERS AND FACILITATORS (BASED ON EXPERIENCE, PAST NEEDS ASSESSMENTS, AND PUBLISHED LITERATURE)	ADDITIONS OR CONFIRMATION FROM THEORIES, MODELS, AND FRAMEWORKS	FINDINGS FROM NEW DATA (IN-DEPTH INTERVIEWS, SURVEYS)	PRIORITIZED LIST
measures for cancer screening and HPV vaccination ▪ SEMM fits well with organizational priorities ▪ SEMM meets the organizational values and norms ▪ Leadership buy-in is critical for the success of SEMM ▪ SEMM can be adapted, tailored, refined to meet specific clinic and community needs ▪ Expectations (*e.g., SEMM will increase screening rates/reduce cancer related mortality; SEMM serves community needs*)	▪ Design quality and package ▪ Networks and communications ▪ Tension for change ▪ External change agents ▪ Reflecting and evaluating ▪ Technical assistance ▪ Planning and executing	for promotion of BCS, CCS, and HPV vaccination services. ▪ Concerns about data protection (e.g., who will be responsible for upkeep of data) and will it flow directly to clinic's EHR system ▪ Concerns about risk management ▪ Implementing SEMM can lessen clinic staff workload and save time ▪ Developing communication strategies facilitates program promotion and implementation among clinic staff ▪ Past experience with successfully implementing similar programs	▪ Staff capacity—for example, staff and CHWs have the knowledge, skills and time to implement SEMM ▪ Outreach coordinator skills and confidence in planning and implementing SEMM ▪ Ability to pilot (trialability)

BCS, breast cancer screening; CCS, cervical cancer screening; CHW, community health worker; EHR, electronic health records; HPV, human papillomavirus; SEMM, Salud en Mis Manos.

(*continued*)

CASE STUDY 5.2 EXPLORING BARRIERS AND FACILITATORS OF IMPLEMENTATION OF *SALUD EN MIS MANOS*, A BREAST AND CERVICAL CANCER SCREENING INTERVENTION FOR HISPANIC WOMEN (*continued*)

listening sessions with members of the Community Advisory Board (CAB) with years of community engagement experience and knowledge of community clinic structures also helped to confirm and validate the factors. Next the team conducted in-depth interviews and surveys with medical directors, CHWs and clinic program managers, clinic outreach coordinators in the clinics. They used a measure to assess CFIR inner setting constructs (Fernandez et al., 2018) and structured the in-depth interviews to explore whether certain constructs that had come up in the brainstorming session and additional ones from CFIR, Social Cognitive Theory, organizational readiness) were relevant. These findings from the new data collection activities were analyzed using mixed methods approaches, compared with listing of potential barriers and facilitators in the other two columns (Table 5.5) and prioritized based on an assessment of importance and changeability. The team decided to enter the prioritized list of contextual factors framed positively—that is, that even when a barrier was identified (e.g., clinic leadership did not believe that SEMM implementation was a high priority), it would be stated in terms of the change that needed to happen to improve implementation outcomes (as done in IM step 2).

Using the four core processes described in this chapter to ensure that barriers and facilitators were identified using engagement, theories and frameworks were engaged, and new data were collected gave the team confidence that they had considered the range of factors that could influence implementation. Carrying out the prioritization process helped them determine which of these were most important (related to implementation) and changeable (could be modified through implementation strategies). Recognizing that some of the contextual factors identified could not readily be changed, the team decided to measure these during the implementation effort to see how those factors may have modified the impact of implementation strategies on both implementation and effectiveness outcomes.

SUMMARY

The field of implementation science offers guidance to practitioners for considering contextual factors influencing implementation that can augment their own valuable knowledge and experience. This chapter has described the importance of understanding potential barriers and facilitators of implementation and a process for identifying them through the application of practical implementation science approaches. Although implementation science theories and frameworks can be complex, understanding their basic components (constructs), definitions, and why or how they can inform implementation practice can ensure that implementation efforts address or at least are aware of the many factors that can influence implementation success or failure.

There is no one correct way to identify, document, and understand all potential factors that influence implementation in each setting. However, using a combination of experience, published evidence, stakeholder engagement, theories and frameworks, and new data can help generate a robust list of barriers and facilitators that are likely to influence implementation in a specific context. Critically evaluating the resulting list and using a prioritization process to focus efforts will help ensure that the factors targeted are the most impactful. Ultimately, to go beyond simply understanding what happened or predicting what might happen, knowledge of the contextual factors present must be used to inform implementation strategies to achieve optimal implementation outcomes. This will result in better implementation and sustainment of new practices, policies, interventions, or other innovations that improve well-being.

KEY POINTS FOR PRACTICE

1. Implementation science frameworks can help guide both researchers and practitioners in the systematic assessment of context. By systematic, we mean that a well-developed framework can help you step through the broad range of barriers or facilitators that have potential to negatively or positively influence your ability to achieve your implementation goals. Without this assessment, you may be "going in blind" and then hit unexpected challenges that can lead to failure. With this assessment, you'll be in a much stronger position for success.
2. Practitioners should look at the constructs under one or more determinant frameworks prior to brainstorming about potential barriers and facilitators. For example, using the CFIR, they can ask themselves (and other stakeholders) about all of the possible barriers and facilitators across the domains.
3. After listing all possible contextual factors, engage key stakeholders and partners in helping prioritize and identify the most important contextual factors that could either facilitate or hinder implementation.
4. Using both quantitative (survey) and qualitative (interviews) data and integrating information gleaned from both sources can provide both breadth (across a team or organization) and depth of understanding of contextual factors related to implementation.
5. Following the core processes described in the chapter using theory, experience, community input, and new data can provide a greater awareness of all factors influencing implementation (even if they are not all addressed with the implementation strategy).
6. Using logic models can help illustrate how various factors influence implementation and health outcomes.

COMMON PITFALLS IN PRACTICE

1. Many people are not sure how to choose among the many available frameworks to help guide assessment of context. Don't let yourself get paralyzed by the wide range of choices. We have described a few examples in this chapter. Read about these frameworks and visit any associated technical support websites to learn a bit more about the ones that interest you the most. Then talk with your mentors and peers about their experiences and recommendations. Then you can decide based on the framework or frameworks (you can use more than one) that gives you the most clarity about how to proceed. There is no one "right" framework; you can feel good about your choice if it makes sense and is valuable in helping you navigate the work of identifying barriers and facilitators.
2. When considering context, implementers often think of just organizational factors (size, location, accreditation status, etc.) but often miss individual and team factors (such as leadership, readiness to change, skills, self-efficacy, and trust).
3. Failure to prioritize the most salient barriers and facilitators that will be targeted with the implementation strategies is a common pitfall. Considering importance and changeability can help prioritize factors.

DISCUSSION QUESTIONS

1. Which framework would you choose and why? Consider using the T-CaST tool to help you think about usability, testability, applicability, and acceptability of your chosen framework.
2. Based on your chosen framework, which constructs do you think might be most important to assess based on your past experiences or based on a project you are planning? Why?
3. How would you determine which factors are changeable (and thus could be a target of the implementation strategy) versus other factors that may be important to measure because they could impact implementation outcomes?
4. Why does it make sense to use both qualitative and quantitative methods to assess contextual factors?
5. How does prioritizing contextual factors help with implementation?

REFERENCES

Attipoe-Dorcoo, S., Chattopadhyay, S. K., Verughese, J., Ekwueme, D. U., Sabatino, S. A., & Peng, Y. (2021). Engaging community health workers to increase cancer screening: A community guide systematic economic review. *American Journal of Preventive Medicine*, *60*, e189–e197. https://doi.org/10.1016/j.amepre.2020.08.011

Balasubramanian, B. A., Heurtin-Roberts, S., Krasny, S., Rohweder, C. L., Fair, K., Olmos-Ochoa, T. T., Stange, K.C., Gorin, S.S., & MOHR Study Group. (2017). Factors related to implementation and reach of a pragmatic multisite trial: The my own health report (MOHR) study. *The Journal of the American Board of Family Medicine*, *30*, 337–349. https://doi.org/10.3122/jabfm.2017.03.160151

Bamuya, C., Correia, J. C., Brady, E. M., Beran, D., Harrington, D., Damasceno, A., Crampin, A.M., Magaia, A., Levitt, N., Davies, M. J., & Hadjiconstantinou, M. (2021). Use of the socio-ecological model to explore factors that influence the implementation of a diabetes structured education programme (EXTEND project) in Lilongwe, Malawi and Maputo, Mozambique: A qualitative study. *BMC Public Health*, *21*, 1355. https://doi.org/10.1186/s12889-021-11338-y

Bartholomew-Eldredge, L. K, Markham, C., Ruiter, R. A., Fernandez, M. E., Kok, G., & Parcel, G. (2016). *Planning health promotion programs: An intervention mapping approach* (4th ed.). Jossey Bass.

Bergström, A., Skeen, S., Duc, D. M., Blandon, E. Z., Estabrooks, C. A., Gustavsson, P., Hoa, D. T. P., Källestål, C., Målqvist, M., Nga, N. T., Persson, L.-Å., Pervin, J., Peterson, S., Rahman, A., Selling, K., Squires, J. E., Tomlinson, M., Waiswa, P., & Wallin, L. (2015). Health system context and implementation of evidence-based practices—Development and validation of the context assessment for community health (COACH) tool for low- and middle-income settings. *Implementation Science*, *10*, 120. https://doi.org/10.1186/s13012-015-0305-2

Birken, S. A., Bunger, A. C., Powell, B. J., Turner, K., Clary, A. S., Klaman, S. L., Yu, Y., Whitaker, D. J. Self, S. R., Rostad, W. L. Shanley Chatham, J. R., Kirk, M. A., Shea, C. M., Haines, E., & Weiner, B. J. (2017). Organizational theory for dissemination and implementation research. *Implementation Science*, *12*, 62. https://doi.org/10.1186/s13012-017-0592-x

Birken, S. A., Rohweder, C. L., Powell, B. J., Shea, C. M., Scott, J., Leeman, J., Grewe, M. E., Alexis Kirk, M., Damschroder, L., Aldridge II, W. A., Haines, E. R., Straus, S., & Presseau, J. (2018). T-CaST: An implementation theory comparison and selection tool. *Implementation Science*, *13*, 143. https://doi.org/10.1186/s13012-018-0836-4

Blachman-Demner, D. R., Wiley, T. R. A., & Chambers, D. A. (2017). Fostering integrated approaches to dissemination and implementation and community engaged research. *Translational Behavioral Medicine*, *7*, 543–546. https://doi.org/10.1007/s13142-017-0527-8

Bronfenbrenner, U. (2009). *The ecology of human development: Experiments by nature and design*. Harvard University Press.

Brownson, R. C., Kumanyika, S. K., Kreuter, M. W., & Haire-Joshu, D. (2021). Implementation science should give higher priority to health equity. *Implementation Science*, *16*, 28. https://doi.org/10.1186/s13012-021-01097-0

Butler, M., Epstein, R. A., Totten, A., Whitlock, E. P., Ansari, M. T., Damschroder, L. J., Balk, E., Bass, E. B., Berkman, N. D., Hempel, S., Iyer, S., Schoelles, K., & Guise, J.-M. (2017). AHRQ series on complex intervention systematic reviews – paper 3: Adapting frameworks to develop protocols. *Journal of Clinical Epidemiology*, *90*, 19–27. https://doi.org/10.1016/j.jclinepi.2017.06.011

Buunk, A. P., & Van Vugt, M. (2013). *Applying social psychology: From problems to solutions* (2nd ed.). Sage.

CFIR Research Team-Center for Clinical Management Research. (2021). *Consolidated framework for implementation research—Quantitative data*. [cited 2021 May 30]. https://cfirguide.org/evaluation-design/quantitative-data/

Dale, J., Caramlau, I. O., Lindenmeyer, A., & Williams, S. M. (2008). Peer support telephone calls for improving health. *Cochrane Database Systematic Reviews, 2008*, Cd006903. https://doi.org/10.1002/14651858.CD006903.pub2

Damschroder, L. J., Aron, D. C., Keith, R. E., Kirsh, S. R., Alexander, J. A., & Lowery, J. C. (2009). Fostering implementation of health services research findings into practice: A consolidated framework for advancing implementation science. *Implementation Science, 4*, 50. https://doi.org/10.1186/1748-5908-4-50

Damschroder, L. J., Reardon, C. M., AuYoung, M., Moin, T., Datta, S. K., Sparks, J. B., Maciejewski, M. L., Steinle, N. I., Weinreb, J. E., Hughes, M., Pinault, L. F., Xiang, X. M., Billington, C., & Richardson, C. R. (2017). Implementation findings from a hybrid III implementation-effectiveness trial of the Diabetes Prevention Program (DPP) in the Veterans Health Administration (VHA). *Implementation Science, 12*, 94. https://doi.org/10.1186/s13012-017-0619-3

Damschroder, L. J., Reardon, C. M., Sperber, N., Robinson, C. H., Fickel, J. J., & Oddone, E. Z. (2016). Implementation evaluation of the Telephone Lifestyle Coaching (TLC) program: Organizational factors associated with successful implementation. *Translational Behavioral Medicine, 7*, 233–241. https://doi.org/10.1007/s13142-016-0424-6

Desveaux, L., Ivers, N. M., Devotta, K., Ramji, N., Weyman, K., & Kiran, T. (2021). Unpacking the intention to action gap: A qualitative study understanding how physicians engage with audit and feedback. *Implementation Science, 16*, 19. https://doi.org/10.1186/s13012-021-01088-1

Dissemination & Implementation Models in Health Research & Practice. (2021). *Measure constructs*. [cited 2021 Oct 16]. https://dissemination-implementation.org/content/measures.aspx.

Domlyn, A. M., Scott, V., Livet, M., Lamont, A., Watson, A., Kenworthy, T., Talford, M., Yannayon, M., & Wandersman, A. (2021). R = MC(2) readiness building process: A practical approach to support implementation in local, state, and national settings. *Journal of Community Psychology, 49*, 1228–1248. https://doi.org/10.1002/jcop.22531

Domlyn, A. M., & Wandersman, A. (2019). Community coalition readiness for implementing something new: Using a Delphi methodology. *Journal of Community Psychology, 47*, 882–897. https://doi.org/10.1002/jcop.22161

Donnelly, J. E., Goetz, J., Gibson, C., Sullivan, D. K., Lee, R., Smith, B. K., Lambourne, K., Mayo, M. S., Hunt, S., Lee, J. H., Honas, J. J., & Washburn, R. A. (2013). Equivalent weight loss for weight management programs delivered by phone and clinic. *Obesity, 21*, 1951–1959. https://doi.org/10.1002/oby.20334

Drzensky, F., Egold, N., & van Dick, R. (2012). Ready for a change? A longitudinal study of antecedents, consequences and contingencies of readiness for change. *Journal of Change Management, 12*, 95–111. https://doi.org/10.1080/14697017.2011.652377

English, M. (2013). Designing a theory-informed, contextually appropriate intervention strategy to improve delivery of paediatric services in Kenyan hospitals. *Implementation Science, 8*, 39. https://doi.org/10.1186/1748-5908-8-39

Ezezika, O., Gong, J., Abdirahman, H., & Sellen, D. (2021). Barriers and facilitators to the implementation of large-scale nutrition interventions in Africa: A scoping review. *Global Implementation Research and Applications, 1*, 38–52. https://doi.org/10.1007/s43477-021-00007-2

Fernandez, M. E., Gonzales, A., Tortolero-Luna, G., Williams, J., Saavedra-Embesi, M., Chan, W., & Vernon, S. W. (2009). Effectiveness of Cultivando la Salud: A breast and cervical cancer screening promotion program for low-income Hispanic women. *American Journal of Public Health, 99*, 936–943. https://doi.org/10.2105/AJPH.2008.136713

Fernandez, M. E., Ten Hoor, G. A., van Lieshout, S., Rodriguez, S. A., Beidas, R. S., Parcel, G., Ruiter, R. A. C., Markham, C. M., & Kok, G. (2019). Implementation mapping: Using intervention mapping to develop implementation strategies. *Frontiers in Public Health, 7*, 158. https://doi.org/10.3389/fpubh.2019.00158

Fernandez, M. E., Walker, T. J., Weiner, B. J., Calo, W. A., Liang, S., Risendal, B., Friedman, D. B., Tu, S. P., Williams, R. S., Jacobs, S., Herrmann, A. K., & Kegler, M. C. (2018). Developing measures to assess constructs from the inner setting domain of the consolidated framework for implementation research. *Implementation Science, 13*, 52. https://doi.org/10.1186/s13012-018-0736-7

Foster, T. C., Johnson, J. K., Nelson, E. C., & Batalden, P. B. (2007). Using a Malcolm Baldrige framework to understand high-performing clinical microsystems. *Quality & Safety in Health Care, 16*, 334–341. https://doi.org/10.1136/qshc.2006.020685

Funnell, S., & Rogers, P. (2011). *Purposeful program theory: Effective use of theories of change and logic models*. Jossey-Bass.

Gagliardi, A. R., Webster, F., Brouwers, M. C., Baxter, N. N., Finelli, A., & Gallinger, S. (2014). How does context influence collaborative decision-making for health services planning, delivery and evaluation? *BMC Health Services Research, 14*, 545. https://doi.org/10.1186/s12913-014-0545-x

Glandon, D., Paina, L., Alonge, O., Peters, D. H., & Bennett, S. (2017). 10 Best resources for community engagement in implementation research. *Health Policy and Planning, 32*, 1457–1465. https://doi.org/10.1093/heapol/czx123

Gold, D. B., Anderson, D. R., & Serxner, S. A. (2000). Impact of a telephone-based intervention on the reduction of health risks. *American Journal of Health Promotion, 15*, 97–106. https://doi.org/10.4278/0890-1171-15.2.97

Green, L. W., Gielen, A. C., Peterson, D. V., Kreuter, M. W., & Ottoson, J. M., (Eds.) (2022). *Health program planning, implementation, and evaluation: Creating behavioral, environmental, and policy change*. Johns Hopkins University Press.

Green, L. W., & Kreuter, M. W. (Eds.). (1999). *Health promotion planning: An educational and ecological approach* (3rd ed.). Mayfield Publishing Company.

Green, L.W., & Kreuter, M.W. (Eds.). (2005). *Health promotion planning: An educational and ecological approach* (3rd ed., 621 pp). Mayfield Publishing Company.

Gyamfi, J., Allegrante, J. P., Iwelunmor, J., Williams, O., Plange-Rhule, J., Blackstone, S., Ntim, M., Apusiga, K., Peprah, E., & Ogedegbe, G. (2020). Application of the consolidated framework for implementation research to examine nurses' perception of the task shifting strategy for hypertension control trial in Ghana. *BMC Health Services Research, 20*, 65. https://doi.org/10.1186/s12913-020-4912-5

Harvey, G., & Kitson, A. (2016). PARIHS revisited: From heuristic to integrated framework for the successful implementation of knowledge into practice. *Implementation Science, 11*, 33. https://doi.org/10.1186/s13012-016-0398-2

Helfrich, C. D., Li, Y. F., Sharp, N. D., & Sales, A. E. (2009). Organizational readiness to change assessment (ORCA): Development of an instrument based on the promoting action on research in health services (PARIHS) framework. *Implementation Science, 4*, 38. https://doi.org/10.1186/1748-5908-4-38

Holt, D. T., & Vardaman, J. M. (2013). Toward a comprehensive understanding of readiness for change: The case for an expanded conceptualization. *Journal of Change Management, 13*, 9–18. ttps://doi.org/10.1080/14697017.2013.768426

Jones, D. L., Rodriguez, V. J., Butts, S. A., Arheart, K., Zulu, R., Chitalu, N., & Weiss, S. M. (2018). Increasing acceptability and uptake of voluntary male medical circumcision in Zambia: Implementing and disseminating an evidence-based intervention. *Translational Behavioural Medicine, 8*, 907–916. https://doi.org/10.1093/tbm/iby078

Kegler, M. C., Liang, S., Weiner, B. J., Tu, S. P., Friedman, D. B., Glenn, B. A., Herrmann, A. K., Risendal, B., & Fernandez, M. E. (2018). Measuring constructs of the consolidated framework for implementation research in the context of increasing colorectal cancer screening in federally qualified health center. *Health Services Research, 53*, 4178–4203. https://doi.org/10.1111/1475-6773.13035

Kellogg Foundation. (2004). *Using logic models to bring together planning, evaluation, and action—Logic model development guide*. Battle Creek, Michigan.

Kilbourne, A. M., Switzer, G., Hyman, K., Crowley-Matoka, M., & Fine, M. J. (2006). Advancing health disparities research within the health care system: A conceptual framework. *American Journal of Public Health, 96*, 2113–2121. https://doi.org/10.2105/AJPH.2005.077628

King, D. K., Shoup, J. A., Raebel, M. A., Anderson, C. B., Wagner, N. M., Ritzwoller, D. P., & Bender, B. G. (2020). Planning for implementation success using RE-AIM and CFIR frameworks: A qualitative study. *Frontiers in Public Health, 8*, 59. https://doi.org/10.3389/fpubh.2020.00059

Kirk, M. A., Kelley, C., Yankey, N., Birken, S. A., Abadie, B., & Damschroder, L. (2016). A systematic review of the use of the consolidated framework for implementation research. *Implementation Science, 11*, 72. https://doi.org/10.1186/s13012-016-0437-z

Kitson, A. L., Rycroft-Malone, J., Harvey, G., McCormack, B., Seers, K., & Titchen, A. (2008). Evaluating the successful implementation of evidence into practice using the PARiHS framework: Theoretical and practical challenges. *Implementation Science, 3*, 1. https://doi.org/10.1186/1748-5908-3-1

Komalasari, R., Wilson, S., & Haw, S. (2021). A social ecological model (SEM) to exploring barriers of and facilitators to the implementation of Opioid Agonist Treatment (OAT) programmes in prisons. *International Journal of Prisoner Health*, ahead-of-print. http://hdl.handle.net/1893/32314

May, C., Mair, F., Finch, T., MacFarlane, A., Dowrick, C., Treweek, S., Rapley, T., Ballini, L., Ong, B. N., Rogers, A., Murray, E., Elwyn, G., Légaré, F., Gunn, J., & Montori, V. M. (2009). Development of a theory of implementation and integration: Normalization process theory. *Implementation Science, 4*, 29. https://doi.org/10.1186/1748-5908-4-29

May, C., Murray E., Finch T., Mair, F., Treweek S., Ballini, L., Macfarlane A., Girling, M., & Rapley, T. (2015). *Normalization process theory–NPT Toolkit*. http://www.normalizationprocess.org/npt-toolkit/

McDonald, K. M. (2013). Considering context in quality improvement interventions and implementation: Concepts, frameworks, and application. *Academic Pediatrics, 13*, S45–S53. https://doi.org/10.1016/j.acap.2013.04.013.

McKay, J. R., Lynch, K. G., Shepard, D. S., & Pettinati, H. M. (2005). The effectiveness of telephone-based continuing care for alcohol and cocaine dependence: 24-month outcomes. *Archives of General Psychiatry, 62*, 199–207. https://doi.org/10.1001/archpsyc.62.2.199

McLeroy, K. R., Bibeau, D., Steckler, A., & Glanz, K. (1988). An ecological perspective on health promotion programs. *Health Education Quarterly, 15*, 351–377. https://doi.org/10.1177/109019818801500401

Means, A. R., Kemp, C. G., Gwayi-Chore, M.-C., Gimbel, S., Soi, C., Sherr, K., Wagenaar, B. H., Wasserheit, J. N., & Weiner, B. J. (2020). Evaluating and optimizing the consolidated framework for implementation research (CFIR) for use in low- and middle-income countries: A systematic review. *Implementation Science, 15*, 17. https://doi.org/10.1186/s13012-020-0977-0

National Institute of Allergy and Infectious Diseases. (2020). *CFAR/ARC ending the HIV epidemic supplement awards*. Author.

Nilsen, P. (2015). Making sense of implementation theories, models and frameworks. *Implementation Science, 10*, 53. https://doi.org/10.1186/s13012-015-0242-0

Norris, J. M., White, D. E., Nowell, L., Mrklas, K., & Stelfox, H. T. (2017). How do stakeholders from multiple hierarchical levels of a large provincial health system define engagement? A qualitative study. *Implementation Science, 12*, 98. https://doi.org/10.1186/s13012-017-0625-5

O'Reilly, P., Lee, S. H., O'Sullivan, M., Cullen, W., Kennedy, C., & MacFarlane, A. (2017). Assessing the facilitators and barriers of interdisciplinary team working in primary care using normalisation process theory: An integrative review. *PLoS One, 12*, e0177026. https://doi.org/10.1371/journal.pone.0177026

Perri, M. G., Limacher, M. C., Durning, P. E., Janicke, D. M., Lutes, L. D., Bobroff, L. B., Dale, M. S., Daniels, M. J., Radcliff, T. A., & Martin, A. D. (2008). Extended-care programs for weight management in rural communities: The treatment of obesity in underserved rural settings (TOURS) randomized trial. *Archives of Internal Medicine, 168*, 2347–2354. https://doi.org/10.1001/archinte.168.21.2347

Pinto, R. M., Park, S., Miles, R., & Ong, P. N. (2021). Community engagement in dissemination and implementation models: A narrative review. *Implementation Research and Practice, 2*. https://doi.org/10.1177/2633489520985305

Plsek, P. E., & Wilson, T. (2001). Complexity, leadership, and management in healthcare organisations. *BMJ, 323*, 746–749. https://doi.org/10.1136/bmj.323.7315.746

Porter, M. E. (2010). What is value in health care? *The New England Journal of Medicine, 363*, 2477–2481. https://doi.org/10.1056/nejmp1011024

Ramaswamy, R., Shidhaye, R., & Nanda, S. (2018). Making complex interventions work in low resource settings: Developing and applying a design focused implementation approach to deliver mental health through primary care in India. *International Journal of Mental Health Systems, 12*, 5. https://doi.org/10.1186/s13033-018-0181-7

Rimer, B. K., & Glanz, K. (Eds.). (2005). *Theory at a glance: A guide for health promotion practice* (2nd ed.). National Institutes of Health.

Rogers, L., De Brún, A., & McAuliffe, E. (2020). Defining and assessing context in healthcare implementation studies: A systematic review. *BMC Health Services Research, 20*, 591. https://doi.org/10.1186/s12913-020-05212-7

Ruiter, R. A. C., & Crutzen, R. (2020). Core processes: How to use evidence, theories, and research in planning behavior change interventions. *Frontiers in Public Health, 8*, 247. https://doi.org/10.3389/fpubh.2020.00247

Ruiter, R., Massar, K., Vugt, M., & Kok, G. (2013). Applying social psychology to understanding social problems. In A. Golec & A. Cichoka (Eds.), *Social Psychology of Social Problems - The intergroup context*. Palgrave MacMillan.

Sabatino, S. A., Lawrence, B., Elder, R., Mercer, S. L., Wilson, K. M., Devinney, B., Melillo, S., Carvalho, M., Taplin, S., Bastani, R., Rimer, B. K., Vernon, S. W., Melvin, C. L., Taylor, V., Fernandez, M., Glanz, K., & Community Preventive Services Task Force. (2012). Effectiveness of interventions to increase screening for breast, cervical, and colorectal cancers: Nine updated systematic reviews for the guide to community preventive services. *American Journal of Preventive Medicine, 43*, 97–118. https://doi.org/10.1016/j.amepre.2012.04.009

Scaccia, J. P., Cook, B. S., Lamont, A., Wandersman, A., Castellow, J., Katz, J., & Beidas, R. S. (2015). A practical implementation science heuristic for organizational readiness: $R = MC^2$. *Journal of Community Psychology, 43*, 484–501. https://doi.org/10.1002/jcop.21698

Shaw, E. K., Ohman-Strickland, P. A., Piasecki, A., Hudson, S. V., Ferrante, J. M., McDaniel, R. R., Nutting, P. A., & Crabtree, B. F (2013). Effects of facilitated team meetings and learning collaboratives on colorectal cancer screening rates in primary care practices: A cluster randomized trial. *The Annals of Family Medicine, 11*, 220–228. https://doi.org/10.1370/afm.1505

Stange, K. C., & Glasgow, R. E. (2013). *Considering and reporting important contextual factors in research on the patient-centered medical home*. Agency for Healthcare Research and Quality. Publ. No. 13-0045-WF.

Stead, L. F., Hartmann-Boyce, J., Perera, R., & Lancaster, T. (2013). Telephone counselling for smoking cessation. *Cochrane Database of Systematic Reviews*. https://doi.org/10.1002/14651858.CD002850.pub4

U.S. Preventive Services Task Force. (2003). Behavioral counseling in primary care to promote a healthy diet: Recommendations and rationale. *American Journal of Preventive Medicine, 24*, 93–100. https://doi.org/10.1016/s0749-3797(02)00581-0

Wandersman, A., & Scaccia, J. P. (2017). *Organizational readiness: Measurement and as a predictor of progress: Final report*. Robert Wood Johnson Foundation.

Wandersman Center. (2019). *Prevention readiness building guide©*. Author.

Washington, Uo. (2021). The state of measurement in implementation science. [cited 2021 Oct 16]. https://impsciuw.org/implementation-science/research/measures/.

Weiner, B. J., Amick, H., & Lee, S. Y. (2008). Conceptualization and measurement of organizational readiness for change: A review of the literature in health services research and other fields. *Medical Care Research and Review, 65*, 379–436. https://doi.org/10.1177/1077558708317802

Weiner, B. J., Lewis, M. A., & Linnan, L. A. (2009). Using organization theory to understand the determinants of effective implementation of worksite health promotion programs. *Health Education Research: Theory and Practice, 24*, 292–305. https://doi.org/10.1093/her/cyn019

Weiner, B. J., Mettert, K. D., Dorsey, C. N., Nolen, E. A., Stanick, C., Powell, B. J., & Lewis, C. C. (2020). Measuring readiness for implementation: A systematic review of measures' psychometric and pragmatic properties. *Implementation Research and Practice, 1*. https://doi.org/10.1177/2633489520933896

Wold, B., & Mittelmark, M. B. (2018). Health-promotion research over three decades: The social-ecological model and challenges in implementation of interventions. *Scandinavian Journal of Public Health, 46*, 20–26. https://doi.org/10.1177/1403494817743893.

Woodward, E. N., Matthieu, M. M., Uchendu, U. S., Rogal, S., & Kirchner, J. E. (2019). The health equity implementation framework: Proposal and preliminary study of hepatitis C virus treatment. *Implementation Science, 14*, 26. https://doi.org/10.1186/s13012-019-0861-y

6

Engaging Stakeholders

Melanie Pellecchia, Kimberly T. Arnold,
Liza Tomczuk, and Rinad S. Beidas

Learning Objectives

By the end of this chapter, readers will be able to:

- Define implementation stakeholders and stakeholder engagement
- Describe types of stakeholders and types of engagement
- Identify stakeholders and conduct a stakeholder analysis
- Identify potential challenges in engaging stakeholders
- Select one or more stakeholder engagement strategies relevant to your implementation initiative
- Describe how and when to meaningfully engage stakeholders

CASE STUDY 6.1A IMPLEMENTING A PARENT-MEDIATED INTERVENTION FOR YOUNG CHILDREN WITH AUTISM

Big City Early Intervention (EI) System provides publicly funded early intervention services for infants and toddlers from birth to 3 years of age with developmental delays or other disabilities who live in Big City, USA. Like many other large mental health and early intervention service systems, Big City EI is made up of many independent agencies that provide services to children throughout the city. Many of the clinicians working in the Big City EI System operate independently, each with their own approach to working with young children with autism spectrum disorder (ASD) and their families. Cassandra D., Director of Strategic Planning for the EI System, believes many of the clinicians are "stuck" in outdated approaches to intervention and may be resistant to change. Cassandra wants to improve the use of evidence-based interventions for young children with ASD throughout the system, but she wants to learn more about current research on best practices in intervention for this population. Cassandra has read about the effectiveness of parent-mediated interventions, but there are several manualized parent-mediated interventions for this population, and she is not sure which would be the best fit for the Big City EI System. Of critical importance to Cassandra and the leadership team in Big City EI is that the intervention selected is feasible for implementation within a large urban service system serving mostly under-resourced families and aligned with the system's priorities for engaging and supporting caregivers of young children with disabilities.

INTRODUCTION

Systems change and implementation of evidence-based interventions (EBI) affects many individuals and groups. In Case Study 6.1A the implementation process affects administrators, like Cassandra, who lead the system, along with agency leaders who oversee provision of services, clinicians who deliver services to children and families, and the families who receive these services. Given that implementation initiatives affect a range of stakeholder groups, successful implementation often relies on successfully engaging these stakeholders. Cassandra is motivated to learn more about best practices for young children with ASD to inform her implementation initiative, but it would also be important for her to gather information about stakeholders' perspectives toward various treatment options. Some important questions that Cassandra will need to ask are: How do providers currently work with families of young children with ASD? What are their perspectives toward implementing a parent-mediated intervention? What kinds of supports will providers need from the Big City EI system and from agency leaders to use this treatment approach? How do parents and caregivers view parent-mediated interventions? Thoughtful consideration of each of these questions and a deeper understanding of how each stakeholder group is affected by the implementation initiative will help Cassandra develop an implementation plan that is more likely to be successful.

WHO ARE STAKEHOLDERS?

Stakeholders are groups or individuals who can affect or are affected by an issue (Schiller et al., 2013). Within implementation efforts, stakeholders are individuals affected by the implementation process. A range of individuals are involved, each with a different stake or vested interest in the outcomes of the project. Stakeholders comprise a wide range of individuals or groups with varying degrees of involvement and can provide critical insights into the factors which influence effectiveness and implementation outcomes.

Concannon and colleagues (2012) developed the **7 Ps Framework** to offer a clear and simple taxonomy for identifying stakeholders involved within comparative effectiveness research and this framework can be readily applied to implementation efforts. The 7 Ps Framework categorizes stakeholders into seven groups. The first group includes **patients and the public**, or users or recipients of healthcare and population-focused public health initiatives. This group also includes patients' caregivers, families, and patient and advocacy organizations. The second group of stakeholders includes **providers**; providers are individuals and organizations that deliver healthcare to patients and populations. The third stakeholder group includes **purchasers**. Purchasers are those responsible for underwriting healthcare costs, such as employers and other agencies in charge of sponsoring healthcare costs. The fourth group, **payers**, including insurers, Medicare, and Medicaid among others, are responsible for reimbursement for care. **Policy makers**, including those associated with governmental and nongovernmental agencies, comprise the fifth group of stakeholders. The sixth group of stakeholders, **product makers,** consists of drug and device manufacturers and intervention developers. Lastly, **principal investigators**, researchers, and their funders make up the seventh stakeholder group (Concannon et al., 2012). Each of these stakeholder groups must be considered and engaged with throughout implementation efforts (Table 6.1).

TABLE 6.1 The 7 Ps Framework for Identifying and Classifying Stakeholders

STAKEHOLDER GROUP	DESCRIPTION	EXAMPLE
Patients and the public	Current users of healthcare, including their caregivers, families, and advocacy organizations	Parents and children with autism receiving early intervention services
Providers	Individuals and organizations that provide care to patients and populations	Therapists and special educators working with those parents
Purchasers	Individuals and other agencies that underwrite healthcare costs	The Early Intervention System within the county
Payers	Insurers and others responsible for reimbursement	The State Office of Child Development and Early Learning
Policy makers	Government entities, professional associations, and other policy-making entities	Administrators and leadership within the county government office
Product makers	Device and drug manufacturers and intervention developers	Early intervention treatment manual developer
Principal investigators	Researchers and their funders	University researcher

Source: Adapted from Concannon, T. W., Meissner, P., Grunbaum, J. A., McElwee, N., Guise, J.-M., Santa, J., Conway, P. H., Daudelin, D., Morrato, E. H., & Leslie, L. K. (2012). A new taxonomy for stakeholder engagement in patient-centered outcomes research. *Journal of General Internal Medicine*, 27(8), 985–991. https://doi.org/10.1007/s11606-012-2037-1.

WHAT IS STAKEHOLDER ENGAGEMENT?

Implementation science has produced robust evidence about the importance of relying heavily on engaging stakeholders throughout the implementation process that can be applied in implementation practice. Yet stakeholder engagement can take many forms and the level of engagement from stakeholders often varies across implementation efforts. To successfully engage stakeholders in the implementation of EBIs, a clear definition and understanding of the construct of stakeholder engagement are needed. Multiple definitions and descriptions of stakeholder engagement have been offered in recent years. One such definition highlights the importance of creating a shared understanding with a range of individuals or groups to improve decision-making within implementation efforts. Deverka and colleagues define **engagement** as "an iterative process of actively soliciting the knowledge, experience, judgment and values of individuals selected to represent a broad range of direct interest in a particular issue, for the dual purposes of creating a shared understanding and making relevant, transparent and effective decisions" (Deverka et al., 2012, p. 6). Similarly, stakeholder engagement in implementation research has been defined as a "bi-directional relationship between the stakeholder and researcher that results in informed decision-making about the selection, conduct, and use of research" (Concannon et al., 2012, p. 986). While this second definition describes engagement between a stakeholder and researcher, it can also be readily applied to practical implementation efforts between a stakeholder and EBI implementer through careful attention to the key constructs described within this working definition.

A critical aspect of this definition relates to the *bi-directional* nature of the relationship between the stakeholder and implementer. The implementer shares information related to the practice or innovation, while the stakeholder shares information related to the practice's fit, feasibility, and appropriateness for the setting. Successful stakeholder engagement involves shared learning through a continuous feedback loop for all involved in the implementation effort, with bi-directional sharing of knowledge and experiences across groups to inform implementation (Pellecchia et al., 2018). This stands in notable contrast to traditional training efforts that involve a unidirectional approach to knowledge sharing, in which an implementer shares knowledge about a practice with stakeholders through didactic instruction with little opportunity for stakeholders to share insights about contextual factors that will influence implementation of the practice. When stakeholders are engaged successfully, this bi-directional relationship results in collaboration and shared decision-making that meaningfully influences the implementation process. At its core, stakeholder engagement extends beyond simply going through the motions of obtaining stakeholders' feedback to a more nuanced relationship which takes care to ensure that stakeholders have actual power to affect the implementation process and implementation outcomes (Goodman & Sanders Thompson, 2017).

The level of stakeholder engagement within implementation efforts often falls on a broad continuum, with varying levels of participation among stakeholders. Levels of stakeholder engagement have been described within three broad categories: (a) non-participation, (b) symbolic participation, and (c) engaged participation (Goodman & Sanders Thompson, 2017). **Non-participation** involves efforts to inform stakeholders, rather than to engage stakeholders in the planning or decision-making of implementation efforts (Goodman & Sanders Thompson, 2017).

Activities involved in non-participating engagement include those found in traditional dissemination efforts such as *outreach* (targeted efforts to reach stakeholders and disseminate information about a practice) and *education* (targeted efforts to educate stakeholders about a particular topic). Implementers might choose to involve stakeholders in the non-participation level of engagement during initiatives in which the primary goal is to share information with stakeholders, such as sharing information with school officials about a tobacco prevention program aimed at preventing tobacco use among school-aged children (Brink et al., 1995) or sharing resources for sun safety and skin protection to elementary schools and child-care facilities (Buller et al., 2005).

The next level of engagement, **symbolic participation**, invites stakeholders to participate in discussions about implementation plans and have a voice in the decision-making process. Activities involved in symbolic participation include *coordination* (stakeholders provide feedback which informs implementation decisions but are not involved in designing and carrying out implementation efforts) and *cooperation* (stakeholders provide help with implementation efforts, instead of just providing advice) (Goodman & Sanders Thompson, 2017). In each of these scenarios, stakeholders have a deep understanding of the implementation effort and provide guidance related to implementation. However, there are no assurances that stakeholders' suggestions will ultimately be adopted. Within the symbolic participation level of engagement, stakeholders are encouraged to advise, but the research/implementation team ultimately holds decision-making power related to the implementation efforts. When the primary goal is to solicit advice or feedback about the implementation plan from stakeholders, implementers are using symbolic participation in stakeholder engagement. Examples of symbolic participation include gathering information from a group of school administrators to inform the implementation of a universal reading intervention for elementary students, or convening focus groups with pregnant women to gather information about their perspectives toward changes in prenatal care and screening before implementing the changes.

In the third and highest level of stakeholder engagement, **engaged participation**, stakeholders have shared decision-making authority and collaboratively manage the implementation effort. Implementation projects adopting a model of engaged participation with stakeholders often involve concerted efforts for *collaboration* between the stakeholders and implementers where both groups are actively involved in designing and implementing the project. Stakeholders are more likely to dictate implementation priorities and control the design and implementation of the project in this level of engagement. In this scenario stakeholders take the lead in many or all major decisions related to the implementation effort (Goodman & Sanders Thompson, 2017). Projects assuming engaged participation of stakeholders often strive to adopt *community-based participatory research* principles within the implementation effort. These principles include an emphasis on mutual trust and respect among groups, respect and acknowledgment of each other's expertise, mutual benefit for all parties, and shared decision-making (Goodman & Sanders Thompson, 2017; Wallerstein & Duran, 2006). Implementers adopt an engaged level of stakeholder participation when the primary goal of the implementation project is a sustained partnership that will lead to meaningful long-term implementation of an EBI largely driven by stakeholders' needs and priorities. For example, implementation efforts to adapt and implement a firearm safety promotion program in pediatric primary care require ongoing partnership and shared decision-making to center all voices and ensure that multiple perspectives are represented (Benjamin Wolk et al., 2018).

It is important to note that implementation efforts will likely necessitate varying levels of stakeholder engagement. In some scenarios, non-participation methods such as disseminating information about policy changes, outreach, and education may be appropriate and sufficient for the project's goals. For implementation initiatives aiming to enact concrete and sustained implementation of a practice, engaged participation within a stakeholder-centered approach is needed. Identifying the level of stakeholder engagement needed to meet the project goals is an important step which should occur early in the implementation process.

HOW DOES STAKEHOLDER ENGAGEMENT HELP ADVANCE HEALTH EQUITY?

The Robert Wood Johnson Foundation (RWJF) defines health equity as a world in which, "everyone has a fair and just opportunity to be as healthy as possible. This requires removing obstacles to health such as poverty, discrimination, and their consequences, including powerlessness and lack of access to good jobs with fair pay, quality education and housing, safe environments, and health care" (Braverman et al., 2017, p. 2). The National Institutes of Health recommends disseminating scientific discoveries, including EBIs, to reach populations who tend to have worse health outcomes compared to the general population (e.g., people who are socio-economically disadvantaged with lower levels of education or income, people with disabilities; Nápoles & Stewart, 2018). However, most EBIs were developed and tested in academic settings for highly selected, mostly White and/or middle-class populations (Bonevski et al., 2014; McNulty et al., 2019; Nápoles & Stewart, 2018). Fewer EBIs were designed for populations who experience health disparities or have been applied in the settings in which they spend most of their time (i.e., non-clinical community settings); thus, EBIs are not reaching the populations most in need or likely to benefit from them (Bonevski et al., 2014; Chinman et al., 2017; Nápoles & Stewart, 2018). Engaging stakeholders, particularly those who experience health disparities, in implementation research and practice is an essential element to achieving health equity.

Marginalized populations (e.g., Black/African American and Indigenous peoples) have historically been excluded from equitable care from the United States healthcare system (Nelson, 2002; Nuriddin et al., 2020) and have further been exploited in research trials (e.g., Tuskegee Study of Untreated Syphilis in the Negro Male, Henrietta Lacks; Brandt, 1978; Skloot, 2017; Washington, 2006). Inequities in social determinants of health—including housing, education, food security, experiences of racism, and lack of access to high-quality care—continue to drive health inequities today (Crear-Perry et al., 2020; Hardeman & Karbeah, 2020). Racism and the deliberate exclusion of stakeholders at the recipient and community levels of medical and health interventions have both contributed to the development and implementation of numerous interventions that are not culturally appropriate or responsive to the lived experience of those receiving them. The lack of stakeholder engagement, especially stakeholders from marginalized backgrounds, has also contributed to the well-established research-to-practice gap and low rates of uptake, implementation, and sustainability of EBIs in clinical and non-clinical settings (Chinman et al., 2017; McNulty et al., 2019; Nápoles & Stewart, 2018). According to Chinman et al. (2017), equity has not been an explicit goal of implementation science from the start but is becoming increasingly recognized as a critical issue. Additionally, it has been noted that prioritizing the delivery of EBIs to marginalized populations who currently receive high-quality care at lower rates than more privileged populations is a "special case" of implementation challenges, and authors suggest blending methods from health disparities research and implementation science to advance health equity (Chinman et al., 2017; Nápoles & Stewart, 2018).

Various equity-focused implementation frameworks and compilations of implementation strategies (e.g., Baumann & Cabassa, 2020; Chinman et al., 2017; Eslava-Schmalbach et al., 2019; Galaviz et al., 2020; Woodward et al., 2019) have highlighted the importance of engaging stakeholders in implementation research and practice to improve equity in access to high-quality health services and implementation of EBIs. Engaging stakeholders across multiple levels and throughout the intervention planning and design, development and delivery, evaluation, and dissemination processes helps advance health equity through culturally responsive implementation. The contextual fine-tuning enabled through stakeholder engagement increases adoption, enhances implementation, and improves sustainability of EBIs (Baumann & Cabassa, 2020; Chinman et al., 2017; Eslava-Schmalbach et al.,

2019; Galaviz et al., 2020; Nápoles & Stewart, 2018). While it is imperative to engage the stakeholders who make the decision to adopt and sustain EBIs, as well as those who will implement, pay for, promote, and evaluate EBIs, it is of utmost importance to also engage stakeholders who will use or receive care shaped by EBIs (e.g., clients, patients, students) and community members who are directly impacted by targeted health disparities or the specific health problem(s) that EBIs intend to improve.

Baumann and Cabassa (2020) reframed the following five elements of implementation science to address inequities in healthcare delivery: (a) focus on reach from the very beginning; (b) design and select interventions for vulnerable populations and low-resource communities with implementation in mind; (c) implement what works and develop implementation strategies that can help reduce inequities in care; (d) develop the science of adaptations; and (e) use an equity lens for implementation outcomes. Engaging stakeholders (e.g., clients, patients, family members, healthcare organizations and providers, and community members) in each of these elements is key to addressing health disparities and achieving health equity (see Table 6.2). For example, stakeholders' knowledge of local populations and underlying drivers of health disparities can inform the development and implementation of effective programs (McNulty et al., 2019; Nápoles & Stewart, 2018). Since they are part of the community, stakeholders likely have unique perspectives on ways to increase recruitment and engagement of community members in implementation efforts and enhance the reach of EBIs in community settings (Boothroyd et al., 2017). They could also aid in the identification, development, testing, and adaptation of practical implementation strategies and actively participate in adapting EBIs to better fit their setting or population (Baumann & Cabassa, 2020; Gaias et al., 2021; Mance et al., 2010).

TABLE 6.2 Recommendations for Increasing Stakeholder Engagement in Implementation Research and Practice to Address Inequities in Healthcare and Public Health

IMPLEMENTATION STRATEGY	KEY POINTS	RECOMMENDATIONS[a]	ADDITIONAL RECOMMENDATIONS FOR INCREASING STAKEHOLDER ENGAGEMENT
Focus on reach from the very beginning	■ The underrepresentation of vulnerable populations and communities persists in clinical and implementation trials. ■ Equity requires attention to reach and represent vulnerable populations in clinical trials and implementation studies ■ Studies need to mirror the context where vulnerable populations are served and live	■ Increase enrollment and engagement of vulnerable populations in clinical and implementation trials ■ Broaden the settings and communities where implementation studies are conducted	■ Involve vulnerable and marginalized populations in recruitment for clinical and implementation trials ■ Engage community members in implementation efforts to enhance the reach of EBIs in community settings

(*continued*)

TABLE 6.2 Recommendations for Increasing Stakeholder Engagement in Implementation Research and Practice to Address Inequities in Healthcare and Public Health ***(continued)***

IMPLEMENTATION STRATEGY	KEY POINTS	RECOMMENDATIONS[a]	ADDITIONAL RECOMMENDATIONS FOR INCREASING STAKEHOLDER ENGAGEMENT
Design and select interventions for vulnerable populations with implementation in mind	■ The linear process of intervention development contributes to implementation gaps ■ An implementation perspective to intervention development forces developers to consider the fit between the intervention and the implementation context	■ Place implementation outcomes at the forefront of the intervention development process ■ Incorporate user-centered designs and participatory approaches to develop interventions *with*, *for*, and *in* the community	■ Use the Transcreation Framework for Community-engaged Behavioral Interventions to Reduce Health Disparities to develop and implement EBIs with stakeholders in community settings ■ Ask stakeholders which implementation outcomes are most important to them
Implement what works and develop implementation strategies that can help reduce inequities in care	■ EBIs known to reduce inequities in care are not routinely used in real-world settings ■ Implementation strategies can support the adoption of EBIs in vulnerable communities	■ Invest in the identification, development, and testing of implementation strategies for EBIs that can reduce healthcare inequities ■ Implementation strategies in vulnerable communities may need to include additional components (e.g., cultural competence, advocacy)	■ Identify, develop, and test practical implementation strategies for EBIs in partnership with stakeholders that can reduce healthcare and public health inequities ■ Determine how existing implementation strategies may contribute to inequitable implementation ■ Consider adding components to implementation strategies that are culturally relevant and responsive

(continued)

TABLE 6.2 Recommendations for Increasing Stakeholder Engagement in Implementation Research and Practice to Address Inequities in Healthcare and Public Health *(continued)*

IMPLEMENTATION STRATEGY	KEY POINTS	RECOMMENDATIONS[a]	ADDITIONAL RECOMMENDATIONS FOR INCREASING STAKEHOLDER ENGAGEMENT
Develop the science of adaptation	■ Attention to the unique contextual factors that influence healthcare inequities is critical to implement EBIs in vulnerable populations ■ A broader conceptualization of adaptation is critical for addressing healthcare inequities as it expands the purview of adaptations to consider the EBI, implementation strategies, and the context of practice	■ Adaptations need to be done systematically and be guided by frameworks ■ A common data platform can be used to track and help identify optimal adaptations across different contexts and populations ■ Adaptations can be used as an implementation strategy	■ Make adaptations to EBIs in collaboration with stakeholders to better fit their setting or population ■ Adapt implementation strategies to explicitly center the goals of reducing disparities and promoting health equity
Use an equity lens for implementation outcomes	■ Implementation outcomes are important because they are inter-related with services and client outcomes ■ Limited attention has been given to examining issues of equity in implementation outcomes	■ Descriptive and explanatory studies are needed to identify the factors and mechanisms that contribute to inequities in implementation outcomes ■ Conduct studies to develop, test, and refine implementation strategies to achieve equity in implementation outcomes	■ Use qualitative and mixed methods to learn from stakeholders about the factors and mechanisms that contribute to inequities in implementation outcomes from their perspective ■ Conduct studies using participatory approaches to develop, test, and refine implementation strategies to achieve equity in implementation outcomes

EBI, evidence-based intervention.

[a]From Baumann, A. A., & Cabassa, L. J. (2020). Reframing implementation science to address inequities in healthcare delivery. *BMC Health Services Research*, *20*(1), 190. https://doi.org/10.1186/s12913-020-4975-3

The Transcreation Framework for Community-engaged Behavioral Interventions to Reduce Health Disparities (referred to as **the transcreation framework** for short) goes beyond adapting and translating EBIs for delivery in new settings to the co-design of new interventions with community members that better fit community needs and contexts than original EBIs (Nápoles & Stewart, 2018). The Transcreation Framework promotes evidence building with interventions that are initially tested in community settings and with populations who experience health disparities instead of traditional efficacy trials conducted under constrained circumstances with predominantly White populations (Nápoles & Stewart, 2018). The Framework also involves engaging community stakeholders throughout the entire research and implementation processes (including planning, recruitment, intervention delivery, and evaluation) to transcreate EBIs to be meaningful, useful, and deliverable with fidelity in community settings to address health disparities (Nápoles & Stewart, 2018). Overall, stakeholder engagement models of health equity include concepts of fairness and justice—which are key components of health equity—and involve engaging individuals who have directly experienced obstacles to health as well as those who may work with them or make decisions that could help remove the obstacles they face.

HOW DO WE IDENTIFY STAKEHOLDERS?

Stakeholder Analysis

The use of stakeholder analysis as a tool to identify, evaluate, and understand stakeholders has become increasingly popular in the fields of management and health policy (Table 6.3; Newcombe, 2003; Walker et al., 2008). A **stakeholder analysis** aims to "evaluate and understand stakeholders from the perspective of an organization, or to determine their relevance to a project or policy" (Brugha & Varvasovszky, 2000, p. 239). When conducting a stakeholder analysis within implementation efforts, questions are asked about a stakeholder's position, influence, interest, and networks and how each of those relate to the implementation effort. A stakeholder analysis is an iterative and ongoing process that can be conducted prior to and during the implementation process. It is often used during the planning and preparation phases of the implementation process to improve the chances of implementation success by identifying and gathering information about the key stakeholders most likely to influence the implementation effort. It can also be conducted during or after the implementation process as part of ongoing evaluation and quality improvement efforts (Varvasovszky & Brugha, 2000). Stakeholder analysis provides an in-depth understanding of who has a stake in an implementation initiative, each group's vested interest, and their interrelationships with each other—all of which have been described as critical to effective decision-making (Reed et al., 2009).

The first step of a stakeholder analysis is to identify key stakeholders, those with a vested interest in the implementation effort. Soliciting expert opinions, focus groups, structured interviews, and snowball sampling are common methods for identifying stakeholders within a stakeholder analysis (Dougill et al., 2006; Reed et al., 2009). After a core group of stakeholders have been identified, the next step is to gather information on stakeholders' perspectives and potential influence on key issues related to the implementation effort. This involves thoughtful consideration of each potential stakeholder's power, position, and interest related to the implementation effort (Gilson et al., 2012). Group discussions, interviews, and surveys can be used to gather information about stakeholders' power, position, and interest in a stakeholder analysis (Schmeer, 1999). Questions asked during the discussions and interviews should solicit information about stakeholder's experience with and perspectives toward the EBI. Open-ended questions that allow the stakeholder to discuss their views are preferred because they are more likely to yield rich information during the

TABLE 6.3 Steps of a Stakeholder Analysis

STEP	PROCESS
1. Identify potential stakeholders	Solicit expert opinions Conduct focus groups Conduct structuredinterviews Use snowball sampling
2. Gather information through interviews or surveys	Assess perspectives on key issues (power, position, influence)
3. Compile a list of stakeholders for engagement	Incorporate information from previous steps to compile a list of stakeholders for engagement Iteratively update the stakeholder group based on new findings or feedback throughout the implementation process

TABLE 6.4 Key Factors Assessed in a Stakeholder Analysis

CONSTRUCT	DEFINITION	SAMPLE INTERVIEW QUESTIONS
Position	Whether the stakeholder supports, opposes, or is neutral to the implementation effort	How would implementing (insert EBI) help your organization? What would have to change in order to implement (insert EBI)? Who do you think would support/oppose implementing (insert EBI) in your organization? Why would they support/oppose it?
Interest	Advantages or disadvantages the implementation effort may present to the stakeholder	What are the advantages/disadvantages to implementing (insert EBI)? How would implementing (insert EBI) improve your clients'/patients' outcomes? What would make it hard to implement (insert EBI)?
Power	Stakeholder's ability to influence the implementation process or outcome	How do you demonstrate your support/opposition to implementing (insert EBI)? What resources do you have available to support implementing (insert EBI)? How would you communicate your support/opposition to implementing (insert EBI) to others?

interview. The information gathered through the stakeholder analysis leads to a working description of relevant stakeholders and their potential influence on the implementation effort. It is important to engage stakeholders with diverse or discordant positions regarding the implementation effort, as these opposing views can add rich and nuanced perspectives related to potential barriers and facilitators to implementation. Engaging stakeholders with power to effectively influence the implementation process is also critical to successful implementation (Gilson et al., 2012). Stakeholders with power to influence implementation may not always be those in leadership roles. For example, a beloved and long-tenured teacher may have more influence over their fellow teachers' attitudes toward an EBI than the school principal. It would be essential to engage that influential teacher early in the implementation plan to understand their perspectives about the EBI (Table 6.4).

HOW ARE STAKEHOLDERS INVOLVED IN IMPLEMENTATION?

Stakeholder involvement in implementation often varies based on the project needs and stakeholder priorities. Stakeholder involvement also may vary depending on the phase of implementation. The **EPIS framework of implementation** (Aarons et al., 2011) provides a conceptual model that maps the implementation process across four distinct phases of implementation: Exploration, Preparation, Implementation, and Sustainment. Engaging stakeholders across each phase of implementation can lead to more meaningful and sustained implementation. Stakeholder involvement during the **Exploration** phase of implementation includes identifying a practice gap or conducting a needs assessment to identify a potential implementation need. Stakeholder involvement during the **Preparation** phase includes selecting an EBI to implement, identifying the implementation setting, identifying implementers, identifying consumers, selecting outcomes of interest, and providing input on the implementation plan. During the **Active Implementation** phase stakeholders often provide feedback about the implementation plan and guide adaptations to the plan when needed. Stakeholders also may be responsible for deploying implementation strategies themselves during the active implementation phase and they can provide feedback when interpreting implementation outcomes to inform ongoing implementation. Finally, the end goal of most implementation efforts is ongoing sustainment of the EBI within the community. Therefore, stakeholders have a critical role in the **Sustainment** phase of implementation. Stakeholders can be instrumental in disseminating implementation findings to larger audiences to enhance sustainment. They can also be influential in garnering support for implementation and long-term buy-in from consumers. The goal of most implementation initiatives is to transfer implementation oversight and responsibility to the community. Engaging key stakeholders who are positioned to assume control of the implementation initiative, and partnering with them throughout the implementation process, can facilitate sustained implementation of an EBI in community practice.

Stakeholder involvement throughout all phases of implementation improves the likelihood that the implementation plan will be feasible, acceptable, and appropriate for the setting. However, specific stakeholder groups may not need to be involved during all phases of implementation. For example, an implementation initiative aimed at implementing a mental health screening tool in schools involved different stakeholder groups at different phases of implementation. School district administrators were engaged during the Exploration phase to learn about the district's needs, priorities related to identifying mental health risks in their student population, and current practices. District level administrators, principals, school psychologists, and school counselors were engaged during the Preparation phase to develop the implementation plan. School psychologists, school counselors, and teachers were engaged during the Active Implementation phase to partner in implementing the screening tool and provide feedback about the feasibility, acceptability, and appropriateness of the screening tool and the implementation plan. Finally, all stakeholder groups were engaged during the Sustainment phase to disseminate information about the screening tool to families and school personnel, as well as inform adaptations to the implementation plan. Engaging multiple stakeholder groups from one system or organization, like the school district described in this example, requires careful consideration of inter-personal dynamics and power differentials among stakeholders. For example, supervisees may not feel comfortable providing open feedback about implementation challenges if their supervisors are present. Convening stakeholder groups of teachers separate from principals provided a forum for open discussion and feedback about the screening tool, which may have been suppressed if teachers were queried in front of their supervising principals (Table 6.5).

TABLE 6.5 Stakeholder Involved Activities Across EPIS Implementation Phases

EPIS FRAMEWORK IMPLEMENTATION PHASE	EXAMPLES OF STAKEHOLDER INVOLVEMENT
Exploration	Identifying practice gap Conducting a needs assessment
Preparation	Selecting innovation to implement Identifying implementation setting Identifying implementers Identifying consumers/patients Selecting outcomes of interest Providing input on the implementation plan
Active Implementation	Providing feedback on the implementation process Guiding implementation adaptations Interpreting implementation outcomes
Sustainment	Disseminating implementation findings Taking over ongoing implementation

DISCRETE IMPLEMENTATION STRATEGIES FOR STAKEHOLDER ENGAGEMENT

Stakeholder engagement can take many forms, from soliciting brief feedback to developing stakeholder-driven implementation plans. The spectrum of possibilities for engaging stakeholders can be conceptualized as discrete implementation strategies. The Expert Recommendations for Implementing Change (ERIC) framework provides a discrete compilation used to define commonly adopted implementation strategies (Powell et al., 2015). An extension of the ERIC framework used concept mapping to categorize these discrete implementation strategies and highlighted two distinct categories of stakeholder-related implementation strategies: develop stakeholder interrelationships and train and educate stakeholders (Waltz et al., 2015). These categories highlight the breadth of discrete implementation strategies that can be used to engage stakeholders throughout the implementation process. Some implementation strategies focused on stakeholder engagement provide concrete approaches for sharing information and resources with stakeholders during the Exploration and Preparation phases of the implementation process. These include *identify and prepare champions, recruit, designate and train for leadership, build a coalition, conduct local consensus discussions,* and *conduct educational meetings*. The goal of these implementation strategies is to engage stakeholders during the initial phases of implementation to garner support for the implementation plan and ultimately improve implementation readiness and implementation climate. Discrete implementation strategies involving stakeholders are also often implemented during the Active Implementation phase of the implementation process. These include *conduct educational outreach visits, capture and share local knowledge, use advisory boards and workgroups,* and *obtain and use patient/consumer feedback*. The goal of these implementation strategies is to obtain feedback from stakeholders actively involved in the implementation process and then use that feedback to iteratively inform adaptations to the implementation plan. Use of these implementation strategies during the Active Implementation phase can improve the feasibility, acceptability, appropriateness, and contextual fit of the implementation plan (Table 6.6).

TABLE 6.6 Implementation Strategies Focused on Stakeholder Engagement

ERIC IMPLEMENTATION STRATEGY	DEFINITION[a]
Capture and share local knowledge	Capture local knowledge from implementation sites on how implementers and clinicians made something work in their setting and then share it with other sites
Identify and prepare champions	Identify and prepare individuals who dedicate themselves to supporting, marketing, and driving through an implementation, overcoming indifference or resistance that the intervention may provoke in an organization
Conduct educational meetings	Hold meetings targeted toward different stakeholder groups (e.g., providers, administrators, other organizational stakeholders, and community, patient/consumer, and family stakeholders) to teach them about the clinical innovation
Conduct educational outreach visits	Have a trained person meet with providers in their practice settings to educate providers about the clinical innovation with the intent of changing the provider's practice
Conduct local consensus discussions	Include local providers and other stakeholders in discussions that address whether the chosen problem is important and whether the clinical innovation to address it is appropriate
Obtain and use patient/consumer feedback	Develop strategies to increase patient/consumer and family feedback on the implementation effort
Use advisory boards and workgroups	Create and engage a formal group of multiple kinds of stakeholders to provide input and advice on implementation efforts and to elicit recommendations for improvements
Build a coalition	Recruit and cultivate relationships with partners in the implementation effort

[a]From Powell, B. J., Waltz, T. J., Chinman, M. J., Damschroder, L. J., Smith, J. L., Matthieu, M. M., Proctor, E. K., & Kirchner, J. E. (2015). A refined compilation of implementation strategies: Results from the Expert Recommendations for Implementing Change (ERIC) project. *Implementation Science, 10*(1), 21. https://doi.org/10.1186/s13012-015-0209-1

CASE STUDY 6.1B IMPLEMENTATION STRATEGIES USED TO ENGAGE EARLY INTERVENTION STAKEHOLDERS

Cassandra D. used a series of implementation strategies to engage stakeholders in the Big City EI System. A series of **local consensus discussions** were held with stakeholders including administrators, agency leaders, and service providers to better understand the service needs for young children with ASD across the system and select an EBI that was aligned with stakeholders' priorities, needs, and the system's infrastructure. Once the intervention was selected, Cassandra **obtained feedback from families** through focus groups where she shared videos and excerpts describing the intervention. She also shared simple concrete information comparing

(*continued*)

CASE STUDY 6.1B IMPLEMENTATION STRATEGIES USED TO ENGAGE EARLY INTERVENTION STAKEHOLDERS (*continued*)

parent-mediated intervention approaches to traditional child-directed intervention approaches and open-ended inquiry to learn about parents and caregivers' perspectives toward both approaches to treatment. Cassandra and her team also **conducted educational meetings** with providers, agency leaders, and administrators across the Big City EI System to share information about the intervention with them. She held **educational outreach visits** with providers who worked in the agencies selected for implementation to teach those providers and staff about the intervention prior to training. A **community advisory board** made up of providers, administrators, agency leaders, and parents was convened to guide the implementation plan development and provide feedback about implementation throughout the process. This community advisory board met monthly and provided valuable feedback about the appropriateness and feasibility of the implementation plan. As implementation was underway, Cassandra **identified and prepared champions** from agencies throughout the city who not only implemented the intervention with high fidelity but advocated for use of the intervention within their agencies. She then supported those local champions in becoming certified trainers in the intervention and publicly recognized them for their implementation efforts. Importantly, Cassandra also connected those champions with providers who were reluctant or struggling with implementing the intervention, to promote social norms around using the intervention with their clients. When implementation challenges were observed in some agencies, she convened meetings with agency leaders to **capture and share local knowledge** related to successes with implementing the intervention to overcome observed implementation barriers. Throughout all these activities, Cassandra **built a coalition** with stakeholders across Big City EI System focused on developing a feasible and acceptable plan to improve the implementation of an evidence-based intervention for young children with ASD.

WHAT ARE THE BENEFITS OF STAKEHOLDER ENGAGEMENT IN IMPLEMENTATION?

There are many benefits of engaging stakeholders in implementation efforts. First, stakeholder engagement can enhance implementation outcomes (Goodman & Sanders Thompson, 2017; Jones et al., 2009; Martinez et al., 2018). Baumann and Cabassa (2020) noted that implementation outcomes are interrelated with effectiveness outcomes. Thus, stakeholder engagement can inherently improve effectiveness outcomes, which is the ultimate goal of implementation efforts. However, limited empirical attention has been devoted to fully examining the underlying mechanisms of increasing stakeholder engagement in implementation efforts to advance health equity and achieve beneficial implementation outcomes. Proctor et al. (2011) defined implementation outcomes as, "the effects of deliberate and purposive actions to implement new treatments, practices, and services" (p. 65). Implementation outcomes are key intermediate outcomes to and necessary prerequisites for achieving subsequent clinical and service outcomes (including equity). The implementation outcomes defined by Proctor et al. (2011) include *acceptability, adoption, appropriateness, cost, feasibility, fidelity, penetration (reach),* and *sustainability.* Engaging stakeholders in implementation efforts can positively impact all implementation outcomes.

Previous studies have demonstrated that engaging stakeholders in the development, adaptation, and implementation of interventions can lead to improvements in appropriateness, feasibility, and/or acceptability of EBIs (e.g., Goodkind et al., 2012; Mance et al., 2010; Shelef et al., 2016). For example, engaging stakeholders in the development or adaptation of EBIs may lead to more positive attitudes toward EBIs and increased willingness of stakeholders to implement or participate in the interventions. When stakeholders who are implementing EBIs find the intervention to be acceptable or appropriate, they are typically more committed to implementing it with fidelity. When community stakeholders are actively engaged in developing or adapting interventions, they can advocate for what they deem to be culturally relevant, appropriate for their setting, and/or for the intended users of the interventions (Nápoles & Stewart, 2018). Community stakeholders are also able to provide important insight on what actions or resources are needed to increase penetration (reach) or facilitate sustainability of EBIs in their specific setting. Bolstering community resources and capacity increases the likelihood of success and sustainability of EBIs, but communities should be engaged throughout the entire process to take full advantage of these resources and address disparities in a sustainable way (Nápoles & Stewart, 2018). Meaningful partnerships with stakeholders who are funders, agency administrators, or policy makers may also lead to increased uptake or EBIs and/or reduced implementation costs through grants, donations, or allocation of agency funding to EBIs.

Second, stakeholder engagement can lead to better selection and utilization of implementation strategies. Oftentimes, implementation strategies are selected by researchers and/or practitioners who are not receiving EBIs or directly involved in implementing or paying for EBIs. Involving stakeholders through coalitions, advisory boards, and obtaining their feedback on implementation efforts could aid in better selection of implementation strategies that are acceptable, appropriate, and feasible for the intended implementation setting and population, and better utilization of implementation strategies by relevant stakeholders. For example, when implementing EBIs in schools, school stakeholders (e.g., principals, teachers, guidance counselors) have deep knowledge and understanding of their school's setting and student population. Practitioners and researchers seeking to implement EBIs in schools should work with school stakeholders to co-select implementation strategies to enhance implementation and increase the likelihood of sustaining EBIs. However, it is also important to note that stakeholders tend to focus on issues of cost or feasibility of implementation strategies that, while important, should be rounded out with perspectives on the potential impact of the strategies to enhance implementation outcomes and how critical the strategies are to a successful implementation effort. Lyon et al. (2019) engaged school stakeholders (e.g., administrators, school mental health providers, behavior specialists) in an evaluation of the importance and feasibility of the *School Implementation Strategies, Translating ERIC Resources* (SISTER) compilation of 75 implementation strategies that were adapted from the ERIC implementation strategies compilation for use in the education sector. Although many of the strategies (33 of 75) were rated by school-based implementation practitioners as highly feasible and important, 24 of the 75 strategies were rated low for feasibility and importance (Lyon et al., 2019). These findings suggest that is crucial to engage stakeholders in the selection of implementation strategies and consider both the feasibility *and* importance of the strategies for improving implementation efforts.

Third, stakeholder engagement can facilitate future collaborative implementation research and practical efforts that are of mutual importance to the community, practitioners, and researchers/evaluators. Practical implementation efforts can and should unearth gaps in the evidence base. By meaningfully engaging stakeholders, the evidence gaps can be appropriately prioritized by elevating those of greatest relevance to community partners. Engaging various stakeholders in implementation efforts can also contribute to ongoing partnerships between stakeholders that result in more robust and impactful research projects and practices to improve the public's health. For example, in Philadelphia, partnerships between the University of Pennsylvania Center for Mental Health and local public policy, behavioral health, and educational institutions have contributed to numerous community-partnered implementation research studies and increased adoption and implementation of EBIs by practitioners in clinical and community settings (Pellecchia et al., 2018; Stewart et al., 2021).

WHAT ARE THE CHALLENGES WITH STAKEHOLDER ENGAGEMENT IN IMPLEMENTATION?

Although stakeholder engagement provides many benefits, there are challenges. First, it is important to remember that identifying stakeholders and building relationships with them takes time. Researchers/evaluators and implementation practitioners who are partnering with and/or implementing EBIs within communities may face challenges with timing if the community is eager to get a new EBI delivered before implementers have had the opportunity to engage all relevant stakeholders, gain buy-in and support for the EBI from relevant stakeholders, conduct a contextual inquiry to understand barriers and facilitators of implementation for the EBI in the intended setting, or assess organizational readiness to implement the EBI. To mitigate these challenges, it may be helpful for researchers/evaluators and implementation practitioners to clearly communicate with community stakeholders in advance about the pre-implementation activities that will be conducted and an estimated timeline for the activities so that everyone will be on the same page about timing of implementation of the EBI; or engage in more rapid approaches to accomplish the objectives to align timelines.

In addition to considering the balance of stakeholder priorities with the priorities of funders, the competing priorities of stakeholders involved in implementation may also present challenges and must be considered. For example, when stakeholders whose primary role is not to deliver EBIs are required to or volunteer to implement EBIs in addition to their primary role in their workplace or other setting, certain effectiveness and implementation outcomes such as fidelity may be negatively impacted. For instance, in the context of schools, teachers are sometimes trained to deliver EBIs for mental health in addition to their primary role of educating their students. If protected time in the school schedule is not devoted to their delivery of mental health EBIs, curriculum demands may impede their ability to successfully implement the EBIs. Additionally, stakeholder turnover is frequent and is sometimes linked with competing priorities within or outside of their organization. When layering the implementation of EBIs on top of existing responsibilities of stakeholders, actions should be taken to reduce competing demands that may serve as barriers to implementation and keep stakeholders engaged in a changing landscape. Providing incentives, revising professional roles, and improving the well-being of implementers are examples of implementation strategies that could be used to prevent professional burnout and reduce implementers' burden of delivering EBIs (Cook et al., 2019; Powell et al., 2015).

Just as stakeholders may have competing priorities, various stakeholders may also value different implementation outcomes (Proctor et al., 2011). Those bearing the financial cost for EBIs (payers) may be concerned with budgetary impact and implementation costs, while providers and evaluators of EBIs may be most concerned with fidelity and penetration. Adopters of EBIs, who may or may not be involved in implementation, may be concerned with impact, costs, and acceptability of EBIs among providers in their organization who will be involved in implementing EBIs. Recipients of EBIs may be concerned with the appropriateness of interventions for addressing their needs and improving their health.

CASE STUDY 6.1C CHALLENGES WITH ENGAGING STAKEHOLDERS IN EARLY INTERVENTION

Cassandra faced many challenges implementing a parent-mediated intervention in the Big City EI System. The EI System serves all young children with disabilities, not just those with ASD, which meant agency leaders and providers had many competing priorities and service needs to meet. Effectively partnering with this group required persistence and patience while they worked to ensure equitable and fair service delivery for all children served by the system. Cassandra also faced challenges with gaining buy-in from some providers who were hesitant to change their intervention approach. Many providers held existing beliefs about how to best support young children with ASD, and these beliefs were at times in conflict with the intervention selected for implementation. Gaining buy-in from stakeholders who held treatment beliefs that did not align with the intervention approach required careful planning and repeated attempts at engagement. While implementing the intervention within this large service system, the need for adaptations and flexibility became apparent. For example, adapting the number of intervention sessions provided each week and simplifying the data collection plan were needed to reduce provider burden. Listening to providers' concerns during the rollout and making systematic adaptations based on these concerns led to improved provider fidelity and buy-in. Last, Cassandra faced challenges engaging stakeholders across multiple stakeholder groups. Throughout this process Cassandra involved administrators in the EI System, agency leaders across the System, providers employed by those agencies, and parents who receive service from the agencies in the EI System. Navigating relationships across these stakeholder groups required a deep understanding of the priorities and values held by each stakeholder group, and how to best support each group's priorities, even when the priorities differed or were in conflict. Persistence, flexibility, and frequent open communication with stakeholders helped to overcome many of these challenges to implementing this EBI within a large urban service system.

Community-partnered initiatives have been described as following three major stages: the *vision*, the *valley*, and the *victory* (Jones et al., 2009). The *vision* is the process of developing a shared view of the project's overarching goals and the strategy to accomplish those goals. A clear and shared vision is essential for successful community-based implementation. Developing a compelling vision and reminding each other of the vision when implementation challenges arise can be powerful tools in community-based implementation efforts. The *valley* describes the process of doing the work to achieve the vision. The word *valley* was selected in this framework to "emphasize that a lot of hard work is needed to climb the hill to success" (Jones et al., 2009, p. 5). The valley of engaging stakeholders is a continuous and iterative process that often involves overcoming many challenges and assuming a level of humility and flexibility throughout the process. *Victory* within community-partnered work is coming together to celebrate and acknowledge success. Successful meetings, mutually agreed upon compromises, and completed action steps are all reasons for victory (Jones et al., 2009). The ultimate victory is to position the partnership with stakeholders as a platform for continued work and broader impact beyond the current implementation project.

CASE STUDY 6.1D STAKEHOLDER ENGAGEMENT: PUTTING IT ALL TOGETHER

Throughout this chapter we highlighted case examples illustrating the process of engaging stakeholders in the implementation of an evidence-based intervention for young children with ASD within a large urban early intervention system. Stakeholders were engaged throughout all phases of implementation. This project was driven by the EI System's need to improve the implementation of EBIs for young children with ASD across the system. Equitable delivery of best practices throughout the system drove the implementation plan, which was developed in partnership with administrators, providers, and families within the system. Stakeholders selected an intervention aligned with both best practice in treatment for young children with ASD as well as the Big City EI System's needs, priorities, and infrastructure. Ongoing feedback from a community advisory board informed potential adaptations to the implementation plan. Throughout the implementation process, interviews with administrators, providers, and parents, as well as direct observations of practice-informed adaptations to the training and implementation plans, enabled real-time decisions about the best ways to improve the adoption of the intervention. The stakeholders' needs and priorities continue to drive the plans for long-term sustainment of this intervention for young children with ASD within this service system.

SUMMARY

In this chapter, strategies for engaging stakeholders in implementation efforts were discussed. This chapter also provided an overview of the benefits and challenges to engaging stakeholders in implementation efforts. Meaningfully engaging stakeholders is essential to reducing disparities in health equity and removing barriers to high-quality healthcare and education for marginalized groups.

KEY POINTS FOR PRACTICE

1. Stakeholders can positively or negatively impact implementation success.
2. Historically and contemporarily marginalized populations should be engaged in implementation efforts to advance health equity.
3. A stakeholder analysis provides information that could be used to better understand stakeholders (including their interests, influence, and resources), and facilitate successful implementation of interventions (e.g., policies, programs, services).
4. Stakeholders should be engaged throughout all stages of implementation (e.g., exploration, planning, implementation, and sustainment).
5. Stakeholder engagement can advance health equity, lead to better selection of implementation strategies, and improve implementation and effectiveness outcomes.

COMMON PITFALLS IN PRACTICE

1. Only engaging stakeholders with power, influence, and resources (e.g., policy makers, payers, providers) while leaving out stakeholders with less implementation

decision-making power or influence (e.g., patients and the public) can exacerbate inequities and health disparities in access to EBIs.
2. Underestimating the amount of time that it takes to build and maintain relationships with stakeholders.
3. Prioritizing the needs of stakeholders paying for, implementing, or evaluating implementation efforts over the needs of stakeholders receiving the intervention.
4. Not setting clear and realistic expectations with stakeholders about implementation efforts.
5. Stakeholders may favor strategies that are familiar and feasible and not necessarily offer the greatest impact.

DISCUSSION QUESTIONS

1. Why is it important to engage stakeholders in the implementation process?
2. How can stakeholder engagement advance health equity?
3. How can stakeholders be engaged throughout the implementation process?
4. How could you engage stakeholders in your implementation effort?
5. Which stakeholders do you plan to engage in your implementation effort and why?
6. How can stakeholder engagement enhance implementation outcomes?
7. What are some strategies that could be used to overcome stakeholder engagement challenges?

REFERENCES

Aarons, G. A., Hurlburt, M., & Horwitz, S. M. (2011). Advancing a conceptual model of evidence-based practice implementation in public service sectors. *Administration and Policy in Mental Health, 38*(1), 4–23. https://doi.org/10.1007/s10488010-0327-7

Baumann, A. A., & Cabassa, L. J. (2020). Reframing implementation science to address inequities in healthcare delivery. *BMC Health Services Research, 20*(1), 190. https://doi.org/10.1186/s12913-020-4975-3

Benjamin Wolk, C., Van Pelt, A.E., Jager-Hyman, S., Ahmedani, B. K., Zeber, J., Fein, J. A., Brown, G. K., Gregor, C. A., Lieberman, A., & Beidas, R.S. (2018). Stakeholder perspectives on implementing a firearm safety intervention in pediatric primary care as a universal suicide prevention strategy: A qualitative study. *JAMA Network Open, 1*(7), e185309. https://doi.org/10.1001/jamanetworkopen.2018.5309

Bonevski, B., Randell, M., Paul, C., Chapman, K., Twyman, L., Bryant, J., Brozek, I., & Hughes, C. (2014). Reaching the hard-to-reach: A systematic review of strategies for improving health and medical research with socially disadvantaged groups. *BMC Medical Research Methodology, 14*, 42. https://doi.org/10.1186/1471-2288-14-42

Boothroyd, R. I., Flint, A. Y., Lapiz, A. M., Lyons, S., Jarboe, K. L., & Aldridge, W. A., 2nd. (2017). Active involved community partnerships: Co-creating implementation infrastructure for getting to and sustaining social impact. *Translational Behavioral Medicine, 7*(3), 467–477. https://doi.org/10.1007/s13142-017-0503-3

Brandt, A. M. (1978). Racism and research: The case of the tuskegee syphilis study. *The Hastings Center Report, 8*(6), 21–29. https://doi.org/10.2307/3561468

Braverman, P., Arkin, E., Orleans, T., Proctor, E., & Plough, A. (2017). *What is health equity? And what difference does a definition make?* Robert Wood Johnson Foundation. https://www.rwjf.org/en/library/research/2017/05/what-is-health-equity-.html

Brink, S. G., Basen-Engquist, K. M., O'Hara-Tompkins, N. M., Parcel, G. S., Gorrlieb, N. H., & Lovato, C. Y. (1995). Diffusion of an effective tobacco prevention program. Part I: Evaluation of the dissemination phase. *Health Education Research, 10*, 283–295.

Brugha, R., & Varvasovszky, Z. (2000). Stakeholder analysis: A review. *Health Policy and Planning, 15*(3), 239–246. https://doi.org/10.1093/heapol/15.3.239

Buller, D. B., Buller, M. K., & Kane, I. (2005). Web-based strategies to disseminate a sun safety curriculum to public elementary schools and state-licensed child-care facilities. *Health Psychology, 24*(5), 470–476.

Chinman, M., Woodward, E. N., Curran, G. M., & Hausmann, L. R. M. (2017). Harnessing implementation science to increase the impact of health disparity research. *Medical Care, 55*(Suppl 9 2), S16–S23. https://doi org/10.1097/MLR.0000000000000769

Concannon, T. W., Meissner, P., Grunbaum, J. A., McElwee, N., Guise, J.-M., Santa, J., Conway, P. H., Daudelin, D., Morrato, E. H., & Leslie, L. K. (2012). A new taxonomy for stakeholder engagement in patient-centered outcomes research. *Journal of General Internal Medicine*, *27*(8), 985–991. https://doi.org/10.1007/s11606-012-2037-1

Cook, C. R., Lyon, A. R., Locke, J., Waltz, T., & Powell, B. J. (2019). Adapting a compilation of implementation strategies to advance school-based implementation research and practice. *Prevention Science*, *20*(6), 914–935. https://doi.org/10.1007/s11121-019-01017-1

Crear-Perry, J., Maybank, A., Keeys, M., Mitchell, N., & Godbolt, D. (2020). Moving towards anti-racist praxis in medicine. *Lancet*, *396*(10249), 451–453. https://doi.org/10.1016/S0140-6736(20)31543-9

Dougill, A. J., Fraser, E. D. G., Holden, J., Hubacek, K., Prell, C., Reed, M. S., Stagl, S., & Stringer, L. C. (2006). Learning from doing participatory rural research: Lessons from the peak district national park. *Journal of Agricultural Economics*, *57*(2), 259–275. https://doi.org/10.1111/j.1477-9552.2006.00051.x

Dverka, P. A., Lavallee, D. A., Desai, P. J., Esmail, S. C., Ramsey, S. D., Veenstra, D. L., & Tunis, S. R. (2012). Stakeholder participation in comparative effectiveness research: Defining a framework for effective engagement. *Journal of Comparative Effectiveness Research*, *1*(2). https://doi.org/10.2217/cer.12.7

Eslava-Schmalbach, J., Garzón-Orjuela, N., Elias, V., Reveiz, L., Tran, N., & Langlois, E. V. (2019). Conceptual framework of equity-focused implementation research for health programs (EquIR). *International Journal for Equity in Health*, *18*(1), 80. https://doi.org/10.1186/s12939-019-0984-4

Gaias, L. M., Arnold, K. T., Liu, F. F., Pullmann, M. D., Duong, M. T., & Lyon, A. R. (2021). Adapting strategies to promote implementation reach and equity (ASPIRE) in school mental health services. *Psychology in the Schools*. https://doi.org/10.1002/pits.22515

Galaviz, K. I., Breland, J. Y., Sanders, M., Breathett, K., Cerezo, A., Gil, O., Hollier, J. M., Marshall, C., Wilson, J. D., & Essien, U. R. (2020). Implementation science to address health disparities during the coronavirus pandemic. *Health Equity*, *4*(1), 463–467. https://doi.org/10.1089/heq.2020.0044

Gilson, L., Erasmus, E., Borghi, J., Macha, J., Kamuzora, P., & Mtei, G. (2012). Using stakeholder analysis to support moves towards universal coverage: Lessons from the SHIELD project. *Health Policy and Planning*, *27*(suppl_1), i64–i76. https://doi.org/10.1093/heapol/czs007

Goodkind, J., LaNoue, M., Lee, C., Freeland, L., & Freund, R. (2012). Feasibility, acceptability, and initial findings from a community-based cultural mental health intervention for American Indian Youth and their families. *Journal of Community Psychology*, *40*(4), 381–405. https://doi.org/10.1002/jcop.20517

Goodman, M. S., & Sanders Thompson, V. L. (2017). The science of stakeholder engagement in research: Classification, implementation, and evaluation. *Translational Behavioral Medicine*, *7*(3), 486–491. https://doi.org/10.1007/s13142-017-0495-z.

Hardeman, R. R., & Karbeah, J. (2020). Examining racism in health services research: A disciplinary self-critique. *Health Services Research*, *55*(Suppl. 2), 777–780. https://doi.org/10.1111/1475-6773.13558

Jones, L., Wells, K., Norris, K., Meade, B., & Koegel, P. (2009). Chapter 1. The vision, valley, and victory of community engagement. *Ethnicity & Disease*, *19*(4 Suppl. 6), S6-3–7.

Lyon, A. R., Cook, C. R., Locke, J.J., Davis, C., Powell, B. J., & Waltz, T.J. (2019). Importance and feasibility of an adapted set of implementation strategies in schools. *Journal of School Psychology*, *76*, 66–77. https://doi.org/10.1016/j.jsp.2019.07.014

Mance, G. A., Mendelson, T., III, B. B., Jones, J., & Tandon, D. (2010). Utilizing community-based participatory research to adapt a mental health intervention for African American emerging adults. *Progress in Community Health Partnerships: Research, Education, and Action*, *4*(2), 131–140. https://doi.org/10.1353/cpr.0.0112

Martinez, L. S., Carolan, K., O'Donnell, A., Diaz, Y., & Freeman, E. R. (2018). Community engagement in patient-centered outcomes research: Benefits, barriers, and measurement. *Journal of Clinical and Translational Science*, *2*, 371–376. https://doi.org/10.1017/cts.2018.341

McNulty, M., Smith, J. D., Villamar, J., Burnett-Zeigler, I., Vermeer, W., Benbow, N., Gallo, C., Wilensky, U., Hjorth, A., Mustanski, B., Schneider, J., & Brown, C. H. (2019). Implementation research methodologies for achieving scientific equity and health equity. *Ethnicity & Disease*, *29*(Suppl. 1), 83–92. https://doi.org/10.18865/ed.29.S1.83

Napoles, A. M., & Stewart, A. L. (2018). Transcreation: An implementation science framework for community-engaged behavioral interventions to reduce health disparities. *BMC Health Services Research*, *18*, 1–15. https://doi.org/10.1186/s12913-018-3521-z

Nelson, A. (2002). Unequal treatment: Confronting racial and ethnic disparities in health care. *Journal of the National Medical Association*, *94*(8), 666. https://doi.org/10.17226/12875

Newcombe, R. (2003). From client to project stakeholders: A stakeholder mapping approach. *Construction Management and Economics*, *21*(8), 841–848. https://doi.org/10.1080/0144619032000072137

Nuriddin, A., Mooney, G., & White, A. I. R. (2020). Reckoning with histories of medical racism and violence in the USA. *The Lancet*, *396*(10256), 949–951. https://doi.org/10.1016/S0140-6736(20)32032-8

Pellecchia, M., Mandell, D., Nuske, H., Azad, G., Wolk, C., Maddox, B., Reisinger, E., Skriner, L., Adams, D., Stewart, R., Hadley, T., & Beidas, R. (2018). Community-academic partnerships in implementation research. *Journal of Community Psychology*, *46*. https://doi.org/10.1002/jcop.21981

Powell, B. J., Waltz, T. J., Chinman, M. J., Damschroder, L. J., Smith, J. L., Matthieu, M. M., Proctor, E. K., & Kirchner, J. E. (2015). A refined compilation of implementation strategies: Results from the Expert Recommendations for Implementing Change (ERIC) project. *Implementation Science, 10*(1), 21. https://doi.org/10.1186/s13012-015-0209-1

Proctor, E., Silmere, H., Raghavan, R., Hovmand, P., Aarons, G., Bunger, A., Griffey, R., & Hensley, M. (2011). Outcomes for implementation research: Conceptual distinctions, measurement challenges, and research agenda. *Administration and Policy in Mental Health and Mental Health Services Research, 38*(2), 65–76. https://doi.org/10.1007/s10488-010-0319-7

Reed, M. S., Graves, A., Dandy, N., Posthumus, H., Hubacek, K., Morris, J., Prell, C., Quinn, C. H., & Stringer, L. C. (2009). Who's in and why? A typology of stakeholder analysis methods for natural resource management. *Journal of Environmental Management, 90*(5), 1933–1949. https://doi.org/10.1016/j.jenvman.2009.01.001

Schiller, C., Winters, M., Hanson, H. M., & Ashe, M. C. (2013). A framework for stakeholder identification in concept mapping and health research: A novel process and its application to older adult mobility and the built environment. *BMC Public Health, 13*(1), 428. https://doi.org/10.1186/1471-2458-13-428

Schmeer, K. (1999). *Guidelines for conducting a stakeholder analysis*. Partnerships for Health Reform, Abt Associates Inc.

Shelef, D. Q., Rand, C., Streisand, R., Horn, I. B., Yadav, K., Stewart, L., Fousheé, N., Waters, D., & Teach, S. J. (2016). Using stakeholder engagement to develop a patient-centered pediatric asthma intervention. *Journal of Allergy and Clinical Immunology, 138*, 1512–1517. https://doi.org/10.1016/j.jaci.2016.10.001

Skloot, R. (2017). *The immortal life of Henrietta Lacks*. Broadway Paperbacks.

Stewart, R. E., Mandell, D. S., & Beidas, R. S. (2021). Lessons from Maslow: Prioritizing funding to improve the quality of community mental health and substance use services. *Psychiatric Services*. https://doi.org/10.1176/appi.ps.202000209

Varvasovszky, Z., & Brugha, R. (2000). A stakeholder analysis. *Health Policy and Planning, 15*(3), 338–345. https://doi.org/10.1093/heapol/15.3.338

Walker, D. H. T., Bourne, L. M., & Shelley, A. (2008). Influence, stakeholder mapping and visualization. *Construction Management and Economics, 26*(6), 645–658. https://doi.org/10.1080/01446190701882390

Wallerstein, N. B., & Duran, B. (2006). Using community-based participatory research to address health disparities. *Health Promotion Practice, 7*(3), 312–323. https://doi.org/10.1177/1524839906289376

Waltz, T. J., Powell, B. J., Matthieu, M. M., Damschroder, L. J., Chinman, M. J., Smith, J. L., Proctor, E. K., & Kirchner, J. E. (2015). Use of concept mapping to characterize relationships among implementation strategies and assess their feasibility and importance: Results from the Expert Recommendations for Implementing Change (ERIC) study. *Implementation Science, 10*, 109. https://doi.org/10.1186/s13012-015-0295-0

Washington, H. A. (2006). *Medical apartheid: The dark history of medical experimentation on Black Americans from colonial times to the present*. Doubleday Books.

Woodward, E. N., Matthieu, M. M., Uchendu, U. S., Rogal, S., & Kirchner, J. E. (2019). The health equity implementation framework: Proposal and preliminary study of hepatitis C virus treatment. *Implementation Science, 14*(1), 26. https://doi.org/10.1186/s13012-019-0861-y

7

Creating a Structure for Implementation: Building Implementation Teams and Developing Implementation Plans

Kevin Fiori, Hueiming Liu, and Lisa R. Hirschhorn

Learning Objectives

By the end of this chapter, readers will be able to:

- Use implementation research principles to choose strategies to use for implementation, reflecting implementation determinants and targeted outcomes
- Develop an implementation team and plans to get ready to start implementation
- Plan how to monitor implementation to identify areas where adaptation is needed

CASE STUDY 7.1 EXPANDING HIV PRE-EXPOSURE PROPHYLAXIS FOR CISGENDER WOMEN OF COLOR IN THE UNITED STATES

In the United States, cisgender women of color remain at high risk for HIV but their uptake of pre-exposure prophylaxis (PrEP), an evidence-based biomedical prevention intervention, has been low. The team has done work to confirm that this is an effective evidence-based prevention intervention (EBI) for cisgender women. To design an implementation intervention, the team has done some formative work to understand determinants which may help or hinder these efforts. The team is excited to implement a program to address these barriers and expand PrEP uptake by this population, but what needs to be done next? Who should be working on the next steps? What strategies should be chosen to improve implementation of the EBI? How will the process monitor be monitored to identify where adaptations are needed?

INTRODUCTION

To move into and through creating a structure for implementation, the team will start by getting organized so that they can plan and create the structure for implementation. The work outlined builds on the preparation work already done. At this stage of developing the structure for implementation, the EBI to be put into action has already been identified, the determinants that can facilitate or hinder the work to get the EBI into practice have also been identified (e.g., based on the Consolidated Framework for Implementation Research or CFIR; Damschroder et al., 2009), and so it is time to get started planning for and doing the implementation. This chapter goes through steps on how to develop the plan, how to build the team to implement the EBI, and how to monitor implementation once started. The team will use concepts and tools of implementation research to link together the identified determinants with the strategies needed to achieve implementation outcomes (i.e., the desired result as the EBI is put into practice), clinical outcomes (i.e., the expected change the intervention will make on people who are receiving the EBI), and system outcomes (i.e., changes targeted at the clinic or broader care delivery system levels). Implementation outcomes could include uptake by people providing the intervention as planned (i.e., fidelity and adoption) to the right people (i.e., reach) or changes to the clinic or system (i.e., adoption, sustainability). See Box 7.1.

BOX 7.1 Implementing Telemedicine as a Strategy to Maintain HIV Care and Treatment During COVID-19

To illustrate the concepts and steps in this chapter, this section describes work done in a clinic in response to the COVID-19 pandemic to rapidly transition to telemedicine. This clinic project included changing many clinic visits from in-person to telemedicine visits (televisits) with their usual providers. The clinic was worried that providers and the patients would have some barriers to acceptability and feasibility of televisits. The clinic wanted to know what was needed to ensure that the televisits were effective and acceptable and that equity and quality of care were sustained.

GETTING ORGANIZED

The first step is to determine how to use all the important information that has been gathered through the formative work conducted prior to implementation. How will the team get the needed intervention into action and reach the targeted populations? Who will be responsible for which aspects of implementation? And how will the team know if things are happening as anticipated? This may seem overwhelming, but there are tools that can help.

One tool that may be helpful is a modification of a traditional **logic model**, a planning and evaluation tool frequently used to understand what is needed (inputs), what actions should be happening (activities), and how they link to targeted outcomes and longer term impact (W. K. Kellogg Foundation, 2004). Logic models have been used to help design implementation of projects, communicate the planned steps and goals, ensure required resources are available, and determine the methods for measuring progress from start to completion (Figure 7.1). However, logic models do not typically identify determinants that can either facilitate or serve as barriers to moving from the actions taken to the desired results. For example, training is assumed to result in the ability to complete a task correctly, but barriers such as missing supplies, insufficient guidelines needed to put the training content into practice, and prior assumptions that the barrier to implementation is lack of knowledge among trainees may all make training ineffective. Instead, what may actually be needed is motivation or authority to implement, which required different strategies such as incentives or peer support.

The **Implementation Research Logic Model (IRLM)** (Smith et al., 2020) builds on the traditional logic model by more explicitly linking implementation determinants to strategies, calling out the mechanisms through which they will work and identifying which outcomes (implementation and/or clinical and systems) are targeted (see Box 7.2). The model therefore helps to document what actions are planned and why when designing the implementation of the EBI. Start with the knowledge around the facilitators and barriers (called determinants), which may need to be leveraged or addressed, the strategies chosen to bolster implementation of the EBI, and the mechanisms through which these strategies will help to achieve the assigned goals. This IRLM can serve as a blueprint for what needs to be done, as a communication tool to explain how and why the EBI is implemented (what are the aims, and what does success look like in terms of implementation, individual clinical, and systems outcomes), as a guide for selecting implementation strategies, can inform the Monitoring, Evaluation and Learning plan (MEL, described later in the chapter), and can help identify areas where adaptations are needed.

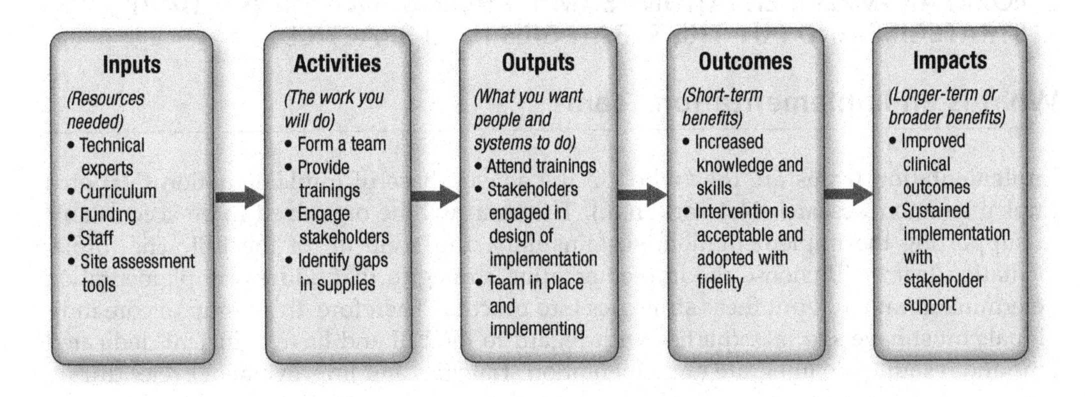

FIGURE 7.1 Example of a simplified logic model to improve delivery of an evidence-based intervention (EBI).

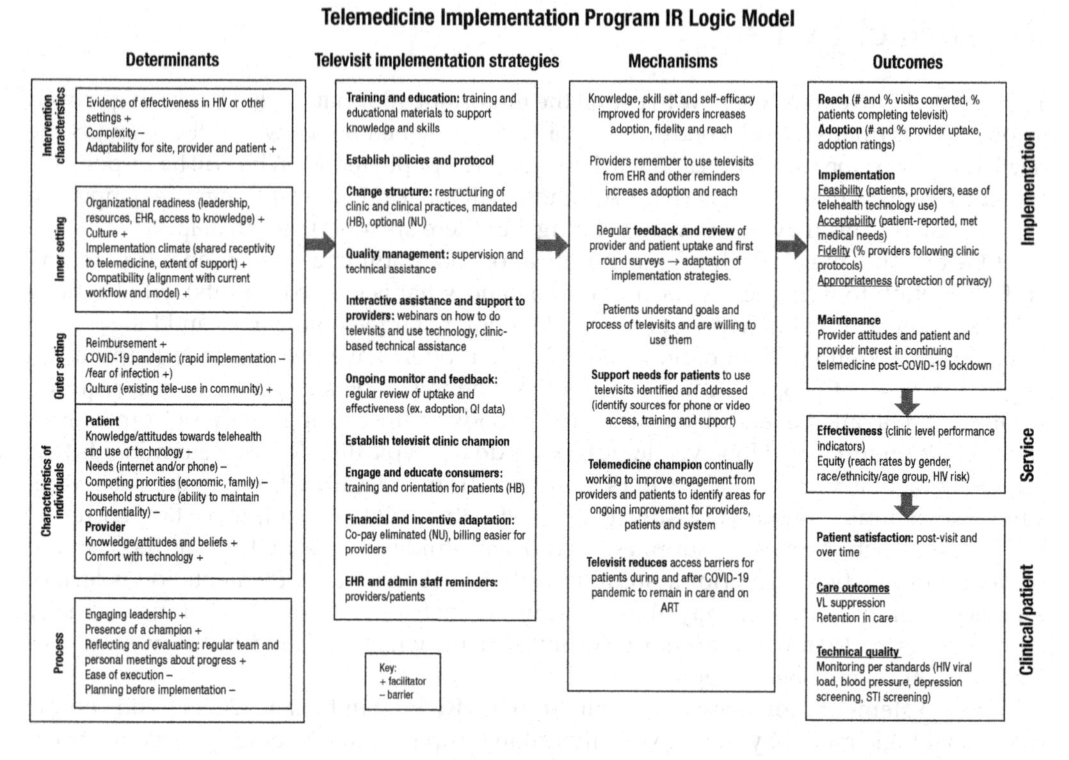

FIGURE 7.2 Example of an implementation research logic model developed for the case study of implementing telemedicine into an HIV clinic during the COVID-19 pandemic.

Figure 7.2 shows an IRLM developed as part of the work to understand the barriers and facilitators and strategies needed to ensure quality, equity, and effectiveness of televisits (C. Hawkins, personal communication).

But the intervention will not happen on its own, and after getting organized, the next steps are to develop a project team who can then specify implementation strategies, determine who will be doing which activities within the team, and specify how the team will know if things are working (or where change is needed).

FORM AN IMPLEMENTATION TEAM TO HELP CHOOSE AND ADAPT STRATEGIES AND PUT THE STRATEGIES INTO PRACTICE

What is an Implementation Team?

Implementation teams are the "who" in the active phase of implementation (National Implementation Research Network, n.d.). The team will be organized to be accountable in supporting the implementation, sustainability, and scale up of the EBI. The implementation team will choose the implementation strategies that address implementation determinants and will put these strategies into practice. Therefore, this group of core individuals must have special expertise with regard to the EBI and have sufficient dedicated time and resources to integrate implementation strategies and improvement cycles during

BOX 7.2 Key Terms Used in the Chapter

Logic Model: Road map that shows the relationships between the resources needed and used for a project or program that will be implemented (activities), predictions of what participants or systems will do (outputs), and the intended effects (outcomes and impacts).

Implementation Research Logic Model: Tool designed to support specifying the conceptual linkages between implementation determinants, implementation strategies and outcomes to increase the rigor and transparency of planning and describing work to better implement EBIs.

Determinants: Factors that might prevent (barriers) or enable (facilitators) implementation of the EBI.

Implementation Strategies: Approaches, techniques and/or methods that are utilized to improve uptake, delivery, and sustainment of EBIs.

Implementation Outcomes: Targeted results derived from the strategies to enhance implementation of an EBI. These are usually indicators of implementation processes, but can also include targeted service, clinical or other individual outcomes.

Examples of implementation outcomes include:

- *Fidelity:* Degree to which an intervention (or strategy) was implemented as planned or as explicitly adapted.
- *Reach (Coverage):* Amount of an intervention-eligible (targeted) population that actually receives the EBI.
- *Adoption:* Intention, initial decision, or action to deliver the EBI at the provider or organizational level.
- *Acceptability:* Opinion (or perception) among targeted populations that the EBI is agreeable and they are willing to use/accept it.
- *Sustainability (Maintenance):* Extent to which the EBI is maintained or institutionalized in a setting.

implementation. The implementation team will be accountable for implementation and will design and lead the implementation strategies across different organizational levels (e.g., state, regional, district, and clinic levels). Importantly, the implementation team is not an advisory group that provides periodic input; instead, they are actively involved on a daily basis in practical decisions and logistics necessary for effective and sustained implementation.

Why is an Implementation Team Needed and What Will it Do?

Implementation teams are essential to achieve desired outcomes using a proactive approach by "making it happen" rather than passively "letting it happen." In tracking outcomes of programs, EBIs are often not used in practice, or are sub-optimally implemented, with a significant time delay. In the experience of comprehensive school reforms in the United States, having implementation teams in place contributed to increased fidelity of the reform, with improved efficiency outcomes (National Implementation Research Network, n.d.). Indeed, implementation teams have become a best practice, as evident in how leading agencies for clinical innovation and heath research have implementation teams to support national rollout of innovations (Agency for Clinical Innovation, 2021).

Implementation teams have three key functions necessary to ensure effective implementation (National Implementation Research Network, n.d.) including: (a) ensure implementation through assessing organizational buy-in/readiness, sustaining implementation drivers, monitoring implementation fidelity, planning, and problem-solving; (b) engage the community to understand their needs, to share information, and co-design solutions to problems; and (c) create enabling environments within the implementation team's sphere of control such as workforce scheduling, professional development, and to work with other teams to address barriers outside the implementation team's sphere of control (e.g., financing structures) through established linkages and feedback systems. In the telemedicine example given earlier, there were many uncertainties with the model, and having a dedicated interdisciplinary implementation team enabled a nimble response to problem solve and enable effective communication with other staff, potentially leading to improved patient and system outcomes.

Identify the Implementation Team

The composition of the implementation team will impact operational decision-making and the overall effectiveness of the implementation and requires careful consideration. Box 7.3 identifies key questions to consider when identifying implementation team members and forming the implementation team. In the example of transitioning to the use of telemedicine in clinics during the COVID pandemic, when forming the implementation team at the clinic level, team members should include individuals who have the clinical expertise, project and workforce management capabilities, information and communication technology knowledge, experience in telemedicine, and a deep understanding of what systems would have to be in place to implement the change in practice. These could potentially be senior nurse unit managers, clinicians from the hospital and the community, community stakeholders, information technology staff, and the district manager/director.

BOX 7.3 Key Questions to Consider in Convening the Implementation Team

- Who will have organizational responsibility for implementation? Identify three to five key individuals to do so.
- Do these individuals have sufficient expertise, knowledge of the innovation, and ability to support front-line workers who are delivering the innovation?
- Do these individuals have adequate capacity (time and resources) to allocate to implementation activities?
- What will be the roles, processes and responsibilities of these team members?
- Do they/can they work well together (e.g., team dynamics based on previous working relationships, personality types, leadership, and, underlying respect of each other's expertise, and team effectiveness)?

An implementation team is usually multidisciplinary, representing different areas of the organization or across organizations involved in implementation. These key stakeholders on the team must be directly involved in the implementation (particularly front-line workers), but the team also needs a diverse set of people with different skills, perspectives, and authority to ensure implementation. Considering the telemedicine example, the implementation team should include administrators or managerial staff who will have influence on implementation, such as access to resources, and have the authority to facilitate adaptation and implementation of strategies that require broader systems-level change. In addition, the team should include data managers who can help with ongoing monitoring and evaluation, as well as data feedback to improve implementation. Other key individuals include champions who are particularly enthusiastic or well-positioned to move implementation forward (such as well-regarded clinical leaders who can demonstrate adoption of telemedicine and address reservations of the quality of care as compared to face-to-face patient care). The strength of the team's composition is in having complementary skills and perspectives, and having an enabling structure with subgroups if there are linked implementation teams across multiple levels (whether within an organization or more broadly such as city, district, and regional levels). For example, for the telemedicine project, some implementation team members would include HIV primary providers, clinic nurses, and other providers, clinic administration including individuals working on reimbursement, and clinic IT staff. In addition, determining how to engage with the targeted population to solicit their input, either directly as part of the team or through an ongoing co-design process, is also important.

Stakeholder mapping can help identify who can help diagnose implementation needs, formulate site-specific implementation strategies, and put them into action. This work can also help identify key champions who can help keep implementation moving forward and opinion leaders who are often important gatekeepers to the adoption of the EBI. In the telemedicine example, other stakeholders besides those on the implementation team may include family physicians and outreach community nurses who may visit patients in the community.

What Tools Can Be Used to Optimize Team Dynamics and Build Effective Teams?

Team dynamics must be taken into account during team selection as it sets the foundation for a well-functioning team. Team dynamics are reliant on mechanisms such as respect and trust, a common mandate, clear communication, and more. These dynamics are especially relevant in interdisciplinary teams, to acknowledge the different skillsets of individuals that are necessary, and to ensure that all contributions are equally valued regardless of position within organizations or across organizations with external stakeholders. For example, perspectives offered by the junior clinician in a team may be as important as the director of an organization, and the statistician on a team is equally important as the qualitative researcher. Accounting for team dynamics requires careful facilitation during team meetings, ensuring open and respectful communication and engaging leaders skilled in conflict resolution. For global health or cross-cultural projects, careful understanding of cultural norms and expectations is another important consideration and includes consideration of seating arrangements in meetings and the use of titles when introducing individuals. Frequently, regularly engaging a cultural mentor or other trusted source to get nuanced advice is beneficial.

After team members have been identified, the team must be built, which includes having clearly defined roles and responsibilities as well as defined processes through which the team will function. This work is important given the diverse backgrounds (cultural, roles, and disciplines) of the team members, especially in international collaborations. This is at times complicated by funding arrangements, such as development aid for resource-poor settings, which comes with an inherent power structure. Therefore, including time, resources, and opportunities for relationship building (such as workshops and opportunities for social interactions) is required. Some other useful structured approaches and tools that can help build teams include:

1. Using a strength-based approach in the allocation of roles, processes and responsibilities to individuals who would be related to the implementation strategies selected. A strength-based approach means to focus and maximize an individual's strengths (e.g., community engagement or project management) that would enable the team members to work synergistically at individual team members' best capacity. There should also be a focus on utilizing team members capacity to solve problems together, rather than focusing on the problem (e.g., lack of clinical know-how), which separates the problem from the person. (State Government of Victoria, 2012, p. 6)
2. Team building modules, such as NuPITA prepared by the United States Agency for International Development (2012), can help organizations and their teams understand and build a high-functioning team. This interactive short-course, to be delivered by a facilitator, outlines what is needed for a team-building workshop and uses case studies, role plays, group discussion, and individual reflection to support team development.
3. The use of operational tools can help build teams. This includes a team charter documenting goals and ethos of the team at the start, which facilitates clear expectations of how everyone on the team can work toward a common vision. Team charters include expectations of leadership (e.g., opportunities to chair meetings), communication mode and frequency, and working norms (e.g., deadlines; University of Otagi, n.d.; University of Washington, 2011). Additionally, teaming agreements developed from the start that outline a conflict resolution process provide a reference for team members to refer back to during times of conflict when emotions may affect decision-making processes (e.g., having a designated third-party arbitrator). Finally, responsibility agreement matrices that outline levels of agency and decision-making power among individual team members for specific tasks (Responsible, Accountable, Consulted, Informed) can enable implementation in the face of ongoing service delivery, limited resources, and competing priorities (Santos, 2021). Tools that help clearly delineate roles and responsibilities are helpful for all teams, and are particularly useful for task shifting approaches where there may be overlap of roles and/or a shift in expectations from before. For example, in the telemedicine model, the overlap occurs as community practitioners may be required to prescribe medications, do a physical exam, and discuss the findings with the specialist who would traditionally provide care in a face-to-face consultation model.

As implementation is a social process, the assignation of roles and responsibilities of the implementation team and addressing team dynamics must take into account the organizational culture. The implementation team's effectiveness will depend on the organizational readiness to adopt a new intervention. In the telemedicine example, the implementation team's effectiveness to meet their designated roles and responsibilities to adapt IT requirements and build infrastructure to facilitate telehealth will be shaped by senior leadership's underlying confidence in or reservations about the quality of care that can be delivered through telemedicine, and the organization's financing structures. Depending on the potential barriers, different implementation team members may be required (e.g., having a senior manager advocate for budgeting requirements and hiring more IT staff to support the telemedicine model of care). Structured tools to assess organizational readiness include the **Checklist Assess Organizational Readiness (CARI) for Evidence-Based Implementation** (Berwick, 2011) to assess domains of system, organizational, staff capacities, functional considerations, organizational culture, senior leadership, and the implementation plan. The use of the CARI tool can enable the implementation team to systematically identify areas of concern, and workshop potential solutions (e.g., gaining the support of managerial sponsorship).

Optimizing the implementation team's performance and effectiveness is a deliberate process to strategically use available resources. For example, the *Team Strategies and Tools to Enhance Performance and Patient Safety (TeamSTEPPS) tool* developed by the Agency for Healthcare Research and Quality provides a training approach to enhance team members' knowledge, attitudes, and performance for quality patient care, while embracing key principles of team structure, communication, leadership, situation monitoring, and mutual support. In the case study of the telehealth medicine model, using TeamSTEPPS can ensure that the implementation team supports front-line clinicians to provide high-quality care through a new telemedicine platform, with everyone having a shared understanding of the aim of the change to implement, as well as their roles and responsibilities in making this change. The work will be further supported with ongoing monitoring and adaption throughout implementation. See Table 7.1.

TABLE 7.1 Examples of Resources to Support Team Building

Team Building Module—Facilitator's Guide (NuPITA, USAID)	This tool, developed for use in lower-resourced settings, outlines what is needed for team-building workshop that will help organizations and their teams understand and build a high-functioning team	https://www.usaid.gov/sites/default/files/documents/1864/Team-Building-Module-Facilitators-Guide.pdf
TeamSTEPPS: Team Strategies and Tools to Enhance Performance and Patient Safety (AHRQ)	TeamSTEPPS is a health care-based training system to create effectively functioning teams. This tool contains brief explanations of key strategies and tools which can used by teams for functions such as communication and leadership	https://www.ahrq.gov/sites/default/files/publications/files/pocketguide.pdf

SELECTING AND DEFINING IMPLEMENTATION STRATEGIES AND OUTCOMES

At this point, the newly constructed team has identified an opportunity and now work can begin to fill a gap in clinical practice or service delivery either from a new EBI or by addressing gaps in delivery of a previously implemented EBI. There have been brainstorming sessions about potential EBIs that have demonstrated efficacy and/or effectiveness in randomized controlled trials that would be relevant to an organization's or health system's gap or to understanding gaps in delivery of existing interventions. There are still several considerations before simply implementing a new EBI or making adaptations of existing interventions in practice that the team needs to develop. First, the EBI that the team identified has likely been implemented in either a controlled setting, like a randomized controlled trial, and/or a setting that is distinct from this case and may require adaption for the organization or health system's context.

Previously, the team should have identified determinants, the enabling and facilitating factors to implementation that affect how and whether the EBI is accepted, delivered with fidelity, sustained, and ultimately whether it is effective in improving health outcomes. At this stage the team needs to consider how these determinants can be leveraged or addressed through implementation strategies, or the "how to" of implementing an EBI in practice. Linking these determinants to the choice of implementation strategies, based on an understanding of the mechanisms through which the strategies will help to achieve the specified goals, can maximize the potential impact of EBIs (Lewis et al., 2018; Waltz et al., 2015). There are two steps to consider in this process.

First, identify the determinants that may help or hinder the implementation (sometimes called contextual factors). These either need to be directly addressed by team strategies or inform which strategies the team chooses and can influence how well the team is able to implement the strategies and the EBI to achieve those goals. For example, in the telemedicine improvement case, the IRLM helped identify important determinants such as internet access among patients, comfort with doing telehealth calls among providers, and reimbursement processes—all of which needed to be addressed through strategies for the intervention to be implemented or be effective (Figure 7.2).

Second, identify the strategies needed to address the identified determinants and put the intervention into practice, and explain how these strategies will work (describe the mechanisms of action). For example, in the telemedicine case, the IRLM helped understand which strategies were needed to address the identified determinants, such as adapting the approach for patients without internet access, training providers on use of the telemedicine platform and confidentiality procedures, and negotiating with payors to facilitate reimbursement. Each of these strategies work to address potential barriers and to increase adoption (e.g., better knowledge and attitudes), acceptability (e.g., technology-appropriate contacts), and sustainability (e.g., reimbursement).

What Is the Difference Between an Evidence-Based Intervention and an Implementation Strategy?

It is important to note the difference between an EBI and the implementation strategies that the team will utilize. A simplified way to think about the EBI is the practice (or "thing") that the team wants people to do or the system to deliver. They are typically programs, practices, principles, procedures, products, pills, and policies (Brown et al., 2017). **Implementation strategies** are the methods or techniques used by a program or clinical team to support the adoption, integration, and sustainability of an EBI in practice. A team may need to include more than one strategy to successfully address multiple determinants. For example, routine vaccination is a key EBI for preventing infectious disease, especially among young children. To improve the effectiveness of this EBI in a rural West African community, a team may include implementation strategies such as stakeholder engagement through working with local opinion leaders like village chiefs, school teachers, and religious leaders; or to increase community knowledge on vaccines through a series of community forums on the importance of vaccinations. A third strategy might involve a new medical record system that automatically identifies children who are behind in their vaccinations and prompts follow-up. These strategies all target improving vaccination uptake, but may have distinct mechanisms that foster acceptability, adoption, and sustainability of the EBI. More information is given in the following about the process of identifying implementation strategies to reflect the determinants and some tips for defining them.

Why Do Implementation Strategies Need To Be Identified For Use In Getting an EBI into Practice or Improving the Delivery of an Existing EBI?

To date there has been ambiguity around how to translate EBIs into real world practice, a gap that implementation science is designed to fill. How an intervention got into practice and why it worked (or did not) is usually an afterthought or secondary aim whether the EBI was effective, which is why a team needs to identify and deploy implementation strategies. The overarching value of these strategies is that they are the ways in which EBI implementation, uptake, and acceptability can be improved. In addition, well-planned and specified implementation strategies contribute to both internal learning for maintaining the ingredients for success (by explaining how success was achieved) as well as informing future work on scaling up the EBI. Strategies are generally not well-described, have inconsistencies in terminology with a lack of precision, and lack adequate detail to inform replication or scale efforts. The vagueness or "black box" around describing implementation strategies continues to serve as a barrier to learning about and disseminating key "how-to" guidance for further implementation. Fortunately, there have been several recent initiatives to provide guidance on both specifying and reporting implementation strategies, as well as important consensus work around terminology. The result of one consensus project, the Expert Recommendation for Implementation Change (ERIC) compilation, includes a standard list and nomenclature of 73 strategies that can be organized in nine conceptual areas (Perry et al., 2019; Powell et al., 2015; Table 7.2). For example, an implementation strategy that works to engage consumers would include the ERIC strategies like *involve patients/consumers, prepare patient/consumers to be active participants*, and *increase demand*.

TABLE 7.2 Nine Conceptual Areas of Implementation Strategies

NINE CONCEPTUAL AREAS	ERIC IMPLEMENTATION STRATEGY EXAMPLE
1. Use evaluative and iterative strategies	Audit and provide feedback
2. Provide interactive assistance	Provide local technical assistance
3. Adapt and tailor to context	Promote adaptability
4. Develop stakeholder interrelationships	Identify and prepare champions
5. Train and educate stakeholders	Conduct ongoing training
6. Support clinicians	Facilitate relay of clinical data to providers
7. Engage consumers	Involve patients/consumers and family members
8. Utilize financial strategies	Access new funding
9. Change infrastructure	Change record systems

Sources: From Powell, B. J., Waltz, T. J., Chinman, M. J., Damschroder, L. J., Smith, J. L., Matthieu, M. M., Proctor, E. K., & Kirchner, J. A. E. (2015). A refined compilation of implementation strategies: Results from the Expert Recommendations for Implementing Change (ERIC) project. *Implementation Science, 10*(1), 1–14. https://doi.org/10.1186/s13012-015-0209-1; Waltz, T. J., Powell, B. J., Matthieu, M. M., Damschroder, L. J., Chinman, M. J., Smith, J. L., Proctor, E. K., & Kirchner, J. A. E. (2015). Use of concept mapping to characterize relationships among implementation strategies and assess their feasibility and importance: Results from the Expert Recommendations for Implementing Change (ERIC) study. *Implementation Science, 10*(1), 1–8. https://doi.org/10.1186/s13012-015-0295-0.

How Are Implementation Strategies Identified?

The team will need to think through how to identify, prioritize, and select strategies based on the identified determinants of implementation. The team may have had informal brainstorming sessions, planning meetings, and/or conducted a formative evaluation to understand the challenges of translating a chosen EBI in the practice context. One approach is to use identified determinants (i.e., facilitators and barriers) to map to specific implementation strategies. For example, some strategies may address a clear barrier such as a lack of training or competency gap. In contrast, some strategies may aim to enhance or leverage an enabling factor such as cohesive team structure, good data infrastructure, or influential leadership within the organization. One concrete approach that may be useful is **implementation mapping**, which is a multi-step process that includes (a) identifying determinants that need to be addressed with a strategy and what change is needed, (b) describing potential mechanisms of change and which implementation strategies could be used, and (c) prioritizing strategies based on team/organizational input or pilot data as well as feasibility. Mapping tools are currently being developed to match potential strategies that address determinants, organized by relevant domains of the CFIR (Lewis et al., 2018). This process of implementation mapping can take time (though it is worth the investment), and will require that the team prioritizes addressing determinants with strategies that are practical given feasibility, acceptability, cost, and sustainment considerations. The team may consider utilizing tools such as a prioritization matrix to help inform discussions and organize this overall process.

How Are Implementation Strategies Named, Specified, and Described?

Once a team has chosen its implementation strategy or strategies, it is important to provide further details by naming, specifying and planning the strategies (Proctor et al., 2013). The rationale behind this approach is to be sure that the team has consensus on what is being done, with whom, and at what frequency. If the team chooses to utilize an established taxonomy like ERIC to name implementation strategies (Powell et al., 2015), it is still important to go through this process as those terms may not quite fit and/or need some adaptation. Using a process developed by Proctor and summarized in Box 7.4 will provide a roadmap that fosters precision and refinement on what the team is planning to do (the "how-to"). This includes detailing the individual strategies by naming and describing them, as well as defining how they will be operationalized (who will do it, what will they be doing, who or what is the target, how often it will be done, when and with what dose). The team will also want to identify which implementation outcomes are expected to see change (e.g., change in provider behavior for adoption or fidelity, or increased acceptability of the EBI for clients), and ideally why the strategy was chosen (i.e., detailing the mechanism of action). Key considerations adapted from a landmark article on detailing strategies (Proctor et al., 2013) include:

1. *Name:* Name the strategy. It can be helpful to start with existing terms from compilations like ERIC, but these may need to be adapted to reflect the terminology familiar with the team setting or strategies which fall outside this list.
2. *Define:* Describe what the strategy involves so that the team and stakeholders know what is planned. This can also help others who may want to learn from this experience understand what is being done.
3. *Specify:* Identify the key components of the strategy including actors, actions, action target, when the strategy is used, dose, outcomes to be affected, and rationale for why this strategy was selected.

In the telemedicine example, one strategy used was audit and feedback, reflecting a mechanism (the belief on why this strategy is important and will help achieve the set goals) that providers will respond to data on how well they are performing in implementing clinical guidelines relative to their peers, and that clinic managers would use the results to identify champions (early and strong adopters) and those for whom additional support is needed. This strategy was also chosen to address issues of equity by monitoring which patients were being offered and able to participate in telemedicine and which were not, in order to identify moderating factors to inform further adaptations of the other strategy components or selection of new strategies to implement. This process is critical for working within teams and organizations and advancing learning across context and health systems.

BOX 7.4 Defining an Audit and Feedback Implementation Strategy for Telemedicine

Strategy Name: Audit and feedback

Strategy Definition: Regular reports were generated on televisit use and shared within the clinic to provide feedback on uptake and reach and to inform discussion where success was happening (high rates of televisits) and where additional support or adaptations were needed (e.g., identifying visits where telemedicine is not felt to be appropriate, patients who may need additional support to complete a televisit, and providers who may need additional coaching)

Actors: Clinic manager

Actions: Provide feedback on different rates of televisit use by provider and patients (preferably disaggregated by key demographic variables such as race/ethnicity, age, and gender)

Action Target: Providers

When Used: Monthly, sent to providers and discussed in clinic meetings (for overall rates)

Dose: Monthly

Outcomes Affected: Adoption, feasibility, acceptability, equity

Rationale (Mechanism): Identify where adaptation or new strategies are needed, remind providers to offer televisits, identify champions to serve as peer mentors for other providers

Choosing and Defining Outcomes

The third step is to identify which outcomes at the implementation, individual, and service levels will be prioritized and targeted by the chosen strategies and how they will be measured. Implementation outcomes include reach (i.e., amount of delivery to the targeted population), fidelity (i.e., the degree to which an EBI is implemented as prescribed in the initial testing or as intended), adoption (i.e., the number, proportion, and representativeness of settings and intervention agents willing to initiate an EBI), acceptability (i.e., the perception among implementation stakeholders that an EBI is agreeable, palatable, or satisfactory), and sustainability (i.e., after a defined period of time, the EBI continues to be delivered and/or individual behavior change is maintained). For example, outcomes from the telemedicine project included Reach (i.e., proportion of eligible patients offered a televisit), Adoption (i.e., proportion of providers offering and delivering telemedicine visits), Acceptability (i.e., proportion of patients who were offered a visit who accepted), and Fidelity (i.e., proportion of televisits that were conducted according to clinic guidelines).

OPERATIONALIZING, MONITORING, AND ADAPTING THE EBI AND IMPLEMENTATION STRATEGIES THROUGH IMPLEMENTATION PLANS

Developing an Implementation Plan

Now that the team is in place, along with the strategies that will help get the intervention into practice, an implementation plan is required to get started. A successful implementation plan will draw from effective program management, adaptive management, and iterative learning, and will enable the team to use their results to inform whether the strategies selected were the right choice, are being done as planned, and quickly identify any surprises (good or bad) which may be emerging. This step may feel familiar, as its core concepts are shared with effective principles of program and project planning and their management. Teams may already have project planning software in use which can help with this step.

The implementation plan should map out the specific steps and responsible individuals or groups needed to put the strategies into place, monitor their implementation (i.e., fidelity and timeliness), and track progress toward the goals (i.e., bringing IRLM to life and staying on track). The plan will also help identify additional resources that are needed and for what, and serves as an organizing and communication tool for the team and broader organization to support coordination and build internal stakeholder engagement and ownership.

There is no one-size-fits all approach to developing an implementation plan, but much of the work will have already been done by defining the team, identifying and specifying the strategies, then identifying the goals. Resources also need to be identified (e.g., financial, time, equipment) that will be needed (which may also be one of the strategies). The IRLM or other implementation blueprints (e.g., logic model, including a list of the strategies and targeted outcomes) can help identify resource needs. Table 7.3 provides an example of an implementation plan that encompasses planning and tracking the progress of the telemedicine implementation. The *Workplan Template* by tools4dev is licensed under a Creative Commons Attribution-ShareAlike 3.0 Unported License

(https://www.tools4dev.org/resources/work-plan-template/).

TABLE 7.3 Example of a Workplan for Monitoring and Evaluation of the Implementation of a Telemedicine Project

Task	Responsible	Status	Year 1				Year 2			
			Q1	Q2	Q3	Q4	Q1	Q2	Q3	Q4
Study preparation										
Develop survey for patients	Pis	Not started								
Develop survey for providers	Pis	Not started								
Develop KII	Qualitative researcher	Not started								
IRB										
Protocol	Pis	Not started								
Submit	RA	Not started								
Prepare request for EMR data	RA	Not started								
Engage stakeholders	Pis	Not started								
Data collection										
Administer survey to patients	RA	Not started								
Administer survey to providers	RA	Not started								
Conduct KIIs	Qualitative researcher	Not started								
Extract EMR data	RA	Not started								
Data analysis										
Analyze surveys	Statistician	Not started								
Analyze KIIs	Qualitative researcher	Not started								
Analyze EMR	Statistician	Not started								
Mixed methods analysis	Pis	Not started								
Dissemination and learning										
Ongoing stakeholder engagement	Pis	Not started								
Feedback to clinic	Pis	Not started								
Publications	Pis	Not started								

Developing a Monitoring, Evaluation, and Learning Plan

The next step is to develop a **Monitoring, Evaluation, and Learning (MEL) plan**, which is a tool that improves overall project performance by helping implementation teams identify where they will need to measure the process of implementation, including what is working or being done and what is not. A MEL plan includes the following three components:

1. Monitoring: How implementation teams know that implementation is happening as planned.
2. Evaluation: How implementation teams know that the outcomes are being reached (and why or why not).
3. Learning: What needs to be adapted if off course, and what lessons learned should be used for implementation in other settings.

Key components of a MEL plan typically include:

1. A plan for how the team will monitor implementation, including indicator measures of activities, outputs, and outcomes. These should be **SMART: Specific, Measurable, Achievable, Relevant, and Timebound) indicators** (see Box 7.5; Kadam, 2021).
2. What evaluations are being planned.
3. When and how these data will be used to identify successes for celebrating and sharing, and emerging barriers which may require change in or new strategies (learning).
4. The resources for these MEL activities.
5. Roles and responsibilities for all proposed MEL actions (accountability).

BOX 7.5 Definitions and Examples of SMART Indicators

SMART indicators are those that are:

- Specific: Defined and understood clearly and measure the targeted area.
- Measurable: Able to be measured reliably and at the level of disaggregation needed given the resources and systems.
- Achievable: Measures an area and target that can be achieved during the project if implemented as planned.
- Relevant: Measures the process of how to implement the EBI or related outcomes, and is reflected in the overall framework (logic model or IRLM, for example).
- Timebound: Describes the time over which the indicators will be measured (e.g., last 30 days, last 6 months).

The details in developing an MEL plan are beyond the scope of this chapter, but some excellent resources are available online (see Table 7.4).

Some of the indicators may have already been identified in the IRLM, detailed strategies, and the identification of relevant implementation outcomes. For example, in the telemedicine project, SMART indicators include: (a) the percent of patients due for a visit

TABLE 7.4 Examples of Resources to Develop a Monitoring, Evaluation and Learning Plan

Monitoring Toolkit: Activity Monitoring, Evaluation, and Learning Plan Template (USAID)	Brief description of the components of an MEL plan following USAID's guidance. This would need to be adapted but is a good resource	https://usaidlearninglab.org/library/activity-monitoring%2C-evaluation%2C-and-learning-plan-template
How to develop an M and E Plan (COMPASS)	Clear description of the steps to create a monitoring and evaluation plan, building from earlier work including developing a logic model. Includes templates for indicators (which can be useful in the work described in the following), although is less specific about the data use/learning steps	https://www.thecompassforsbc.org/how-to-guides/how-develop-monitoring-and-evaluation-plan
Monitoring and evaluation (M&E) plan for NGOs (Toladata)	Practical description of the steps to develop and the components of an M&E plan	https://www.toladata.com/blog/monitoring-and-evaluation-plan/

who are offered a televisit in the last month, both overall and disaggregated by race/ethnicity (Reach and Equity); and (b) the percent of providers who conduct at least one televisit in the last month (Adoption). Notably, the MEL plan may need to be revised in response to changes in the activity or new or changing determinants that occur during the implementation.

Understanding Whether Changes Are Needed in the EBI or Strategies

It also is important to capture adaptations made during implementation and why these changes were made. For example, if training is not effective, how does the strategy need to change (such as moving to a more action-oriented training, or changing the duration and timing)? One framework that has been developed to offer guidance in documenting adaptations to interventions (FRAME; Stirman et al., 2019) or strategies (FRAME-IS; Miller et al., 2021) may be useful for implementation teams. Using these frameworks helps to document what change was made, why, by whom, and which implementation outcome(s) are targeted. Gathering this information ensures that the implementation team knows what was done, understands what worked to help successfully implement the EBI, can identify what helps sustain EBIs, and when efforts are successful can use this information to inform efforts to implement the EBI in new settings. In the telemedicine example, if it is identified that specific populations are not being reached (e.g., an older population), the implementation team may want to adapt the consumer education strategy to call those individuals who have not had a televisit in the last 3 months to understand potential barriers which may need attention (such as access to videoconference technology).

CASE STUDY 7.2 IMPLEMENTING EBIS TO REDUCE UNDER-5 MORTALITY THROUGH COMMUNITY-BASED PRIMARY CARE IN RURAL TOGO

An international, non-governmental organization works in partnership with communities to make quality primary healthcare accessible to all. Since 2004, this organization has worked closely with the government of Togo to identify gaps in healthcare delivery and develop community-based solutions to address these gaps. As part of this approach, the organization strives to be a learning organization, embedding data and pragmatic research within its programs.

In 2014, after the organization had worked for a decade to implement ambulatory HIV/AIDS services, their government partner asked the organization to develop a primary care model that focused on maternal and pediatric healthcare, specifically using the integrated management of childhood illness guidelines. It was felt that the leading causes of premature mortality in this nation at that time could be addressed by this EBI that focuses on improving quality and increasing access to maternal and childhood illness services. The government proposed a partnership starting with four village health centers. The organization started by conducting informational community forums for all locations. Initial meetings with community members revealed interest and motivation for promoting well-being of children and improving birth outcomes.

However, it was also noted that health center staffing was inadequate, with an undertrained workforce, working in facilities without supplies and infrastructure, and with a majority of the community living in extreme poverty. The national health system had a user fee/pay-for-service model that even at subsidized rates was challenging for families to access services. Providers noticed that families often presented to health clinics at a later stage of illness (e.g., with pneumonia), that could have been addressed more effectively if treated earlier. The goal moving forward was to increase access to and quality of EBIs, specifically the integrated management of child illness, into both community and village health centers.

The organization put together a multidisciplinary team that included internal staff from programs, monitoring and evaluation, research team members, and partners from the Ministry of Health. This team worked to refine the intervention elements, develop implementation strategies, and plan timelines for both implementation and evaluation. Engaging stakeholders, they identified specific determinants that might be barriers (inadequate staffing, insufficient training and support, and user fees) and facilitators (community motivation and buy-in and government partnership). Mapping these determinants to strategies through understanding the mechanisms, they choose a number of these. Examples include:

1. *Alter patient fees:* To address barriers related to poverty, user fees for children under 5 and pregnant women (including costs of delivering at a health facility) were eliminated. *Mechanism:* It is possible that by addressing this financial barrier to care families would present more frequently and earlier in the disease course, thus promoting better outcomes and preventing severe disease.
2. *Conduct education outreach and local consensus discussions:* Team members continued meeting with community members and leaders to foster ongoing engagement. *Mechanism:* By continuing to engage community members, the EBI is more likely to be fully integrated. Feedback that informs adaptation and improvement cycles increases the likelihood that the EBI is sustained.

(continued)

CASE STUDY 7.2 IMPLEMENTING EBIS TO REDUCE UNDER-5 MORTALITY THROUGH COMMUNITY-BASED PRIMARY CARE IN RURAL TOGO (*continued*)

3. *Conduct ongoing training and clinical supervision:* This approach included mentorship and enhanced supervision for clinical teams including community health workers. *Mechanism:* Continuous coaching and supervision will address gaps in knowledge and provide accountability and ongoing learning to improve service delivery.

Once consensus was reached around these strategies, the organization put together a monitoring, evaluation, and data use plan and got started.

SUMMARY

Strategically preparing to implement will set teams up for success as they work to get their intervention into practice with fidelity and to reach their targeted populations. This chapter explored the critical steps needed including understanding the determinants of implementation and choosing strategies relevant to these determinants, forming and supporting the team responsible for the work, and giving them the tools such as an implementation plan and MEL plan. The work to support implementation does not end when implementation begins but will require the team to continue to learn what is working or not, why not, and where adaptation is needed. The preparation described in this chapter is needed because implementing interventions is rarely a straight-line journey. Planning, evaluating, and adapting are essential to achieving the outcomes and impact that are envisioned for the implementation.

KEY POINTS FOR PRACTICE

1. Carefully select the implementation team ensuring that key actors with complementary expertise, content knowledge, and sphere of influence are included. Use strength-based approaches and operational tools such as team charters to help establish roles and responsibilities, facilitate a common vision to optimize an effective and dynamic implementation team.
2. An effective implementation team will work synergistically to choose, implement, and evaluate the implementation strategies believed to best engage the community, ensure implementation success, and create an enabling environment for implementation.
3. Engage stakeholders and when needed provide the training to understand the concepts of determinants, strategy mapping, and implementation outcomes. This work may take time but is critical in developing a good implementation plan and MEL plan, and will also allow for more effective adaptation through creating a culture of learning.
4. Distinguish between the evidence-based intervention (EBI) and the implementation strategies that will be used to foster effective uptake of that EBI. The EBI has been demonstrated to be efficacious, so it is critical to focus on effective implementation

which may require multiple strategies that will be influenced by the context and key determinants.

5. Be prepared to adapt the strategies and even the EBIs based on emerging lessons but be sure that these adaptations are done through discussion and are documented and evaluated. By doing so, determinants that drove the changes will be clear and will be able to inform implementation in new settings with similar or different determinants.
6. The development of good implementation plans and MEL plans will ensure that when the team gets started, there will be agreement on what is planned, who is responsible, and an accepted timeline for accountability. There are some great examples online for those who have never done this.

COMMON PITFALLS IN PRACTICE

1. In developing a team, too many people are chosen so as not to offend anyone, so that the team is unable to collaborate effectively.
2. Sometimes key individuals are not included in implementation teams (e.g., leaders or consumers) as there is a sense that it takes too much time. Without these people with key insights and ability to help identify determinants and inform strategies, the plan may not be fully developed and will be less likely to succeed.
3. The implementation team will inadvertently face system challenges and have to think creatively and nimbly to address problems. However, this process can be stressful, with different members having different expectations and perspectives that could lead to conflict. It will be helpful to have conflict resolution processes and strength-based approaches in place (focusing on the problem rather than individuals involved).
4. Understanding determinants and mapping to strategies can take time. But if this is not done carefully, strategies may not reflect barriers or leverage facilitators, either of which will make the implementation less efficient and less effective.
5. There is often a tendency to choose too many indicators to make sure nothing is missed or to include something that might be of interest later. Too many indicators can translate into too many resources being used for measurement and not for reviewing and feedback. In addition, there may be not enough time to define the indicators and make sure they are SMART, leading to problems with quality of the data and values for monitoring evaluation and learning.
6. Implementation strategies are often poorly defined and described or confused with the components of the actual EBI. It is important to use a process to describe in adequate detail how the strategies will be used in order to facilitate learning and knowledge dissemination about the implementation strategies.

DISCUSSION QUESTIONS

1. What are key steps in choosing, building, and supporting a team who will implement the EBI to put into practice (or from one of the case studies)?
2. How determinants be linked that influence the implementation with the implementation strategies? What would be an example of a barrier encountered in a planned project or in Case Study 7.2 ?
3. What are three ways in which using the IRLM can help to plan for implementation and measurement?

4. Why might an implementation strategy need to be adapted and what information should be captured? Who should be involved and how should feedback be provided?
5. Why are MEL plans useful? Describe some SMART indicators that might help monitor the case study organization's implementation. Why is it important for the indicators to be SMART?

REFERENCES

Agency for Clinical Innovation. (2021). *Implementation support*. https://aci.health.nsw.gov.au/make-it-happen/implementation-support

Berwick, M. (2011). *Checklist to Assess Organizational Readiness (CARI) for EIP implementation*. http://melaniebarwick.com/wp-content/uploads/2019/01/CARI-Checklist_for_Assessing_Readiness_for_Implementation-BARWICK.pdf

Brown, C. H., Curran, G., Palinkas, L. A., Aarons, G. A., Wells, K. B., Jones, L., Collins, L. M., Duan, N., Mittman, B. S., Wallace, A., Tabak, R. G., Ducharme, L., Chambers, D. A., Neta, G., Wiley, T., Landsverk, J., Cheung, K., & Cruden, G. (2017). An overview of research and evaluation designs for dissemination and implementation. *Annual Review of Public Health*, *38*, 1–22. https://doi.org/10.1146/annurev-publhealth-031816-044215

Damschroder, L. J., Aron, D. C., Keith, R. E., Kirsh, S. R., Alexander, J. A., & Lowery, J. C. (2009). Fostering implementation of health services research findings into practice: a consolidated framework for advancing implementation science. *Implementation Science*, *4*(1), 50. https://doi.org/10.1186/1748-5908-4-50

Kadam, S. (2021). *What are SMART indicators in monitoring and evaluation*. https://neerman.org/what-are-smart-indicators-in-monitoring-and-evaluation/

Lewis, C. C., Scott, K., & Marriott, B. R. (2018). A methodology for generating a tailored implementation blueprint: An exemplar from a youth residential setting. *Implementation Science*, *13*(1), 1–13. https://doi.org/10.1186/s13012-018-0761-6

Miller, C. J., Barnett, M. L., Baumann, A. A., Gutner, C. A., & Wiltsey-Stirman, S. (2021). The FRAME-IS: A framework for documenting modifications to implementation strategies in healthcare. *Implementation Science*, *16*(1), 1–12. https://doi.org/10.1186/s13012-021-01105-3

National Implementation Research Network. (n.d.). *Active implementation hub, Module 3: Implementation teams*. Retrieved May 1, 2021, from https://nirn.fpg.unc.edu/module-3

Perry, C. K., Damschroder, L. J., Hemler, J. R., Woodson, T. T., Ono, S. S., & Cohen, D. J. (2019). Specifying and comparing implementation strategies across seven large implementation interventions: A practical application of theory. *Implementation Science*, *14*(1), 1–13. https://doi.org/10.1186/s13012-019-0876-4

Powell, B. J., Waltz, T. J., Chinman, M. J., Damschroder, L. J., Smith, J. L., Matthieu, M. M., Proctor, E. K., & Kirchner, J. A. E. (2015). A refined compilation of implementation strategies: Results from the Expert Recommendations for Implementing Change (ERIC) project. *Implementation Science*, *10*(1), 1–14. https://doi.org/10.1186/s13012-015-0209-1

Proctor, E. K., Powell, B. J., & McMillen, J. C. (2013). Implementation strategies: Recommendations for specifying and reporting. *Implementation Science*, *8*(1), 139. https://doi.org/10.1186/1748-5908-8-139

Santos, J. M. (2021). *Understanding responsibility assignment matrix (RACI Matrix)*. Understanding Responsibility Assignment Matrix (RACI Matrix).

Smith, J. D., Li, D. H., & Rafferty, M. R. (2020). The implementation research logic model: A method for planning, executing, reporting, and synthesizing implementation projects. *MedRxiv*, 1–12. https://doi.org/10.1101/2020.04.05.20054379

State Government of Victoria, Department of Education and Early Childhood Development. (2012). *Strength-based approach: A guide to writing transition learning and development statements*. http://www.education.vic.gov.au/earlylearning/transitionschool

Stirman, S. W., Baumann, A. A., & Miller, C. J. (2019). The FRAME: An expanded framework for reporting adaptations and modifications to evidence-based interventions. *Implementation Science*, *14*(1), 1–10. https://doi.org/10.1186/s13012-019-0898-y

University of Washington. (2011). *Team charter*. http://faculty.washington.edu/jwhelan/Documents/Assignments/Samples/Charter Sample.pdf

University of Otagi. (n.d.). *Developing a Team charter*.

United States Agency for International Development. (2012). *Team building module facilitator's guide* (issue September). https://www.usaid.gov/sites/default/files/documents/1864/Team-Building-Module-Facilitators-Guide.pdf

Waltz, T. J., Powell, B. J., Matthieu, M. M., Damschroder, L. J., Chinman, M. J., Smith, J. L., Proctor, E. K., & Kirchner, J. A. E. (2015). Use of concept mapping to characterize relationships among implementation strategies and assess their feasibility and importance: Results from the Expert Recommendations for Implementing Change (ERIC) study. *Implementation Science*, *10*(1), 1–8. https://doi.org/10.1186/s13012-015-0295-0

W.K. Kellogg Foundation. (2004). *Logic model development guide.* https://headwaterslab.files.wordpress.com/2018/01/logicmodel_kellogg.pdf

8

How to Implement an Evidence-Based Intervention

Ryan R. Singh and Lisa Saldana

Learning Objectives

By the end of this chapter, readers will be able to:

- Describe the typical implementation process, from pre-implementation to sustainment
- Understand the goals of process frameworks, compare them based on theoretical and practical considerations, and discuss why each is useful in guiding the implementation process
- Describe the Stages of Implementation Completion (SIC) process model as a roadmap for, and a tool to measure, successful implementations
- Explain the critical steps of EBI implementation following the SIC model

CASE STUDY 8.1 BEGINNING THE IMPLEMENTATION PROCESS

"Imagine" is a community-based organization that has partnered with the regional government to address unmet needs of the families referred to the child welfare system. Imagine will adopt an evidence-based intervention (EBI) aimed to support parents who are living with substance use disorder through harm-reduction strategies, parental skill development, and providing case management for any unmet needs. This multi-component, community-based EBI is delivered by trained providers who work with parents one-on-one. Imagine has determined that this particular EBI addresses the needs of the families in the community, and many staff members have voiced their support for the program.

Imagine wants to ensure that the EBI can be sustained, and has been committed to using an evidence-based implementation process at all points including selecting the intervention. Funding for the implementation of the EBI has been made available through a federal grant, but this financial support is finite. Therefore, Imagine will rely on combining various funding sources to supplement the grant to continue delivering the intervention over time. Beyond securing appropriate funding, Imagine is interested in learning more about the necessary steps to take following program selection to successfully implement and sustain the EBI. Imagine has listed several questions and concerns regarding successful implementation. These include:

- Our dedicated staff are focused on their current work. How can we prepare them for the new EBI?
- Can our staff manage a new EBI or do we need to hire new employees?
- Do we need to adapt the EBI to our local context?
- Once the EBI is running, how can we ensure that that our staff are delivering the intervention effectively?
- What kind of external support can we expect during implementation?

To accomplish its goals, Imagine is working closely with EBI purveyors who provide technical assistance and support to guide a quality implementation process (described in the following).

INTRODUCTION TO IMPLEMENTING AN EVIDENCE-BASED INTERVENTION

Implementing an evidence-based intervention (EBI) into real-world practice requires more than selecting the EBI and then providing EBI services immediately; rather, for successful implementation, it is helpful to conceptualize the process—or steps/stages—that a newly adopting site must go through to effectively deliver the intervention routinely (Nilsen, 2015). This process begins before an EBI delivery site adopts a particular EBI. That is, implementation is initiated when a site begins to consider the need for a new program or practice (Aarons et al., 2011). A "site" is defined as a system, organization, agency, community, or other entity with decision-making power to adopt new programs.

Decision-makers weigh multiple consideration when selecting a new EBI to adopt (Wang et al., 2010). Often the considerations are tied to the reason for seeking a new EBI. Some reasons adoptions are initiated include pursuit of available funding, to address an identified unmet need, or to improve the quality of services being offered. Sites might start by exploring what types of interventions are available that align with the needs of the population served. Sometimes a formal needs assessment is conducted to identify the most suitable intervention for the priority population. In some cases, a needs assessment is completed in conjunction with additional assessments that address the appropriateness, or fit, of an EBI, the resources required, readiness and capacity-building strategies, and adaptations needed (Meyers et al., 2012). Regardless, adopting a new EBI necessitates a set of strategies or implementation activities to facilitate the transition from EBI selection, to preparation, to successful delivery and sustainment.

This chapter focuses on the steps, or stages, that sites typically progress through toward achieving competency in EBI delivery. First, a comparison of different implementation process frameworks will be presented to provide a glance at how the implementation process is conceptualized and how each framework might be useful in practice settings. Then, a description of the Stages of Implementation Completion (SIC) tool will be described, including lessons learned across implementations that have used the SIC. This will be followed by a brief discussion of pre-implementation and then a detailed exploration of the steps sites can take to move from implementation toward sustainment. This chapter concludes with a description of common pitfalls sites might experience during implementation of EBIs.

The Implementation Process

EBI implementation takes considerable effort, but sites that use effective implementation strategies along their journey tend to reap the greatest benefits. Sites that overlook important implementation strategies throughout the process are more likely to experience poor implementation outcomes (Saldana et al., 2012). Thus, it is critical for sites to move through implementation with a plan to support the complex process. This plan should involve consideration of when specific implementation activities should be employed, who should be involved in activity completion, how much time should be spent on each activity, and the order in which the process should be expected to unfold (although real-world implementation might require re-addressing certain activities that were overlooked or that changed over time).

In addition to a commitment of effort, the implementation process takes considerable time. Indeed, from initiation to the point at which an EBI is fully operating within a site, the process can take years! In order to grasp this extensive time commitment, and the timeline through which the activities unfold, implementation frameworks can provide a roadmap of the intermediate outcomes targeted throughout the implementation process.

Guiding the Implementation Process

There are a number of process frameworks and models developed to guide the implementation process (Nilsen, 2015), some of which are prescriptive in nature, offering steps or stages through which to move during implementation. This chapter draws attention to three examples of frameworks and models that, together, encompass pre-implementation, implementation, and sustainment. Newly adopting sites sometimes are supported by an EBI purveyor to become familiar with process frameworks, and select one that is appropriate for their context to guide implementation. An EBI purveyor has expert knowledge of fidelity to a program or practice and takes an active role in supporting the implementation process (Fixsen et al., 2005). Proctor et al. (2019) highlight another widely used term—intermediary. Thus, those individuals or groups that provide implementation support, and are external to the site that is adopting, planning, and implementing an EBI, are likely to identify their role as either purveyors or intermediaries (Corcoran et al., 2015; Franks, 2010; Franks & Bory, 2015; Proctor et al., 2019). For simplicity, we will assume that the two terms can be used interchangeably, and refer to these external individuals and/or organizations that support implementation as purveyors for the remainder of the chapter. Although working with a purveyor is common across a range of health-related programs, it is not a given, nor is it always necessary to partner with an external consultant. Nevertheless, if a site does implement an EBI without external support, there is all the more reason to rely on a theoretical framework or process model to help guide implementation.

The Quality Implementation Framework

The quality implementation framework (QIF) was developed to guide both implementation research and practice in a systematic manner. The framework is based on a body of evidence that cuts across multiple implementation-related fields of study, thus providing a tool that is relevant across a range of real-world practice disciplines. The QIF consists of four temporal phases that include a total of 14 critical steps to consider when implementing an EBI. The framework assumes that an EBI already has been selected by a site. Therefore, pre-implementation begins with developing a strong fit between the EBI and the site in which it will be delivered (i.e., Phase 1). To accomplish this, a newly adopting site is encouraged to consider its needs, resources, capacity, and overall buy-in throughout the site, along with adaptations to the EBI that might be necessary (Meyers et al., 2012). EBI adaptations should be made to improve fit, while maintaining the core components of the intervention (i.e., the intervention components that make it "work"). Phase 2 involves creating a structure for implementation, including a plan for what and when implementation activities occur, and who accomplishes such activities. Pre-implementation (Phases 1 and 2) activities make up the vast majority of steps within the QIF. Phase 3 begins implementation, with a focus on the provision of technical assistance, and monitoring and feedback to track progress. Phase 4 involves evaluation for future implementation with a focus on identifying any necessary improvements for replication as the EBI is implemented in other settings (Meyers et al., 2012). Although Phase 4 highlights the need for ongoing refinements for scale-up, the QIF has limited focus on moving past implementation toward sustainment of a particular EBI once successfully adopted. Throughout the four phases, the QIF assumes ongoing collaboration between EBI developers, adopters, and purveyors (referred to as different "systems" in the QIF; Meyers et al., 2012).

The Exploration, Preparation, Implementation, Sustainment Framework

Exploration, preparation, implementation, sustainment (EPIS) is a process framework (Aarons et al., 2011) that is frequently used throughout the implementation research and practice fields; a recent review identified 762 citations of EPIS, 49 of which represented individual rigorous research trials (Moullin et al., 2019). Similar to the QIF, EPIS is a four-phase framework, with the first two phases focused on pre-implementation. Phase 1 involves Exploration, in which decision-makers and their stakeholders are aware of a need and seek to find an EBI to address that need. Once the decision is made to adopt an EBI, implementers move to Phase 2—Preparation. This phase involves identification of potential barriers and facilitators of implementation and the development of a detailed plan to support implementation including identification of what is necessary to support a sustainable program. Activities such as planning for training, coaching, and audit and feedback occur during this phase. Additionally, during Phase 2, sites are encouraged to create a plan for generating a supportive environment within the workforce to implement the EBI—often referred to as implementation climate. Implementation climate is defined as the extent to which implementing site staff perceive that the adoption, implementation, and use of an EBI is expected, rewarded, and supported by the site (Ehrhart et al., 2014).

Phase 3 involves EBI implementation. During this time, a site begins delivering the EBI, while monitoring the dynamic process of intervention delivery and ongoing support for quality implementation. Quality monitoring allows sites to detect potential challenges in EBI delivery, and to realign implementation strategies as necessary. Finally, Phase 4 of the EPIS framework—Sustainment—details the ongoing strategies that are necessary to support maintenance of service delivery and implementation processes (i.e., leadership, supportive coaching, fidelity monitoring). Within each of the four EPIS phases, the importance of inner context (organizational-level factors known to influence implementation, including leadership, culture, and climate, as well as individual-level factors related to EBI delivery) and outer context (factors that influence implementation that fall outside of the delivery site, such as policies that inhibit or facilitate implementation, and characteristics of the priority population) is considered. Of note, adaptation is conceptualized to be possible and sometimes necessary across all four EPIS phases at both the EBI level, and at the level of inner and outer contexts of the implementation environment.

Finally, the EPIS framework emphasizes bridging factors that link the outer and inner context. Bridging factors include relationships among partners, policies, and adopting sites. The processes by which these relationships are fostered are complex but essential to support the sustainment of EBIs in new settings. EPIS includes determinants that influence the inner context (e.g., provider characteristics), as well as the outer context (e.g., available funding) at all four phases of implementation (Aarons et al., 2011; Moullin et al., 2019). Thus, the framework helps practice settings get a better sense of where to focus effort during the phases of implementation. Although EPIS provides a roadmap for the implementation process as a whole (i.e., pre-implementation through to sustainment), as well as determinants that might relate to implementation success, in their systemic review of research application of EPIS, Moullin et al. (2019) found that the framework most often has been applied to the implementation phase (i.e., Phase 3). Though an incredibly helpful framework for implementers, the EPIS framework is not intended to provide specific guidance on specific strategies, or measurement of those strategies, needed to implement an EBI.

The Stages of Implementation Completion Process Model

The SIC (Figure 8.1) is a tool for planning and tracking EBI implementation within healthcare programs, and functions as a measure of implementation fidelity. That is, the SIC is an empirically derived tool that can measure implementation process and milestones. It has demonstrated success in predicting implementation outcomes through consideration of a site's implementation behavior assessed during pre-implementation and implementation phases. The tool can be used by purveyors and newly adopting sites to monitor, guide, and predict implementation success based on adherence to, and quality completion of, the implementation plan (i.e., implementation fidelity). The activities that are represented on the SIC define the implementation strategies and considerations that are recommended for completion for quality implementation, and thus, the SIC tool has been used with increasing frequency as a roadmap for implementation between purveyors and newly adopting sites.

The SIC is comprised of eight key stages of implementation activities spanning three phases of the implementation process including pre-implementation, implementation, and sustainment (Figure 8.1). Across each of the eight stages there are implementation activities that are common across any EBI implementation (e.g., planning meeting, contracting, hiring or selecting providers, training providers) and there might be activities that are EBI-specific (e.g., community partner stakeholder meeting, set-up and test technology

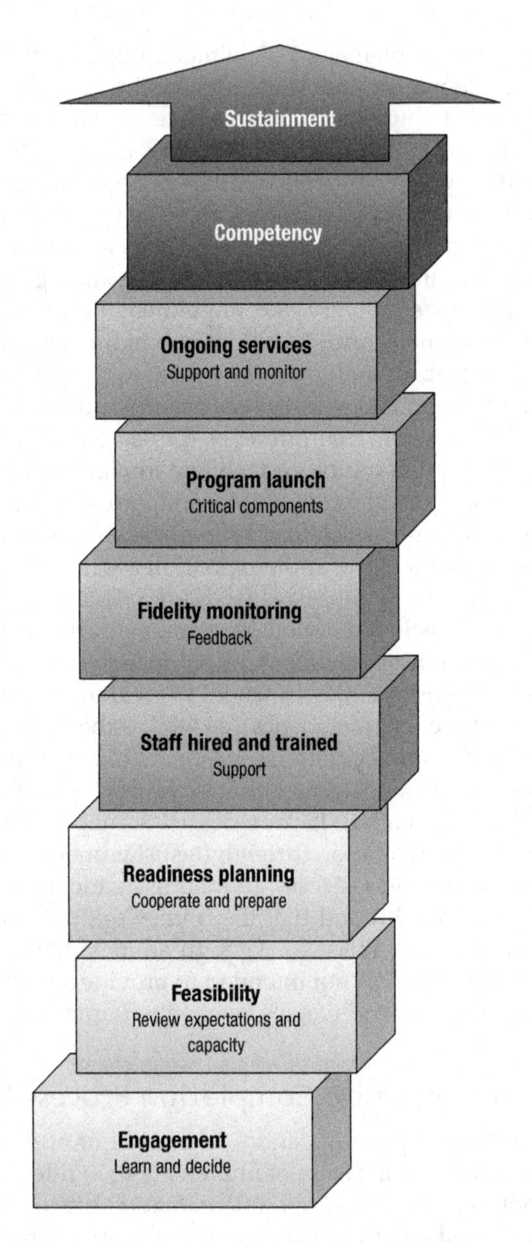

FIGURE 8.1 The stages of implementation completion process model for implementing an EBI. Stages build on one another across three phases—pre-implementation (light gray), implementation (medium gray), and sustainment (dark gray).

equipment). In this way, the SIC allows for adaptation of activities within the stages of implementation to enable accurate measurement of the proposed implementation process (Saldana et al., 2020). Completion of activities is documented by the purveyor or outside observer of the site moving through the implementation process of the EBI. Tracking implementation activities and milestones enables purveyors to identify, and correct for, specific barriers that impede the implementation process, and to encourage sites to maintain a positive implementation path. The SIC has been used across a range of practices with consistent outcomes pointing to the role of completion of key pre-implementation and implementation activities as essential for implementation success. Table 8.1 presents a comparison of the QIF, EPIS and SIC for use in implementation planning.

TABLE 8.1 Comparison of Different Implementation Process Frameworks and Models

	QUALITY IMPLEMENTATION FRAMEWORK (QIF)	EXPLORATION, PREPARATION, IMPLEMENTATION, SUSTAINMENT (EPIS)	THE STAGES OF IMPLEMENTATION COMPLETION (SIC)
Similarities	Provide a phasic approach to implementation Point to the value of pre-implementation Identify the recursive and non-linear process for implementation Can be used to map the process of a given implementation Conceptualize moving through implementation phases by conducting targeted implementation activities within each phase		
Differences	Developed from theory "Recipe" of activities that influence implementation Focuses on collaboration among developer, adopter, and purveyor Does not acknowledge outer context factors No consideration for sustainment Cannot measure and predict implementation success	Developed from theory Bridging factors that influence implementation Focuses on community collaborators Acknowledges outer context factors Consideration for sustainment Cannot measure and predict implementation success	Data driven construction "Recipe" of activities that influence implementation Focuses on internal and external collaborators Acknowledges outer context factors Consideration for sustainment Can be used as a tool to measure and predict implementation success
Strengths (+) & Limitations (−)	(+) Specify interaction among the developer, the adopter, and purveyors (+) Important questions that can be addressed in real-world settings to help guide implementation (+) Emphasis on pre-implementation activities (10 of the 14 total steps of the QIF) (−) Limited in tracking implementation activities (−) Not all steps supported by strong empirical evidence	(+) Outer and inner context factors that can influence implementation (+) Bridging factors (+) Can inform system-level implementation (+) Emphasizes the process and determinants of implementation (contextual determinants of EPIS supported by a large body of evidence) (+) Focus on implementation within public service sectors (−) No formalized method for tracking implementation activities	(+) Data driven and developed empirically (+) Can track implementation activities and milestones, and can predict implementation success (+) Useful as a roadmap and a tool to measure implementation process (+) Empirically tested (+) General and EBI-specific activities allow for a tailored implementation monitoring process for each EBI implementation (+) Tracking enables detection and correction of implementation problems

(*continued*)

TABLE 8.1 Comparison of Different Implementation Process Frameworks and Models (*continued*)

	QUALITY IMPLEMENTATION FRAMEWORK (QIF)	EXPLORATION, PREPARATION, IMPLEMENTATION, SUSTAINMENT (EPIS)	THE STAGES OF IMPLEMENTATION COMPLETION (SIC)
			(+) Supported by a web-based platform that organizes, displays, and reports implementation progress and outcomes (−) Requires knowledge of the date that implementation activities were completed (−) Customized for each EBI, therefore generalization is a challenge
Selecting a Process Framework			
When the EBI has not yet been selected and several are under consideration		✓	
When developing an implementation plan	✓	✓	✓
When considering pre-implementation	✓		✓
To guide implementation	✓	✓	✓
When creating a protocol to share with stakeholders to set expectations	✓	✓	✓

(*continued*)

When considering how factors at multiple levels influence implementation	✓	✓
To track milestones and predict implementation success		✓
To compare the pace and activity completion between sites		✓
To compare the implementation of one practice to the implementation of another		✓
To consider how systems interact with one another	✓	
When planning for sustainment	✓	✓

How to Implement an Evidence-Based Intervention Using the Stages of Implementation Completion

As described, the SIC provides a process model for the implementation of EBIs, including concrete steps that a site can take to achieve competent EBI delivery (Table 8.2). This section describes the SIC in greater detail, including the reason for its development, its evolution in use over time, and lessons learned from the over 1,900 implementations that have been monitored with the SIC.

The Stages of Implementation Completion Development

The SIC was developed to fill the gap in the ability to measure the implementation process. As part of a large randomized implementation trial, two approaches to implementing the same EBI were examined (Saldana & Chamberlain, 2012). The EBI—Treatment Foster Care Oregon (TFCO; formerly known as Multidimensional Treatment Foster Care)—is an intervention developed as an alternative to out-of-home placement for youth with severe behavioral and mental health problems in foster care (Chamberlain & Mihalic, 1998). The intervention is complex, with a team of interventionists working together on a coordinated treatment plan, led by a Team Lead. This Lead also provides support to foster parents to deliver evidence-based treatment in their homes to the referred youth. TFCO programs are adopted by individual foster care provider agencies, in contract with child welfare, juvenile justice, and mental health systems.

TABLE 8.2 SIC Measure: Stages and Phases With Example Activities

STAGE	ACTIVITY
PRE-IMPLEMENTATION PHASE	
Stage 1: Engagement	Date interest indicated
Stage 2: Feasibility Assessment	Date feasibility questionnaire completed Date program champion identified
Stage 3: Readiness Planning	Date of stakeholder meeting Date of communication plan completed
IMPLEMENTATION PHASE	
Stage 4: Staff Hired and Trained	Date first interventionist selected Date of clinical training
Stage 5: Fidelity Monitoring Established	Date fidelity training conducted Date recording equipment tested
Stage 6: Services and Consultation Begin	Date of first client served Date of first fidelity review
Stage 7: Ongoing Services, Consultation, Fidelity Monitoring, and Feedback	Date clinical team first achieves 80% or higher on fidelity assessment
SUSTAINMENT PHASE	
Stage 8: Competency	Date of site certification Date site providers meet all fidelity standards

Note: The date of activity completion is tracked for each item. Forty-six implementation activities populate the eight stages on the Universal SIC. Stages 1–3 are Pre-Implementation, Stages 4–7 are Implementation, and Stage 8 is achievement of program competency for Sustainment.

In this study, 51 counties were randomized to one of two implementation approaches to support the implementation of TFCO (Brown et al., 2014). Although the TFCO study hypothesized that the experimental implementation strategy would be more effective than the standard approach in guiding sites in a successful implementation process, no tool to measure the implementation process was available at that time. Thus, the SIC was developed as a measure of implementation process and milestones. Because of the multi-component nature of the TFCO intervention, and the non-linear nature of implementation (e.g., changes in funding or staff turnover might cause a pause in some activities, or the need for replacement training), the development process considered how to create a measure that was necessarily time-dependent yet flexible, with the potential to assess varying implementation strategies that might be activated, but within a standardized implementation process. The resulting SIC operationalized key implementation activities that sites conducted across eight stages that span pre-implementation, implementation, and sustainment (see Figure 8.1). Table 8.3 provides examples activities from the TFCO-SIC.

SIC data was collected through purveyor reports of site completion of implementation strategies delineated on the SIC (i.e., SIC activities). Using the SIC codebook to identify when a site had adequately completed a SIC activity, the date of completion was recorded. If a site did not complete an activity, it was coded as not completed. By recording the dates of completion or the failure of a site to complete an activity, patterns emerged of "what" and "when" activities in the implementation process were conducted, and how these patterns differed for successful versus non-successful sites. SIC patterns were summarized with three scores: (a) Duration—time taken for completion of implementation activities, calculated by the date of completion of the first and last activities completed in a stage or

TABLE 8.3 Example TFCO Activities Within the Eight SIC Stages

STAGE	ACTIVITY
Stage 1: Engagement	Date of interest indicated Date agreed to consider implementation
Stage 2: Feasibility Assessment	Date of first county planning contact Date feasibility questionnaire completed
Stage 3: Readiness Planning	Date of cost/funding plan review Date of referral criteria review Date of stakeholder meeting
Stage 4: Staff Hired and Trained	Date first staff hired Date clinical training held
Stage 5: Fidelity Monitoring Established	Date fidelity measure training held Date of first program admin. Call
Stage 6: Services and Consultation Begin	Date of first placement Date of first consult call Date of first clinical meeting video received
Stage 7: Ongoing Services, Consultation, Fidelity Monitoring, and Feedback	Date of site visit #1 Date of implementation review #1 Date of final program assessment
Stage 8: Competency	Date program certified

Note: At the time of the study, there were 35 activities on the SIC. Since this time the tool has been refined and now has 50 activities defined.

phase; (b) Proportion—percentage of activities completed in a stage or phase; and (c) Final Stage—the furthest point in the implementation process achieved. The SIC was used to successfully predict TFCO program start-up from the proportion of activities completed, and the time it took to complete them, predicting whether or not a site served a client (Saldana et al., 2012). Outcomes indicated that there were no differences by condition in the number of counties that adopted TFCO, but that those participating in the experimental implementation approach showed greater quality of implementation as scored by the SIC and, in so doing, served more than twice the number of clients than the standard implementation condition (Brown et al., 2014).

Findings from this trial also demonstrated the SIC's utility as an implementation template on which to map the assessment of implementation costs. By taking the activities defined by the SIC and assessing the direct and indirect resources used by sites to complete them, the implementation costs needed by sites to implement TFCO were identified. This cost mapping—called the Cost of Implementing New Strategies (COINS)—was able to distinguish implementation costs and resources between the two implementation conditions, and showed that the greatest variation in resource use between conditions occurred in pre-implementation (Saldana et al., 2014).

Stages of Implementation Completion Expansion

Despite the critical role that process plays in implementation, there were no standard measures for its assessment. Given the utility of the SIC in the TFCO study in measuring implementation process and predicting outcomes, there was interest in learning if the SIC might be useful for measuring the implementation of other EBIs. Thus, with funding from NIMH, the SIC team conducted a measurement trial to adapt the SIC for other complex behavioral health interventions, involving different public service systems, and to see if the tool replicated its predictive utility (Saldana, 2014). Partnering with the developers of other EBIs including Multisystemic Therapy (MST; Henggeler et al., 2009), Multidimensional Family Therapy (MDFT; Liddle, 2002), and Coping Cat (Kendall, 1994; Kendall & Khanna, 2008), the SIC team operationalized each EBI's implementation approach from the point of Engagement (SIC Stage 1) to Competency (SIC Stage 8). Operationalization procedures followed a qualitative approach whereby the SIC team conducted a site visit to the EBI purveyor agency, reviewed documentation from previous implementations, and conducted semi-structured interviews with the developer and purveyor staff over the course of a 2-day meeting. A concrete set of implementation activities then was outlined by the SIC team, including a definition for completion, and reviewed for accuracy by the purveyors. Outcomes for each of the EBIs replicated the original ability for the SIC scores to reliably distinguish between good and poor implementation process completion, and predict which implementations would be successful versus discontinued.

As the interest in measuring implementation process continued to grow, a number of other EBIs began to request an adaptation of the SIC to help measure their implementation approach. In so doing, the SIC team began to recognize strong overlap in different practices' implementation activities. For example, many practices identified a formal feasibility assessment, a stakeholder readiness meeting, and multiple training activities. Using a team reliability coding approach, verified by practice developer agreement, 46 common implementation activities were identified across different practices. These activities comprise the Universal SIC (Saldana et al., 2015)—a standardized version of the SIC available for practices to customize by labeling the items for their intervention, but not changing the items included. See Table 8.2, which provides example Universal SIC items across each of the eight stages of implementation.

Lessons Learned From Using the Stages of Implementation Completion

As the SIC's utility has continued to grow, it has been used in a range of studies, real-world implementations, and presentations. Currently the SIC either has been fully tailored and adapted from the ground-up, or customized using the Universal SIC template, for over 55 programs and practices, including mental health, school prevention programs, primary care interventions, substance abuse treatments, large state system initiatives, and other efforts. Recent examples include interventions for housing, juvenile justice, substance use treatment, and school (Aalsma et al., 2019; Frank et al., 2021; Nadeem et al., 2018; Powell et al., 2020; Sterrett-Hong et al., 2021; Watson et al., 2020). The standard adaptation process includes a partnership between the SIC team and those implementing the practice, to understand the essential steps in the implementation process that must be followed to successfully scale-up the intervention (Saldana et al., 2020). SIC users can enter their data directly into a SIC website that culls the data into a single Universal SIC mapped data set. This data set provides the opportunity to learn about implementation process across a range of implementation types in a way that observing a single data set (i.e., from one site's implementation) does not allow. Thus, the SIC data provide a rich and unique window into what to consider for successful implementation regardless of the intervention and the setting in which it is being implemented.

As the number of SIC users continues to grow, the SIC team and purveyor partners have learned several lessons that should be considered across implementation in general. These include:

1. Implementations should be as simple as possible while including all of the essential steps to support a new program. That is, it is important that sites go through all eight stages of implementation, but advance through them by completing only activities that have been identified as helpful in supporting implementations relevant to the EBI. Some implementers make the mistake of thinking that implementations need to be complicated to be useful. However, sites that are implementing typically have limited resources and staff time that can go toward a new implementation effort. A strong implementation process should have the goal of making implementation as easy and resource efficient as possible for a new site.
2. It is essential to remember that implementation of a new program most often means that a site has to stop doing something else, do what they have been doing differently, or add another whole new thing to their existing processes and workload. Although the EBI being implemented might ultimately prove to be time- and cost-saving to the site, in the moment of adopting it feels cumbersome. It is important to break down implementation processes into manageable steps, identify the appropriate individuals to complete them, and support adopters to maintain a steady pace and momentum toward program launch (Stage 6).
3. Implementations should draw on the previous success of a site. SIC research and collaboration has highlighted that if a site has already adopted policies and procedures for a previous implementation that are consistent with the new adoption, they can leverage these earlier activities rather than "starting from scratch." As part of a feasibility assessment, it is important to identify what implementation activities the site already is "ready" to conduct, and these activities might be skipped during the readiness planning stage (Stage 3).
4. Pre-implementation (Stages 1–3) is the most important phase of implementation. During this period, the site builds the infrastructure necessary for a successful implementation. Some sites rush through this process because of hurried timelines or the

belief that training staff in the program is enough to get started. Outcomes from the SIC have shown consistently that poor proportion scores during pre-implementation predict a program that is not likely to achieve competency.

5. Stakeholder engagement is essential throughout the implementation process. Sites that launch a program without involving members from the referring community and consumers of the intervention are less likely to understand and effectively address the problem they are trying to solve.

CASE STUDY 8.2 MAPPING OUT THE IMPLEMENTATION PROCESS

Working closely with the EBI purveyor, Imagine outlined the implementation process that would be most efficient for their implementation efforts given their resource and staff limitations. The defined implementation process was tailored to the service delivery and provider expectations for the selected EBI, and mapped to the needs of the Imagine organization and surrounding community. In doing so, Imagine was able to grasp the magnitude of the process—that there are multiple stages and steps to be completed along the way, and that multiple individuals, who already have competing priorities, will be necessary to involve. Recognizing the need for adequate time to properly move through implementation, Imagine contacted their funder and let them know that realistically, they needed several months to fulfill their pre-implementation plan. In the discussion, Imagine advocated that by following the defined implementation roadmap, Imagine would be more likely to effectively implement the EBI and develop a sustainable program that would fit within the local context and benefit the families served. Imagine successfully negotiated this change in timeline, which made them feel confident to embark on implementation!

THE PROCESS OF IMPLEMENTING AN EVIDENCE-BASED INTERVENTION

The following section of the chapter describes the process of implementing an EBI. Guided by the SIC, the pre-implementation phase is briefly described, followed by a more in-depth presentation of the later stages of the implementation process.

Pre-implementation

The SIC model asserts that pre-implementation is the most critical phase of the implementation process. Sites that place emphasis on completing the stages of pre-implementation tend to reap the greatest rewards in terms of implementation outcomes. The first three stages of the SIC process model include site engagement with the EBI (Stage 1), assessment of the feasibility of implementing the EBI (Stage 2), and readiness planning for ensuring a supportive infrastructure for the EBI (Stage 3). Previous SIC research consistently has demonstrated the importance of completing pre-implementation activities (Saldana et al., 2012, 2020; Sterrett-Hong et al., 2021). Thus, the launch of program delivery can be predicted based on a site's successful completion of pre-implementation activities. Sites that complete pre-implementation activities (e.g., identify a program champion, conduct a needs assessment, foster stakeholder engagement, assess readiness) are more likely to successfully progress their implementation to the point of serving the targeted population (i.e., launching the EBI program) with the EBI.

Pre-implementation activities might seem intuitive, but often are overlooked. The reality of what is necessary to conduct a quality pre-implementation sometimes pushes up against other considerations such as the request of funders to begin delivering services rapidly or a fixed timeline. Barriers to completing quality implementation include limited staff resources and limited funding or time to implement the EBI effectively (Crable et al., 2020). SIC outcomes have shown that a program launched in the absence of completing necessary pre-implementation activities has a low likelihood of developing a sustainable EBI program (Frank et al., 2021; Watson et al., 2020).

CASE STUDY 8.3 IMAGINE'S PRE-IMPLEMENTATION EXPERIENCE

Imagine followed the SIC process model, beginning with engagement. Imagine's program director, along with additional staff, including program managers and other community partner stakeholders, met with the purveyors to discuss what it would take to bring in the new EBI. Child welfare representatives from the county health department attended the meeting (SIC Stage 1). The county supervisor of child welfare services was the one who introduced the EBI to Imagine. She felt strongly that the intervention would address a gap in services for the area, and was excited to get to the point of engagement. The program director was excited to move forward, but expressed concern that the organization's current staff might not be able to handle another intervention with their current workload (SIC Stage 2). As a result, Imagine identified a program champion to dedicate time assessing the feasibility of the program with an eye toward identifying ways to make the implementation feasible. The champion led an assessment of the capacity of the workforce, as well as the extent to which current providers who were expected to deliver the new EBI would be able to reach the greatest number of parents in need, while maintaining high fidelity delivery of the EBI. This critical step helped Imagine make the decision to develop plans to hire additional providers, and to outline projections to help maintain the current workload while managing the implementation of the new intervention (SIC Stage 3).

Active Implementation

The active Implementation phase of the SIC consists of four stages of implementation, including hiring and training the EBI provider staff (Stage 4), setting up fidelity monitoring and ongoing evaluation and/or feedback systems (Stage 5), launching service delivery and associated monitoring (Stage 6), and ongoing program delivery, quality assurance monitoring, evaluation, and feedback to develop program competency (Stage 7). Each of these stages interact with each other in a dynamic way as newly developing programs experience changes resulting in recursive activity completion, such as the need for new or replacement hiring and training or modifications in the intensity of feedback provided. Next, the stages of the Implementation phase are described in greater detail.

Hiring and Training the Provider Team

During pre-implementation (Stages 1–3), a site should have garnered an understanding of its current provider capacity and be able to determine the need to bring on additional staff to deliver the EBI. Relying on current staff may be problematic if the implementation of a new EBI adds to their workload. The expectations for delivery of a new EBI, in addition to existing full time commitments can engender reluctance by the provider, and lead to potential negative consequences for both the adoption of the new EBI and execution of the original responsibilities or interventions being delivered. Similarly, some implementing sites misstep by trying to "get by" with using their existing program staff to provide the new EBI without first determining if the fit (e.g., skill, knowledge, motivation) of those staff is appropriate. Implementation with poor staff fit have the potential to fail (Maher et al., 2009). However, sometimes if the new EBI is similar in nature or intended to be delivered to a similar population, existing providers might be a good fit to reassign to the program.

Timing is key to the process of hiring/assigning staff. There is a balance to hiring staff early enough in the process to involve them in the final preparation activities, but not too early so as to have staff without duties. Personnel are a significant expense for a new implementation, and, therefore, placing staff on the budget prematurely risks drawing down resources without the delivery of services for reimbursement. For example, one county in the previously noted TFCO implementation trial hired a full clinical team prior to establishing community partnerships for referrals and completion of other pre-implementation activities. This decision led to two key factors that contributed to their lack of success—providers developed poor and inefficient habits without purposeful work for over 3 months, and they were an additional strain on the budget without contributing to program reimbursement. This example highlights the need for thoughtful consideration of the pace of hiring.

Once staff have been identified who are well suited for delivering the EBI and motivated to do so effectively, a rigorous training process should be provided. Often, EBIs come with their own specially tailored trainings that are provided by the purveyor and/or developer group. It is beneficial to ensure that the provider staff and all the individuals who are going to be a part of the EBI participate in some level of training, including leadership and supervisory teams. Moreover, support staff can benefit from an orientation overview to the EBI and how it might intersect with their workflow. Essential to EBI training is understanding what is expected to try and achieve the same outcomes that were achieved in the clinical trials. Thus, it is important for providers to not only be trained in the mechanics of delivering the EBI, but also in understanding the components of the intervention that make it "work" (i.e., the mechanisms of action). Regardless of the training format (e.g., didactic versus interactive), newly adopting sites are encouraged to make sure the provider staff fully participate.

Training for successful EBI delivery should be conceptualized as a process that ebbs and flows over time. Training does not necessarily end; rather, an initial training phase is followed by consistent supervision to support ongoing provider development (Lyon et al., 2011). Initially, training should make use of best practices, extending beyond didactic learning to include active training strategies that allow for practice in delivering the EBI. Role play, observation, and feedback all have received empirical support for changing behaviors of EBI providers during an initial training (e.g., Burke & Hutchins, 2007; Dolcini et al., 2021; Durlak & DuPre, 2008). The expectation should not be that providers will achieve skill mastery and competency after such training efforts. Most often, even the most effective initial training is insufficient in preparing providers for real-world EBI delivery. Thus, the transition from practice in training to real-world EBI delivery is a point at which additional support for providers is needed (Lyon et al., 2011).

Supervisors who provide direct oversight to EBI providers play a central role in supporting their staff, through fidelity monitoring and responsive feedback. However, to achieve effective supervision practices, supervisors require support as well. Purveyors can play a key role in supporting supervisors through remote coaching. This includes the development of a fidelity monitoring system (see the following) and—perhaps even more important—a feedback mechanism to which providers are responsive. Such coaching practices, established at the beginning of the implementation phase, sometimes transfer from the expert purveyors to local supervisors as a site transitions toward competent EBI delivery (see Program Launch for more information). In other instances, purveyors are absent from the implementation process, leaving it instead up to the site to deliver the EBI as intended following training. In both approaches, it is critical that supervisors receive the necessary training to ensure they are capable of monitoring fidelity using best practices in supervision. Although many trainings conclude with a competency assessment, caution should be taken in assuming that the new EBI providers are prepared to deliver the intervention to clients with high fidelity right from the start. As noted previously, immediate support and fidelity monitoring are essential as providers begin to deliver the program outside of the training environment in real-world practice (Lyon et al., 2011).

Preparing for Fidelity Monitoring

Once there is an understanding of EBI staff expectations and roles through training, it is critical to have a plan in place for ongoing monitoring of EBI delivery, and methods for providing feedback to move EBI delivery toward competency. Similar to the influence that fidelity to implementation activities has on achieving positive implementation outcomes, the delivery of the EBI with strong intervention fidelity is key to positive clinical outcomes. Thus, intervention fidelity monitoring should emphasize the mechanisms of action identified in training as underlying the EBI success and the core components that are necessary to achieve them. Providers within EBI delivery sites should have a solid understanding of what components of the program are essential and why these components are necessary to deliver with high fidelity in order to achieve the anticipated health outcomes. Some newly adopting sites assume that the way that an intervention is delivered cannot be adapted for context without hindering intervention fidelity. Instead, by maintaining the mechanisms of action (i.e., core components), the way in which those mechanisms are activated can sometimes be modified without impacting the EBI itself.

Different EBIs have different fidelity monitoring tools, dashboards, or measures as a part of the implementation process. Some are observationally based, whereas others rely on self- or patient-report. Yet others have no formal process for fidelity monitoring, but encourage sites to develop a method to do so. Regardless, to ensure provider fidelity and prevent program drift from the EBI, it is important to have a system in place for monitoring quality assurance. It is recommended that all individuals who take part in delivering the EBI are aware of how fidelity is being measured, how frequently it is being monitored, and what the expectations are for responding to feedback. Audit and feedback systems provide concrete, data driven feedback about performance of service delivery, with the expectation that feedback is provided in a rapid way that providers can respond to, and adjust their practice accordingly. For example, in a supervisor-targeted intervention focused on changing the behavior of frontline caseworkers, caseworker interactions with their unit supervisors were recorded monthly and uploaded to a secure platform for observation by a remote expert EBI coach. The coach reviewed the supervision meeting, rated the meeting using a standardized intervention fidelity monitoring tool, and provided both written and verbal feedback to the supervisor within a week's time, and prior to the following supervision meeting. This cyclical feedback process allowed the supervisors to receive prompt feedback, act on that feedback, and receive feedback again. Doing so led to the majority of supervisors changing their behavior in alignment with the EBI (Saldana et al., 2016).

Although feedback regarding observation of provider delivery of the EBI is the gold standard, this is not always an option due to costs, lack of capacity by the purveyor for observational assessment, or practical reasons depending on the population being served. For example, if an EBI is being delivered out in the community, it might be challenging to observe a provider in vivo or to record provider-patient interactions. If, on the other hand, an EBI is being delivered in an outpatient clinic, it might be possible to observe the session interactions and assess for quality assurance.

Regardless of the method selected, fidelity monitoring only is as helpful as the feedback that is provided and the subsequent response given in return. Fidelity monitoring for the sake of fidelity monitoring can be useful for research; however, for practical real-world delivery of services, it is critical that once performance is evaluated, the provider is given feedback to improve their ongoing practice. As will be described in the following section, fidelity monitoring serves as a key activity in the supervision process. Once fidelity monitoring and quality assurance systems are established, the EBI provider staff now are prepared to begin delivery of services.

Program Launch

A seemingly obvious but important part of the implementation process is determining at what point the EBI is considered to be "off the ground." Depending on the EBI being delivered, this might begin once clients are referred, once they are screened, or once they begin receiving intervention services. Often, launch is associated with the point in which services are delivered for reimbursement. To successfully launch a program, each of the pre-implementation stages ideally will have been completed. Thus, a referral process, billing procedures, and space considerations will have been resolved through the readiness process. Depending on the EBI and context, marketing materials (e.g., brochures, listserv announcements) and community partner presentations (e.g., child welfare unit meetings) will coincide with program launch to facilitate community knowledge of program availability.

Launching the program often requires not only initiating the delivery of services, but also working closely with the purveyor whenever possible. Program launch will invariably uncover gaps in the implementation process that have not been identified previously. At this point in the process, the newly adopting site should observe the process with a critical eye and share observations with the purveyor. This allows for the EBI to be launched with deliberate focus on adhering to key EBI components, and receiving feedback on how to deliver them well. Thus, at program launch services are delivered from the start with an emphasis on fidelity monitoring for feedback.

Although some EBIs are delivered by individual provider staff, without a supervisory structure between the provider and the purveyor, many healthcare EBIs are provided under the guidance of an attending supervisor. For supervision to be effective, supervisors should be trained in the EBI, and supported in their supervision of providers delivering the intervention. Supervisors often are in the most proximal position to monitor EBI delivery. The goal of transitioning from expert consulting/coaching oversight to intrasite supervision should be to maintain high fidelity EBI delivery in the absence of external support (which for many EBIs is finite). This goal relies on the capacity of supervisors to be able to provide a similar level of support for providers. As noted, decisions on supervision strategies (e.g., direct observation, group-based supervision, one-on-one interaction) depend on site capacity and resources. Best practices in supervision include direct observation (Bertram et al., 2015; Schoenwald et al., 2004), if possible. In addition, observation, whenever possible, should be coupled with strategies to provide feedback in an effective manner that is useful to providers. Active learning strategies (e.g., skill demonstration, role play, behavior rehearsal) help providers improve upon their future EBI delivery (Dolcini et al., 2021; Dorsey et al., 2018). Beyond the use of fidelity monitoring tools and provision of effective feedback, best practices in supervision include following a written coaching plan (Bertram et al., 2015). The written coaching plan can be structured from the fidelity monitoring tool. Fidelity should not be a mystery; strong coaching facilitates the implementer's knowledge of the core components of the intervention, how to deliver them well, and how to identify risks to intervention integrity. The coaching plan should highlight the strengths of the implementer and how they can be leveraged to grow in the areas identified in need of development. A written plan fosters consistency and follow-through for effective provider development and subsequent EBI delivery, and might also be useful for training practitioners who are hired after initial implementation (Durlak & DuPre, 2008).

The point at which a program is launched is a milestone to celebrate. As noted previously, a strong pre-implementation phase is a rigorous process, with many moving parts and individuals involved. By the time the program is launched and the first client is served, there might be pressure to press forward quickly. However, to encourage morale among the adopting staff and promote the value of the intervention throughout the site, it is important to stop and mark the initiation of services by recognizing the hard work prior to launch. Newly adopting sites should also recognize the multiple components necessary to fully launch the new program, and to let all members of the site understand their value in promoting and supporting the EBI, even if they are not directly involved in the provision of EBI services. At this stage of the implementation process, sites are serving the priority population, assessing fidelity, engaging in consultation for feedback, and initiating EBI-specific supervision. With each of these key implementation activities in place, the implementation process can proceed to taking steps toward competent EBI delivery.

Ongoing Program Delivery and Quality Assurance Monitoring for Competency

Whether an EBI is delivered by an individual provider or a team of providers, professional development efforts are needed to encourage ongoing delivery of the EBI with fidelity. Because EBI delivery often is complex and must be matched to a wide range of priority population profiles and needs, it is expected that the quality of service delivery and subsequent fidelity ratings will ebb and flow, as programs develop. As noted previously, achievement of competent program delivery often can take years, and requires consistent motivation toward program growth. This includes consistent provider participation in fidelity monitoring and supervisory activities, and site commitment and motivation toward capacity building.

Implementation strategies often are employed throughout the period of time between launch and development of a competent program. Strategies include ongoing training specific to the EBI (e.g., turnover training, booster training, advanced skills acquisition training), individualized coaching tailored to the needs of the provider, financial planning for sustainment, and assessing capacity for growth, as well as other deliberate efforts to build the EBI and position it for long-term maintenance within the site. These activities often are facilitated by the purveyor organization, but completed by an implementation team (e.g., program champion, fiscal officer) within the site that was developed during the readiness process. Often led by the program champion, this phase of the implementation process encourages assessment of program delivery for fidelity, while observing opportunities for contextual modifications to strengthen the reach and effectiveness of the EBI when delivered under the organizational conditions.

Competent Evidence-Based Intervention Delivery

The parameters for competent program delivery vary widely across EBIs. Some EBIs have a built-in process by which the purveyor organization "certifies" or otherwise rates the newly adopting site as delivering the intervention consistently with fidelity. Other EBIs do not have a formal process, but recognize the site when the intervention is delivered well. Yet others have no process at all, and require the site to evaluate itself for achievement of competent delivery and subsequent positive client outcomes. In any case, sites should have a clear understanding of how they will define competency—this definition should have been determined during the readiness planning stage (SIC Stage 3). Competent program delivery should be measured by some combination of achievement of positive client outcomes and consistent delivery of intervention core components. Some programs define competency based on meeting a certain threshold of positive client case closures, delivery of components with fidelity over a pre-determined amount of time, or a percentage of organizational staff delivering the intervention consistently. Once competency is established, ongoing monitoring is essential as drift in delivery is common (Chambers et al., 2013) without sustained quality checks (Bova et al., 2017). Regardless of the structure, it is important for sites to recognize competent delivery within their own providers, celebrate this success, and provide incentives or acknowledgment for sustained EBI delivery.

CASE STUDY 8.4 UNEXPECTED CHANGE DURING IMAGINE'S IMPLEMENTATION PROCESS

Imagine worked closely with purveyors to successfully transition from pre-implementation to delivering the EBI to referred families involved in their local child welfare system. During pre-implementation it was determined that adaptations to the EBI were not necessary to meet the needs of the priority population, but that adaptations were needed in the infrastructure to deliver the EBI (SIC Stage 3). Specifically, because many families in the priority population lived in rural settings, the site needed to reduce the number of cases on each provider's caseload to account for travel time. Doing so had implications for the number of clients served and thus reimbursement. These challenges were addressed head-on with the funders so that by the time Imagine was through pre-implementation, a feasible caseload and reimbursement plan was established. Thus, the needs of the priority population were the driving force in tailoring non-essential components of the intervention.

Early adaptations and assessing the capacity of the EBI delivery site also helped frame the extent to which the EBI would impact the parents involved with child welfare. Early planning led to maximizing the reach of the EBI to the greatest number of people in need of intervention, while maintaining the ability to deliver the program effectively. It was recognized by Imagine's leadership that staff throughout the site were likely to be uncomfortable with the changes that come with introducing a new EBI. Leadership provided time to help staff recognize the need for the EBI, and participate in expressing a shared vision for adopting the program. As providers were hired and trained to deliver the EBI, the program champion was intentional in introducing the new staff to others within the site and facilitating a climate of welcome and integration.

Once Imagine received their first referral and the assigned provider met with the family (SIC Stage 6), the site held a kick-off celebration. The new provider team was introduced fully to the other Imagine staff over an informal meeting. As EBI delivery became routine, the provider team continued to meet with supervisors providing

(continued)

CASE STUDY 8.4 UNEXPECTED CHANGE DURING IMAGINE'S IMPLEMENTATION PROCESS (*continued*)

routine observation and feedback, who in turn met with the EBI expert coaching staff for support and feedback (SIC Stage 7).

By mid-implementation, the use of implementation monitoring tools helped determine that the EBI was being delivered effectively. Imagine was on its way to achieving competency! At this time, however, the child welfare authority issued new policies that impacted the level of need and capacity within the region. Imagine had the opportunity to reach more individuals, but needed to do so without compromising the early success attained by planning and strategically moving through the implementation process. Imagine used the same approach to expand program capacity. Specifically, the site continued to work closely with child welfare staff at the county level, as well as the purveyor. This involved a reassessment of the capacity of the site and the current EBI providers (SIC Stage 2). Imagine determined that additional staff were needed to increase delivery in response to the new child welfare policies. Leadership within Imagine demonstrated a commitment to expanding the program, while providing support for staff during another period of change. This ongoing support, along with consistent collaboration with the community partners, facilitated the successful expansion of the EBI to reach and impact a larger number of parents in need of comprehensive services.

SUMMARY

Implementing an EBI is a complex and dynamic process. Essential to success is an awareness that deliberate time and resources are necessary to develop the infrastructure within a site to support the EBI over time. Through the use of implementation process frameworks and models, such as the QIF, EPIS, or SIC, newly adopting sites can develop a feasible plan for bringing in a new EBI, with a priori expectations set for potential adaptations needed; supervision, monitoring and support processes to have in place; and outcomes for success defined. Armed with a strong implementation process, sites are well-positioned to help advance the delivery of EBIs for populations in need.

KEY POINTS FOR PRACTICE

1. When an EBI is selected for adoption, determine if there is an existing implementation model that is expected to be followed. If so, it will be important to know if there is purveyor support that is provided.
2. Either with the support of a purveyor or as an individual implementing site, it is important to map out the activities that will be needed to implement the EBI. It is important to consider both when and how the activities will be completed. Developing a plan for when and how activities will be completed also can be useful in assessing whether implementation is progressing too fast or too slow. Not spending enough time completing necessary activities can be detrimental, but spending too much time on certain activities can slow momentum and use resources unnecessarily.
3. When considering the strategies to use to complete implementation activities, it is important to consider the resources that will be needed to do the strategy well. Resources might include monetary costs, people, materials, or physical space. Training

providers, for example, is a critical activity and is important to "get it right." Considerations include deciding who conducts the training, how many days training will take, and the materials necessary for the training. An EBI training that is held by a formal training center will require different resources than one held in-house. Training costs often include more than a one-time training and include additions such as travel, professional consultation, and site visits. Consideration of the necessary resources early in the implementation process provides sites the ability to weigh costs and efforts needed over time.

4. Implementation is a complex set of interactions between different individuals, systems, and policies. Thus, it is beneficial to find simplicity wherever possible, and to develop an implementation plan that is feasible and purposeful. Anticipating how these interactions might unfold as implementation progresses is a proactive approach to mitigating any problems that surface.
5. The transition from training providers to real-world EBI delivery should be met with supportive coaching, monitoring, and feedback. Sites that conceptualize training as a process that unfolds over the period of implementation are likely to build a proficient provider team. Purveyors can provide this level of support, but in their absence, supervisors should be prepared to provide the necessary monitoring and feedback to ensure effective EBI delivery over time. Following feedback, purveyors or supervisors should be able to detect responsive behaviors from providers that improves EBI delivery.
6. Re-evaluation of the implementation plan is worthwhile at the point of program launch. Inevitably, there will be gaps in the plan that will need to be addressed.

COMMON PITFALLS IN PRACTICE

Following a model for implementation, such as the SIC, and attending to each step of the process increases the likelihood of implementation success. There are, however, common pitfalls that occur at points in the process, that ultimately can lead to poor implementation fidelity. Following is a list of some of the most common pitfalls encountered during EBI implementation that organizations should be aware of. Strategies to handle such pitfalls are discussed.

1. **Inadequate fit of provider workforce**

   Failure to address workforce capacity in pre-implementation can result in poor implementation outcomes. As mentioned earlier in the chapter, introducing a new EBI can add to the workload of the provider, which in turn can impact the quality of EBI delivery. This might occur if the expectation is to maintain current programming on top of having the responsibility of delivering a new intervention. Although preparation in the pre-implementation stages can help mitigate issues related to inadequate fit of the provider workforce, consideration of staff size and program reach should be ongoing for an implementing organization.

   Staff turnover is one of the most common factors affecting implementation. Changes in staff—particularly a decrease in staff—can also result in increased workload for providers, especially if providers have to take on the caseloads of others who no longer are delivering the EBI. There are a number of strategies sites can use when changes in the provider workforce occur. For instance, a site can decrease the number of people within the priority population who are served. In doing so, program reach is diminished, which has implications for equity in terms of who is receiving the intervention and who is not. Despite these implications, such changes may be necessary to continue delivering an EBI with high fidelity.

It is also possible that sites have the ability to bring on new staff as the implementation process unfolds. One issue, however, is determining how to train newly hired staff if a formal training is no longer available to the site. Supervisors who receive training and are able to provide supportive coaching can be an effective solution to train new hires in situations when a formal training is not available. Thus, it is critical to prepare supervisors to train others by leveraging supportive implementation strategies described earlier in this chapter (e.g., provision of coaching tools to monitor fidelity and provide constructive feedback).

2. **Inadequate pacing of implementation process**
   It is common that EBI implementation sites are excited to start a new program, and overlook important pre-implementation activities. As noted previously, a poor pre-implementation process can inadvertently lead to poor program delivery and limited chance for sustainment. One key factor in pre-implementation quality is allowing adequate time to work through the feasibility (SIC Stage 2) and readiness (SIC Stage 3) processes thoroughly. Encouraged by funders or imposed timelines, newly adopting sites sometimes move through the stages of implementation too quickly. In other instances, a site might not spend time establishing a shared vision among staff, making the false assumption that everyone is on board. Leadership at the top of an organization tend to hold most, if not all, of the decision-making power. It is important to foster engagement throughout an organization, but particularly among the providers who are expected to deliver the new EBI.

   The pacing of implementation has significant implications for budgeting for the EBI, and thus its financial sustainment. The completion of implementation activities has associated costs including personnel and other direct expenses (Saldana et al., 2014). A priori planning and pacing allow for budgeting within annual organizational fiscal cycles, and can be useful in setting parameters that encourage optimal pacing. Careful planning ensures that the pace of implementation is neither too fast nor too slow. As noted previously, hiring of staff for training too far in advance of service delivery encourages personnel spending prior to delivery of reimbursable services. Similarly, staff motivation to implement the EBI and client interest in receiving the service can wane over time if they are notified of the program too far before the service is offered. Thus, adequate EBI implementation pacing must consider provision of sufficient time for thorough completion of implementation tasks, and the resources needed to compete those tasks.

3. **Poor adherence to fidelity monitoring expectations**
   High fidelity EBI delivery is dependent upon effective monitoring processes. Often, implementation is supported by purveyors who provide coaching support. In such instances, purveyors are able to monitor EBI delivery to ensure the intervention is being delivered as intended. However, purveyor support often is finite. Thus, sites ideally will transition to providing strong supervision practices for optimal EBI delivery that can be sustained. Effective supervision takes considerable time and effort. As stated earlier in the chapter, supervisors also need to be trained and supported to ensure that they can provide the oversight needed for frontline providers.

4. **Lack of reliable measurement system to assess the success of implementation**
   As noted previously, some EBI protocols have established measurement systems to monitor the success of implementation and patient outcomes. Others rely on self-monitoring by the organization. Regardless, a common misstep by implementing sites is to not establish consistent monitoring of implementation and clinical outcomes, often due to a lack of reliable measurement systems. During the readiness process, it is essential that sites come to consensus on how outcomes will be measured, expectations for success, and where opportunities will be provided for improvement.

A particular challenge for EBIs whose objective is to achieve a high reach within a population in order to achieve a public health impact (e.g., preventive interventions, population health programs) is establishing metrics to show growth over time. Thus, key to the pre-implementation process is determining the baseline level of population functioning or reach. Although a formal population level assessment often is not feasible, it is feasible to assess the organization's previous success in meeting the identified metrics. Thus, sites are encouraged to develop rigorous plans for measuring change over time in their organization as a result of the EBI versus relying on anecdotal assessment.

DISCUSSION QUESTIONS

1. An organization would like to replace an existing program with an EBI. What should the organization consider when deciding on the implementation team?
2. An organization has evaluated outcomes of an EBI and determine that it is effective. However, the initial funding for EBI implementation is coming to an end. Discuss strategies that this organization could pursue in order to keep this program running.
3. An organization has succeeded in initial implementation in which staff have been trained in delivering a new EBI. Yet, a decision has been made to end external consultation provided by a purveyor organization prematurely. What are the potential risks of such a decision to the sustainability of the EBI?
4. Describe how an organization might determine whether an EBI implementation was successful or not.

REFERENCES

Aalsma, M. C., Dir, A. L., Zapolski, T. C. B., Hulvershorn, L. A., Monahan, P. O., Saldana, L., & Adams, Z. W. (2019). Implementing risk stratification to the treatment of adolescent substance use among youth involved in the juvenile justice system: Protocol of a hybrid type I trial. *Addiction Science & Clinical Practice, 14*(1), 36. https://doi.org/10.1186/s13722-019-0161-5

Aarons, G. A., Hurlburt, M., & Horwitz, S. M. (2011). Advancing a conceptual model of evidence-based practice implementation in public service sectors. *Administration and Policy in Mental Health, 38*(1), 4–23. https://doi.org/10.1007/s10488-010-0327-7

Bertram, R. M., Blase, K. A., & Fixsen, D. L. (2015). Improving programs and outcomes: Implementation frameworks and organization change. *Research on Social Work Practice, 25*(4), 477–487. https://doi.org/10.1177/1049731514537687

Bova, C., Jaffarian, C., Crawford, S., Quintos, J. B., Lee, M., & Sullivan-Bolyai, S. (2017). Intervention fidelity. *Nursing Research, 66*(1), 54–59. https://doi.org/10.1097/NNR.0000000000000194

Brown, C. H., Chamberlain, P., Saldana, L., Padgett, C., Wang, W., & Cruden, G. (2014). Evaluation of two implementation strategies in 51 child county public service systems in two states: Results of a cluster randomized head-to-head implementation trial [4201704]. *Implementation Science, 9*, 134. https://doi.org/10.1186/s13012-014-0134-8

Burke, L. A., & Hutchins, H. M. (2007). Training transfer: An integrative literature review. *Human Resource Development Review, 6*(3), 263–296. https://doi.org/10.1177/1534484307303035

Chamberlain, P., & Mihalic, S. F. (1998). Multidimensional treatment foster care. In D. S. Elliott (Ed.), *Book eight: Blueprints for violence prevention*. Institute of Behavioral Science, University of Colorado at Boulder.

Chambers, D. A., Glasgow, R. E., & Stange, K. C. (2013). The dynamic sustainability framework: Addressing the paradox of sustainment amid ongoing change. *Implementation Science, 8*(1), 117. https://doi.org/10.1186/1748-5908-8-117

Corcoran, T., Rowling, L., & Wise, M. (2015). The potential contribution of intermediary organizations for implementation of school mental health. *Advances in School Mental Health Promotion, 8*(2), 57–70. https://doi.org/10.1080/1754730X.2015.1019688

Crable, E. L., Biancarelli, D., Walkey, A. J., & Drainoni, M.-L. (2020). Barriers and facilitators to implementing priority inpatient initiatives in the safety net setting. *Implementation Science Communications, 1*(1), 1–11. https://doi.org/10.1186/s43058-020-00024-6

Dolcini, M. M., Davey-Rothwell, M. A., Singh, R. R., Catania, J. A., Gandelman, A. A., Narayanan, V., Harris, J., & McKay, V. R. (2021). Use of effective training and quality assurance strategies is associated with high-fidelity EBI implementation in practice settings: A case analysis. *Translational Behavioral Medicine, 11*(1), 34–45. https://doi.org/10.1093/tbm/ibz158

Dorsey, S., Kerns, S. E. U., Lucid, L., Pullmann, M. D., Harrison, J. P., Berliner, L., Thompson, K., & Deblinger, E. (2018). Objective coding of content and techniques in workplace-based supervision of an EBT in public mental health. *Implementation Science, 13*(1), 1–12. https://doi.org/10.1186/s13012-017-0708-3

Durlak, J. A., & DuPre, E. P. (2008). Implementation matters: A review of research on the influence of implementation on program outcomes and the factors affecting implementation. *American Journal of Community Psychology, 41*(3–4), 327–350. https://doi.org/10.1007/s10464-008-9165-0

Ehrhart, M. G., Aarons, G. A., & Farahnak, L. R. (2014). Assessing the organizational context for EBP implementation: The development and validity testing of the Implementation Climate Scale (ICS). *Implementation Science, 9*(1), 157. https://doi.org/10.1186/s13012-014-0157-1

Fixsen, D. L., Naoom, S. F., Blase, K. A., & Friedman, R. M. (2005). *Implementation research: A synthesis of the literature.* University of South Florida, Louis de la Parte Florida Mental Health Institute, National Implementation Research Network (FMHI Pub No. 231).

Frank, H. E., Saldana, L., Kendall, P. C., Schaper, H. A., & Norris, L. A. (2021). Bringing evidence-based interventions into the schools: An examination of organizational factors and implementation outcomes. *Child & Youth Services.* https://doi.org/10.1080/0145935x.2021.1894920

Franks, R. P. (2010). Role of the intermediary organization in promoting and disseminating best practices for children and youth: The Connecticut center for effective practice. *Report on Emotional & Behavioral Disorders in Youth, 10*(4), 87–93.

Franks, R. P., & Bory, C. T. (2015). Who supports the successful implementation and sustainability of evidence-based practices? Defining and understanding the roles of intermediary and purveyor organizations. *New Directions for Child and Adolescent Development, 2015*(149), 41–56. https://doi.org/10.1002/cad.20112

Henggeler, S. W., Schoenwald, S. K., Borduin, C. M., Rowland, M. D., & Cunningham, P. B. (2009). *Multisystemic therapy for antisocial behavior in children and adolescents* (2nd ed.). Guilford Press.

Kendall, P. C. (1994). Treating anxiety disorders in children: Results of a randomized clinical trial. *Journal of Consulting and Clinical Psychology, 62*(1), 100–110. https://doi.org/10.1037/0022-006X.62.1.100

Kendall, P. C., & Khanna, M. (2008). *Coach's manual for Camp Cope-A-Lot: The Coping Cat CD-ROM.* Workbook Publishing Inc.

Liddle, H. A. (2002). *Multidimensional Family Therapy Treatment (MDFT) for adolescent cannabis users: Vol. 5 Cannabis Youth Treatment (CYT) manual series.* Center for Substance Abuse Treatment, Substance Abuse and Mental Health Services Administration.

Lyon, A. R., Stirman, S. W., Kerns, S. E. U., & Bruns, E. J. (2011). Developing the mental health workforce: Review and application of training approaches from multiple disciplines. *Administration and Policy in Mental Health and Mental Health Services Research, 38*(4), 238–253. https://doi.org/10.1007/s10488-010-0331-y

Maher, E. J., Jackson, L. J., Pecora, P. J., Schultz, D. J., Chandra, A., & Barnes-Proby, D. S. (2009). Overcoming challenges to implementing and evaluating evidence-based interventions in child welfare: A matter of necessity. *Children and Youth Services Review, 31*(5), 555–562. https://doi.org/10.1016/j.childyouth.2008.10.013

Meyers, D. C., Durlak, J. A., & Wandersman, A. (2012). The Quality Implementation Framework: A synthesis of critical steps in the implementation process. *American Journal of Community Psychology, 50*(3–4), 462–480. https://doi.org/10.1007/s10464-012-9522-x

Moullin, J. C., Dickson, K. S., Stadnick, N. A., Rabin, B., & Aarons, G. A. (2019). Systematic review of the Exploration, Preparation, Implementation, Sustainment (EPIS) framework. *Implementation Science, 14*(1). BioMed Central Ltd. https://doi.org/10.1186/s13012-018-0842-6

Nadeem, E., Saldana, L., Chapman, J., & Schaper, H. (2018). A mixed methods study of the stages of implementation for an evidence-based trauma intervention in schools. *Behavior Therapy, 49*(4), 509–524. https://doi.org/10.1016/j.beth.2017.12.004

Nilsen, P. (2015). Making sense of implementation theories, models and frameworks. *Implementation Science, 10.* https://doi.org/10.1186/s13012-015-0242-0

Powell, B. J., Haley, A. D., Patel, S. V., Amaya-Jackson, L., Glienke, B., Blythe, M., Lengnick-Hall, R., McCrary, S., Beidas, R. S., Lewis, C. C., Aarons, G. A., Wells, K. B., Saldana, L., McKay, M. M., & Weinberger, M. (2020). Improving the implementation and sustainment of evidence-based practices in community mental health organizations: A study protocol for a matched-pair cluster randomized pilot study of the Collaborative Organizational Approach to Selecting and Tailoring I. *Implementation Science Communications, 1*(1), 9. https://doi.org/10.1186/s43058-020-00009-5

Proctor, E., Hooley, C., Morse, A., McCrary, S., Kim, H., & Kohl, P. L. (2019). Intermediary/purveyor organizations for evidence-based interventions in the US child mental health: Characteristics and implementation strategies. *Implementation Science, 14*(1), 1–14. https://doi.org/10.1186/s13012-018-0845-3

Saldana, L. (2014). The stages of implementation completion for evidence-based practice: Protocol for a mixed methods study. *Implementation Science, 9*(1), 43. https://doi.org/10.1186/1748-5908-9-43

Saldana, L., Bennett, I., Powers, D., Vredevoogd, M., Grover, T., Schaper, H., & Campbell, M. (2020). Scaling implementation of collaborative care for depression: Adaptation of the Stages of Implementation Completion (SIC). *administration and policy in mental health and mental health services research*, *47*(2), 188–196. https://doi.org/10.1007/s10488-019-00944-z

Saldana, L., & Chamberlain, P. (2012). Supporting implementation: The role of community development teams to build infrastructure. *American Journal of Community Psychology*, *50*(3–4), 334–346. https://doi.org/10.1007/s10464-012-9503-0; 10.1007/s10464-012-9503-0

Saldana, L., Chamberlain, P., Bradford, W. D., Campbell, M., & Landsverk, J. (2014). The cost of implementing new strategies (COINS): A method for mapping implementation resources using the stages of implementation completion. *Children and Youth Services Review*, *39*, 177–182. https://doi.org/10.1016/j.childyouth.2013.10.006

Saldana, L., Chamberlain, P., & Chapman, J. (2016). A supervisor-targeted implementation approach to promote system change: The R3 Model. *Administration and Policy in Mental Health and Mental Health Services Research*, *43*(6), 879–892. https://doi.org/10.1007/s10488-016-0730-9

Saldana, L., Chamberlain, P., Wang, W., & Brown, C. H. (2012). Predicting program start-up using the stages of implementation measure. *Administration and Policy in Mental Health and Mental Health Services Research*, *39*(6), 419–425. https://doi.org/10.1007/s10488-011-0363-y

Saldana, L., Schaper, H., Campbell, M., & Chapman, J. E. (2015). Standardized measurement of implementation: The Universal SIC. 7th Annual Conference on the Science of the Dissemination and Implementation in Health. [PMC4551722]. *Implement Science*, *10*(S1), A73. https://doi.org/10.1186/1748-5908-10-s1-a73

Schoenwald, S. K., Sheidow, A. J., & Letourneau, E. J. (2004). Toward effective quality assurance in evidence-based practice: Links between expert consultation, therapist fidelity, and child outcomes. *Journal of Clinical Child and Adolescent Psychology*, *33*(1), 94–104. https://doi.org/10.1207/S15374424JCCP3301_10

Sterrett-Hong, E. M., Saldana, L., Burek, J., Schaper, H., Karam, E., Verbist, A. N., & Cameron, K. (2021). An exploratory study of a training team-coordinated approach to implementation. *Global Implementation Research and Applications*, *1*(1), 17–29. https://doi.org/10.1007/s43477-020-00003-y

Wang, W., Saldana, L., Brown, C. H., & Chamberlain, P. (2010). Factors that influenced county system leaders to implement an evidence-based program: A baseline survey within a randomized controlled trial. *Implementation Science*, *5*(1), 72. https://doi.org/10.1186/1748-5908-5-72

Watson, D. P., Snow-Hill, N., Saldana, L., Walden, A. L., Staton, M., Kong, A., & Donenberg, G. (2020). A longitudinal mixed method approach for assessing implementation context and process factors: Comparison of three sites from a Housing First implementation strategy pilot. *Implementation Research and Practice*, *1*, 263348952097497. https://doi.org/10.1177/2633489520974974

9

An Introduction to Evaluation and Learning in Implementation Science

Arianna Rubin Means, Bradley H. Wagenaar, Sarah J. Masyuko, and Anjuli D. Wagner

Learning Objectives

By the end of this chapter, readers will be able to:

- Develop implementation science evaluation questions that are appropriate for different stages of implementation and varying contexts
- Select and apply an appropriate framework to guide evaluation
- Select appropriate implementation, process, and health impact outcomes to address an evaluation question of interest
- Identify tradeoffs that must be considered in the design of an implementation research evaluation to balance validity and feasibility
- Describe the relative strengths and weaknesses of different evaluation study designs and what they mean for implementation practice

CASE STUDY 9.1A DECIDING TO CONDUCT AN EVALUATION OF A SCHOOL HEALTH INTERVENTION

A group of city-level public health officials in the United States sit around a conference table, discussing an emerging public health challenge in their area. Over the past 5 years, school performance has been declining and disciplinary activities have been increasing among school-age children in the city, particularly within under-resourced schools, affecting student mental health and quality of life. The public health officials excitedly discuss a new school-based social support peer-mentoring intervention that proved to be very effective in improving academic and mental health outcomes in a neighboring state. As they consider adapting and implementing the intervention locally, the public health officials are faced with two primary questions: (a) How can they determine if this intervention is acceptable or feasible in their schools? And (b) How will they know that the intervention is effective, and worth the investment to continue implementing or scaling the peer-mentoring intervention across the city? The questions faced by these public health officials highlight key challenges in evaluating the implementation of programs in real-world contexts.

INTRODUCTION

In this chapter, readers are introduced to the basics of designing an evaluation, including identifying an evaluation question, identifying variables to measure in the evaluation, and steps for deciding which type of evaluation study design to employ to answer different evaluation questions across the stages of implementation and scale-up.

WHAT IS AN IMPLEMENTATION EVALUATION QUESTION?

Evaluating implementation is necessary for improving program effectiveness and optimizing efficiency, which facilitates the investment of finite resources in implementation efforts that are high performing. Evaluating implementation also helps in the adaptation of programs, policies, or interventions to maximize population health. Implementation science is primarily focused on evaluating the effectiveness of *implementation strategies* used to deliver evidence-based clinical care or public health interventions, as opposed to assessing the effectiveness of **evidence-based interventions (EBIs)** themselves. EBIs include programs, practices, principles, procedures, policies, and the use of new pills and products (Hendricks-Brown et al., 2017). Evaluation of EBIs might include testing the clinical efficacy of a new vaccine in a controlled setting or evaluating the real-world effectiveness of a clinical procedure. Evaluations of implementation strategies, on the other hand, include understanding if and by how much an implementation strategy improves delivery of the EBI. For example, in Case Study 9.1 implementers have identified an effective social support EBI, and plan to evaluate a peer-mentoring implementation strategy to increase adoption of the social support practices in schools.

This chapter references different stages of implementation, including pre-implementation, early or mid-implementation, and late implementation (Chamberlain et al., 2011). Relevant *implementation evaluation questions* will differ across these stages of implementation as objectives range from initial adoption of an EBI to long-term sustainability of a program or policy. During the preimplementation stage, evaluators seek to understand if their proposed implementation strategy is well suited to overcome the implementation challenges that prevent widespread or effective use of an EBI. Evaluators can conduct *formative implementation research* to understand the barriers and facilitators to EBI implementation. Evaluators might ask, "What is the acceptability of the EBI or of the implementation strategy, and how might the strategy need to be tailored for this setting?" For example, during formative research, evaluators might learn that a major barrier to implementation of an EBI is that the EBI has low acceptability, and health providers do not believe that the EBI is sufficiently evidence-based. In this scenario, evaluators could use this information to develop or adapt an implementation strategy that could help overcome this barrier within the specific context.

During early implementation, the focus of an evaluation question may be related to increasing adoption of the EBI of interest. An evaluation question might ask: "Does a given implementation strategy increase use of the EBI by a key stakeholder group?" At mid-implementation, evaluators might ask "How does the local context influence fidelity in delivery of the implementation strategy or the EBI of interest?" To answer these questions, implementation science often requires monitoring of *process indicators*, which are used to describe how program activities are delivered, if activities were implemented as intended, and if there is a relationship between implementation activities and targeted outcomes (such as a "dose-response" relationship). Evaluation questions related to late implementation might ask: "How can sustainability or maintenance of this strategy be achieved?"; "How can this program continue to be implemented with fidelity while reducing costs?"; or "What are specific modifications to the implementation strategy that can help the EBI reach specific subgroups of the population that are underserved by the current delivery system?" As described subsequently in this chapter, implementation science typically evaluates changes in *implementation outcomes* to determine if a strategy is effective. Implementation outcomes include the acceptability of an EBI or the implementation strategy used to deliver it, fidelity to implementation protocols, costs of implementation, and sustainability over the long term.

This chapter presents two overarching case studies, applied throughout the chapter to characterize the different components of an implementation evaluation. The first case study characterizes efforts to improve delivery of evidence-based social support interventions for youth exhibiting behavioral challenges in schools in the United States. The second case study spotlights implementation efforts in Kenya to improve tuberculosis (TB) treatment outcomes by increasing access to treatment and support for medication adherence. Across both case studies, this chapter presents key evaluation concepts, including common variables to measure in an implementation evaluation, implementation frameworks that can be applied to guide an evaluation, opportunities to apply mixed methods, and important evaluation design considerations such as the budget, scale, data collection methods, and data sources available for the evaluation.

CASE STUDY 9.2A OPTIMIZING TUBERCULOSIS MANAGEMENT IN KENYA

TB is an infectious disease caused by bacteria that are spread through the air via coughs or sneezes. Children, the elderly, or individuals with compromised immune systems are particularly at risk for developing TB. It is important that people who have TB are treated and take medicine exactly as prescribed. If they do not, they are at risk of severe illness or harboring TB bacteria that can become drug resistant. Kenya

(*continued*)

CASE STUDY 9.2A OPTIMIZING TUBERCULOSIS MANAGEMENT IN KENYA (*continued*)

has a high burden of TB, and patients with TB face challenges accessing TB care due to the costs of medical services, transportation challenges to reach medical care, and mistrust between patients and healthcare providers (Enos et al., 2018; Kadota et al., 2020). A clinical evaluation question in this context might include an investigation of the efficacy of different TB drug regimens. However, an implementation evaluation refocuses the evaluation on the implementation strategy as opposed to the EBI. For example, evaluators have strong evidence from randomized trials that TB medications such as isoniazid and rifapentine are effective at treating TB if taken according to protocols. Implementation evaluations may focus on determining the acceptability of new strategies to deliver TB medications, identifying contextual determinants of effective or ineffective TB program implementation, or evaluating the costs and cost-effectiveness of implementation strategies used to improve care access or medication adherence.

CASE STUDY 9.1B IMPROVING DELIVERY OF SOCIAL SUPPORT INTERVENTIONS FOR YOUTH IN THE UNITED STATES

Social support is effective for promoting positive academic and psychosocial outcomes for school-age youth who are at risk of or experiencing behavioral health challenges (Turley et al., 2017). Thus, social support programs are an EBI for improving student mental health, school attendance, quality of life, and other behavioral health outcomes. However, underserved communities, including ethnic and racial minorities, are less likely to have access to social support interventions in schools. Implementation strategies for delivering social support include peer mentoring, but it can be challenging to effectively integrate peer mentoring into the routine implementation context of schools. To determine if peer mentoring is an appropriate strategy for delivering and strengthening social support in schools, an implementation evaluation could focus on determining the feasibility of the new peer-mentoring strategy, adapting the strategy to perform in different cultural or geographic contexts than those in which they were originally developed, or scaling strategies for delivering social support throughout a school district. In addition to implementation outcomes such as adoption, coverage, and sustainability of school-based peer mentoring, evaluators might also choose to measure student-level outcomes such as changes in student absenteeism, academic performance, and health outcomes, including improvements in student mental health.

HOW DO IMPLEMENTATION SCIENCE FRAMEWORKS CONTRIBUTE TO AN EVALUATION?

Implementation science often draws from established theories, models, or frameworks to evaluate implementation and help guide the process of translating research into practice. Theories, models, and frameworks (henceforth referred to only as frameworks) help implementers and evaluators focus their attention on the essential elements of implementation, providing guidance for how and why implementation succeeds or fails. In this way, frameworks serve as a tool for evaluators to identify factors that are likely to predict implementation success and to develop or refine implementation strategies (Nilsen, 2015). The standardized terminology provided by frameworks also helps to facilitate the comparison of findings from evaluations conducted in different settings. For example, when constructs included in an evaluation framework show differential effects across settings, implementers may have new insight regarding the influence of context on implementation success. There are several implementation science frameworks that can be utilized for an evaluation. This chapter discusses two specific frameworks of interest, the Implementation Outcomes Framework and the RE-AIM framework.

The *Implementation Outcomes Framework* proposes eight discrete implementation outcomes (acceptability, adoption, appropriateness, feasibility, fidelity, implementation cost, penetration/coverage, and sustainability) that reflect "the effects of deliberate and purposive actions to implement new treatments, practices, and services" (Proctor et al., 2011, p. 65). These outcomes can be used to evaluate the success of implementation activities and to compare the effectiveness of strategies to enhance implementation of EBIs within routine public health practice. For example, implementation outcomes such as *acceptability*, *feasibility*, and *appropriateness* offer insight into why individuals do or do not utilize an EBI. Outcomes such as *fidelity* and *penetration* offer insight into why an EBI does or does not achieve desired effects. And outcomes such as implementation *cost* and *sustainability* offer insights into the likelihood that an EBI will be maintained within an organization or health system (Lewis et al., 2018).

The Implementation Outcomes Framework also asserts that implementation outcomes are precursors to service and health outcomes, such as efficiency of service delivery, financial risk protection, patient satisfaction, and changes in health status. Thus, implementation outcomes are not only primary evaluation outcomes themselves but are also considered intermediate outcomes in health services and clinical outcome effectiveness research, helping evaluators to understand the process of implementation and the influence of context on clinical outcomes (Proctor et al., 2011). As a result, implementation outcomes, summarized in Table 9.1, are considered essential elements of an implementation evaluation. For example, if an EBI is adopted but with low fidelity to the clinical protocols, it likely will not achieve targeted health outcomes. Alternatively, if an EBI is adopted and implementers have perfect fidelity to delivery protocols, but it is not acceptable to the local population and thus achieves low population-level coverage, the population-level effect will be limited.

TABLE 9.1 Implementation Outcomes

IMPLEMENTATION OUTCOME	DEFINITION	RELATED TERMS	EXAMPLE QUESTIONS
Acceptability	The perception among implementation stakeholders that an EBI is agreeable, palatable, or satisfactory	Comfort, relative advantage, credibility	How acceptable is a new TB preventive medication to TB providers?
Adoption	The absolute number, proportion, and representativeness of settings and intervention agents who are willing to initiate an EBI	Uptake, utilization, intention to try	Do stakeholder engagement workshops increase the likelihood of adopting regional policies recommending this intervention?

(*continued*)

TABLE 9.1 Implementation Outcomes (*continued*)

IMPLEMENTATION OUTCOME	DEFINITION	RELATED TERMS	EXAMPLE QUESTIONS
Appropriateness	The perceived fit or relevance of the intervention in a particular setting or for a particular provider/consumer	Relevance, perceived fit, compatibility, trialability, suitability, usefulness, practicability	How suitable do providers perceive reduced frequency TB preventive medication to be for people living with HIV, taking daily HIV medication?
Feasibility	The extent to which an EBI can be successfully used or carried out within a given agency or setting	Practicality, actual fit, utility, suitability for everyday use	How practical do working adults find directly observed therapy to ensure adherence to TB medication?
Fidelity	The degree to which an EBI was implemented as it was prescribed in the original testing or as it was intended by its developers	Adherence, delivery as intended, treatment integrity, quality of program delivery, intensity or dosage of delivery	How does a new national policy switching from traditional TB treatment regimens to reduced duration and frequency impact patient treatment completion and appropriate adherence?
Implementation Cost	The incremental cost of the implementation strategy (e.g., how the services are delivered in a particular setting). The total cost of implementation would also include the cost of the EBI itself	Marginal cost	What is the cost of a lower frequency TB preventive medication?
Penetration (provider-level) or coverage (population-level)	The degree to which the population that is eligible to benefit from an intervention actually receives it	Reach, access, service spread or effective coverage	How does a provider incentivization program impact the proportion of individuals who receive TB preventive therapy, among those eligible?
Sustainability	The extent to which the EBI continues to be delivered and/or individual behavior change (i.e., clinician, patient) is maintained; the program and individual behavior	Maintenance, continuation, durability, institutionalization,	Do TB treatment reminders continue to be effective in

(*continued*)

TABLE 9.1 Implementation Outcomes (*continued*)

IMPLEMENTATION OUTCOME	DEFINITION	RELATED TERMS	EXAMPLE QUESTIONS
	change may evolve or adapt while continuing to produce benefits for individuals/the system	routinization, integration, incorporation	maintaining treatment adherence over time?

EBI, evidence-based intervention; HIV, human immunodeficiency virus; TB, tuberculosis.

Sources: Adapted from Proctor, E., Silmere, H., Raghavan, R., Hovmand, P., Aarons, G., Bunger, A., Griffey, R., & Hensley, M. (2011). Outcomes for implementation research: Conceptual distinctions, measurement challenges, and research agenda. *Administration and Policy in Mental Health, 38*(2), 65–76. https://doi.org/10.1007/s10488-010-0319-7; and Peters, D. H., Tran, N. T., & Adam, T. (2013). *Implementation research in health: A practical guide.* World Health Organization.

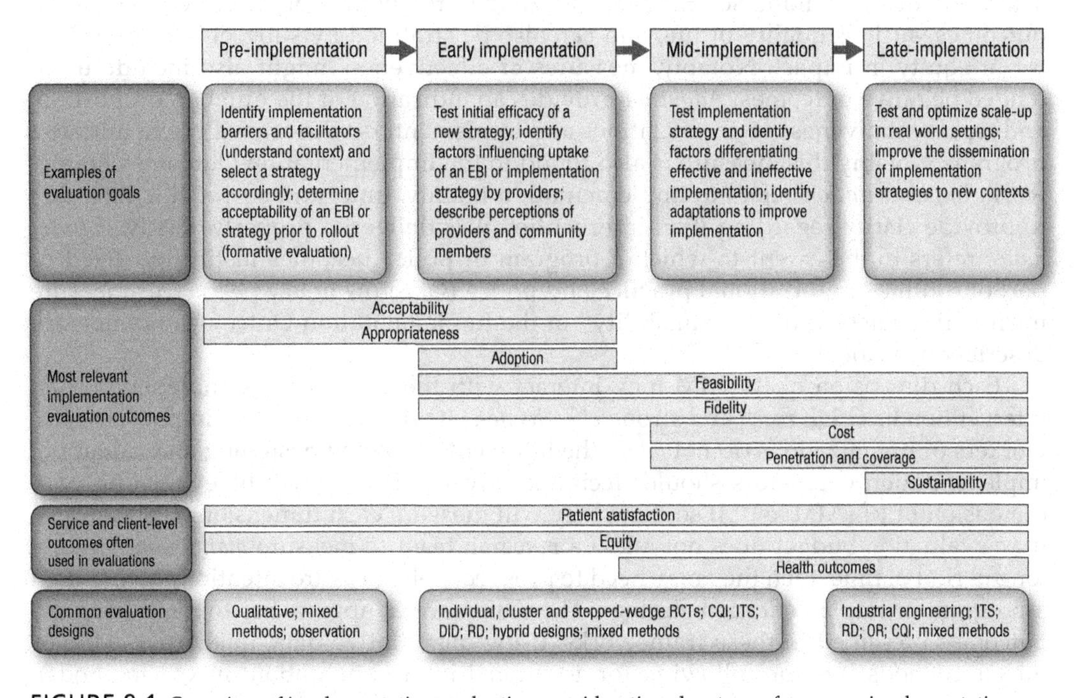

FIGURE 9.1 Overview of implementation evaluation considerations by stage of program implementation.

CQI, continuous quality improvement; DID, difference in differences; EBI, evidence-based intervention; ITS, interrupted time series; OR, operations research; RD, regression discontinuity; RCT, randomized controlled trial.

Not all implementation outcomes will be relevant for every evaluation, and there are at least three factors that should be considered when selecting outcomes from the Implementation Outcomes Framework. First, the stage of implementation influences what outcomes may be relevant. For example, evaluators may wish to study the outcome of *acceptability* early in implementation to understand stakeholder satisfaction with a treatment, service, or innovation. Conversely, within evaluations focused on scale-up, evaluators may employ the outcome of implementation *cost* later in the implementation process, to determine the overall cost-effectiveness of implementation at scale (Figure 9.1). Second, evaluators should consider the level of analysis for the outcomes, as some outcomes may be better suited for individual-level analysis (e.g., *acceptability*) while others may be more appropriate for an aggregate analysis at the level of the healthcare organization (e.g., *penetration*). Third, evaluators should consider the interrelationships between implementation outcomes. For example, the *acceptability* of an innovation may influence the degree to which it is successfully *adopted* (Proctor et al., 2011). It is also important to specify if you are applying outcomes to an EBI, an implementation strategy, or both. For example, you might seek to determine both the cost of an EBI and of the implementation strategy used to deliver it.

The *RE-AIM framework* (Reach, Effectiveness, Adoption, Implementation, Maintenance) was developed to inform program scale-up and maximize the public health impact of an EBI (Glasgow et al., 2019). RE-AIM is one of the most frequently used frameworks for implementation evaluations and has been used for over 20 years, applied in both high- and low-resource settings. The *reach* in RE-AIM describes the absolute number, proportion, and representativeness of individuals who are willing to participate in a program or intervention. Measuring *reach* helps evaluators determine if they have successfully engaged key populations within their intervention and achieved equity in doing so. *Effectiveness* refers to the impact of an EBI on individual outcomes, such as quality of life, and can also be stratified by subgroup as an indicator of equity in impact. Notably, measures of effectiveness might also include unintended negative outcomes. *Adoption* provides an indication of the number, proportion, and representativeness of organizations and implementers who are willing to initiate a program. Notably this measure is also found in the Implementation Outcomes Framework. *Implementation* refers to implementation fidelity, time, and cost and is intended to provide clarity regarding if an intervention was delivered properly. Lastly, *maintenance* refers to the extent to which a program or policy becomes institutionalized or part of routine organizational practice and policy (Glasgow et al., 1999). This measure mirrors the outcome of "sustainability" in the Implementation Outcomes Framework described previously.

Each dimension of RE-AIM may interact with the other. For example, even if an intervention has high *reach* and strong *effectiveness*, it will have minimal impact if health workers or organizations do not *adopt* the intervention. When designing an evaluation, implementation evaluators should decide in advance if they will be evaluating each dimension of RE-AIM and, if so, how they will measure each dimension. For example, if an evaluation budget does not allow a research team to measure *maintenance* over a long period of time, then they may need to prospectively measure intentions to maintain a program or implementation strategy. There are several approaches to measuring the outcomes presented in these frameworks, using quantitative data, qualitative data, or mixed methods (see the following for additional information about mixed methods). For any given approach, it is important that these outcomes are measured accurately and consistently.

CASE STUDY 9.2B APPLYING AN EVALUATION FRAMEWORK TO A TB SERVICES EVALUATION IN KENYA

In this fictional case study, a District Health Office in Kenya has decided to implement a new motivational interviewing strategy to improve medication adherence among adult patients with TB. They have designed an implementation strategy that includes training on motivational interviewing for nursing staff and 1 year of ongoing supervisory support, and they offer it to hospitals throughout the

(*continued*)

CASE STUDY 9.2B APPLYING AN EVALUATION FRAMEWORK TO A TB SERVICES EVALUATION IN KENYA (*continued*)

district to see if they are interested in participating. The evaluators in the District Health Office decide to use the RE-AIM framework to structure their evaluation. The proportion of hospitals and nurses within hospitals that agree to participate in the program and, separately, the proportion of estimated active TB cases in the community accessing this program together represent the *reach* of the program. To determine the *effectiveness* of the program, evaluators track the proportion of patients who successfully adhere to treatment over a 1-year period. *Adoption* is measured as the proportion of trained nurses who incorporate the new motivational interviewing technique into their clinical service. Evaluators measure *implementation* as the cost of the motivational interviewing and supervisory strategy, including both the financial costs of the program as well as the opportunity costs borne by nurses, supervisors, and hospitals that participate. Lastly, the evaluators determine the *maintenance* of the program based upon the proportion of trained nurses who adopted the motivational interviewing in the first year of the pilot program and continue to utilize the technique in the second year of implementation. Together, these measures provide the District Health Office with an overview of the overall effectiveness of implementation, and opportunities to improve implementation to increase public health impact.

HYBRID EFFECTIVENESS-IMPLEMENTATION EVALUATIONS

In some scenarios, implementers may wish to evaluate an EBI and an implementation strategy together, rather than sequentially one at a time. For example, implementers conducting primarily clinical research may wish to know if there are contextual factors influencing the effectiveness of an EBI and may thus incorporate implementation outcomes such as acceptability or fidelity as process outcomes. Likewise, implementation evaluators may need to ensure that an EBI continues to be safe and effective at improving population health in a new setting. "Hybrid" implementation science and clinical effectiveness studies can be used to integrate clinical and implementation research (Curran et al., 2012). In a *hybrid effectiveness-implementation study*, evaluators aim to simultaneously understand the clinical effectiveness of an EBI as well as the effectiveness of implementation strategies used to deliver it. This is accomplished by collecting data on implementation outcomes such as acceptability, fidelity, or costs, while also collecting clinical health outcomes at the level of the patient or population. These designs may be particularly important to address potential health equity concerns when an EBI is adapted, implemented, and/or scaled-up within a different context than it was originally tested.

Hybrid effectiveness-implementation studies can take several forms; for example, they can have a primary aim of testing EBI effectiveness while simultaneously gathering information on the acceptability or feasibility of an implementation strategy. This approach would be taken when there is limited data on EBI clinical effectiveness. Alternatively, a hybrid effectiveness-implementation study can have the primary aim of testing different implementation strategies and their effect on implementation outcomes, while also collecting data on patient-level health outcomes as a "check" that modification of the implementation strategy did not negatively impact the effectiveness of the EBI. This approach would be taken when there is already robust existing data on EBI clinical effectiveness.

CASE STUDY 9.2C STRUCTURING A HYBRID EFFECTIVENESS-IMPLEMENTATION TRIAL TO IMPROVE TB CARE

In this fictional case study, a Kenyan District Health Office has an urgent need to improve the proportion of TB patients living with HIV who initiate and adhere to TB treatment. The District Health Office decided to launch a new program to determine if an implementation strategy, direct text messaging of medication reminders to patients, improves treatment uptake and sustained adherence. However, the District Health officials were concerned about broadly rolling out the program because there was no existing evidence about treatment effectiveness in their specific setting. As a result, local evaluators designed a hybrid effectiveness-implementation study to evaluate both implementation and clinical outcomes in the newly launched program. The evaluators selected primary implementation outcomes of *adoption* (the proportion of providers who send at least one medication reminder text message to patients within the first month of the program) and *fidelity* (the proportion of providers who follow the implementation strategy protocol in all text messages). Secondary clinical effectiveness outcomes included adverse events and treatment success (incidence of active TB). By measuring both outcomes together, the evaluators were able to work with public health officials to maximize the acceptability of the text messaging strategy while also affirming that the treatment continues to be safe and effective in their district.

HOW ARE MIXED METHODS INCORPORATED WITHIN AN EVALUATION DESIGN?

An evaluation may include quantitative data, qualitative data, or a mix of both. Quantitative data (e.g., binary, categorical, or continuous variables) and analysis can be used to answer evaluation questions such as: "Does this implementation strategy influence the targeted outcome, and if so by how much?" or, "What is the comparative effectiveness of this implementation strategy, and how does it differ by setting or population?" Qualitative data on the other hand include text transcripts from individual interviews or focus group discussions, document review, photography, or other non-quantitative data. Qualitative data can be used to answer evaluation questions that might be more explanatory than quantitative questions, such as: "Why does this implementation strategy influence or not influence the targeted outcome?" When evaluators design a mixed methods evaluation, they purposefully integrate quantitative and qualitative data within the evaluation's design, development of data collection instruments, or analysis. Mixed methods combine the power of stories (qualitative data) with the power of numbers (quantitative data; Pluye & Hong, 2014).

There are many reasons why implementation evaluators may wish to conduct a mixed methods evaluation. First, evaluators may wish to *triangulate* findings to identify whether the two sources of data support the same conclusion, also known as convergence or corroboration. When findings do corroborate each other, evaluators might feel more confident in their conclusions. When findings diverge from each other, evaluators may wish to understand the divergence, and use the conflicting findings to drive additional data collection or to develop hypotheses that explain the divergence. Mixed methods can provide an *explanation* of evaluation findings, by elaborating, enhancing, illustrating, or clarifying the results from one method with the results from the other method. Mixed methods can be used to inform *sampling* by refining or identifying key population(s) of interest. For example, quantitative data may elucidate who key adopters and non-adopters of an EBI might be, and evaluators could separately interview individuals from each group to better understand their implementation behaviors. Lastly, *instrument development* is often aided by mixed methods when, for example, qualitative data collection is used to improve the wording of survey items or, conversely, findings from a survey are used to develop specific questions on qualitative interview guides (Creswell & Clark, 2017). For these reasons mixed methods help address the complexities of implementation more comprehensively than a single data source alone.

Sometimes quantitative and qualitative data are collected at the same time. In this case, typically evaluators analyze the data independently but compare, contrast, and interpret the findings together. For example, an evaluator might conduct a survey of facility staff to develop a complete understanding of their use of an EBI, and conduct focus group discussions with the health workers in the facility on the same topic. The evaluator would analyze the data separately but merge the results to assess how the quantitative and qualitative findings converge or diverge.

Quantitative and qualitative data may also be collected at different times (e.g., sequentially). Sometimes quantitative data are collected first. In this case, findings from quantitative data can be used to inform the sampling of participants for qualitative data collection, whose stories can provide important context for implementation successes or challenges. For example, an evaluator might conduct a survey of hospital staff to develop a complete understanding of their use of an EBI. After analyzing the quantitative findings, the evaluator could follow up with focus group discussions, using the resulting qualitative data to help clarify or explain any surprising findings from the quantitative results.

Sometimes qualitative data are collected first, followed by quantitative data. For example, an evaluator might conduct qualitative focus group discussions with health workers about their perceptions of a specific EBI. The evaluator can then use those findings to develop a quantitative survey instrument to assess the overall prevalence of certain behaviors that surfaced during the qualitative phase of the research. Similarly, qualitative methods can also be used to develop a conceptual model and hypotheses, and quantitative methods can be used to validate the model by testing the hypotheses.

Mixed methods combine the strengths of quantitative and qualitative data, while also compensating for the specific limitations of each method alone. Notable challenges of using mixed methods include the complexity of collecting multiple types of data and, as a result, the need for more resources; drawing from more analytical approaches requires more time to conduct the evaluation and more personnel with a variety of skillsets.

CASE STUDY 9.1C A MIXED METHODS EVALUATION OF A SOCIAL SUPPORT INTERVENTION IN SCHOOLS

In this fictional case study, a school board is evaluating a new evidence-based social emotional learning curriculum targeted at middle school students. Over the past 2 years, the school district has trained a small group of teachers in each school to serve as local "teacher champions" for the curriculum. The teacher champions train their colleagues and provide ongoing support on how to integrate the new curriculum into the classroom or troubleshoot challenging situations after the curriculum is launched. The evaluation team working with the school board has decided to collect quantitative data first, followed sequentially by qualitative data. First, the evaluators designed a survey that is administered to all teachers in the district to learn about their experiences working with the teacher champions and adopting the curriculum in their classroom. The evaluators analyzed the survey results and identified schools that they consider "high adopters," where most teachers reported working with a teacher champion to integrate the social emotional learning curriculum into their classroom. Likewise, the evaluators identified schools that were "low adopters," where less than half the teachers implemented the new curriculum. Then, they used the survey results to design questions for an interview guide to be used in focus group discussions with teachers in a subset of "high adopter" and "low adopter" schools. The qualitative evidence from the focus group discussions helped explain why some schools excelled at launching the new curriculum, while others struggled. The focus groups also provided an opportunity to learn from the stories and experiences of the teachers in implementing the curriculum, and for teachers to make suggestions on how to improve the teacher champion program and curriculum implementation process.

WHAT ARE KEY CONSIDERATIONS FOR CHOOSING AN EVALUATION DESIGN?

Selecting a Counterfactual

When choosing an evaluation design, evaluators must balance desire for strong evidence that shows that the intervention causes or leads to the improvements (causality) with practical considerations, such as timing, study feasibility, and budget. A strong *counterfactual* increases the strength of the evidence about causality. A counterfactual is what would have happened if implementation had not taken place. While it is impossible for an evaluator to know the true counterfactual, it is possible to craft an approximation of the counterfactual by using a comparison group. The term "counterfactual" is used in this chapter to refer to this approximation. A counterfactual comparison group can provide a strong approximation of the true counterfactual through several design considerations, many of which are discussed in the following sections. A strong counterfactual thus provides confidence that evaluators are measuring the effects of an implementation strategy, and not effects related to chance or other trends happening over time.

An evaluator's approach to establishing a counterfactual is often driven by practical considerations, such as the *degree of control* over the program that will be evaluated. When public health officials are conducting a small study or launching a new program, they can often control the location, target population, and sequencing of program launch. This allows them to develop a counterfactual by deliberately selecting areas that do not receive the program and observing targeted outcomes over the same time period that a program is delivered in other areas. During evaluations of large policies or natural events such as public health emergencies, there is often less control over implementation and thus it may be more challenging for evaluators to exert control over a counterfactual. Another key practical consideration is the *time available* to conduct the evaluation. If an evaluation must be conducted in a short period of time, evaluators should select process indicators and outcome indicators that can feasibly be observed during a short implementation period. When time is limited, evaluators can use retrospective data (e.g., data that were previously collected for other purposes, such as past medical records), instead of prospective data (e.g., data that are collected as the participants are followed over time). Similarly, *budget constraints* influence the choice of a counterfactual by limiting the sample size available for an evaluation (e.g., how many individuals or health facilities can be included in an evaluation). When budgets are tight, evaluators may need to use previously collected data from publicly available datasets to develop a counterfactual and estimate the potential effects of implementation in areas that were not exposed to an intervention.

Weighing the Balance Between Internal and External Validity

In addition to establishing a counterfactual, implementation evaluators must carefully consider the balance between internal and external validity. In an implementation evaluation, *internal validity* refers to the extent to which the observed relationship between an implementation strategy and an outcome is causal and not influenced by other external factors. Threats to internal validity include: (a) lack of clarity regarding whether implementation precedes the observed changes in the outcome, an issue that occurs when evaluators simply collect data at one point in time rather than prospectively across time; (b) fundamental differences in the groups who do and do not receive implementation, which might be responsible for any differences in changes in outcomes; and (c) external events occurring between the start of implementation and outcome measurement that differ between groups, among others.

External validity refers to the extent to which the results of an evaluation are generalizable beyond the specific setting of a given implementation effort. For example, if implementers demonstrate that a strategy can improve fidelity to an EBI in private well-funded clinics, an example of external validity could be the extent to which this strategy could also improve fidelity in public lower-resourced clinics. External validity can be enhanced by selecting diverse groups of participants as well as organizational units that are representative of the context to which evaluation results will be generalized. A common threat to external validity includes sampling bias (e.g., the selected populations and settings are not representative of the populations and settings to which the evaluation will be generalized), among others.

To summarize: When an evaluation has high internal validity, the evaluator can be confident that the relationship between the implementation strategy and the implementation outcome is "real" and unlikely to simply be explained by other factors. When an evaluation has high external validity, the findings are more generalizable and apply to a broad range of populations and settings. However, there is often an inherent tradeoff between internal and external validity; the more representative an evaluation is of broader populations and contexts, the more challenging it may be to control for extraneous factors that influence the implementation-to-outcome relationship of interest.

Choosing a Randomized or Nonrandomized Study Design

Early in the evaluation design process, one of the first questions evaluators must answer is whether they will conduct a *randomized evaluation design* or a *nonrandomized evaluation design*. Randomized evaluations assign individuals or groups to an implementation strategy or comparison group using a random process, such as a die roll or a random number generator. Randomized evaluations are typically considered the gold standard for establishing causality with higher internal validity because, when exposure to the implementation strategy is randomly assigned, there are fewer opportunities for bias. However, randomized evaluations often have lower external validity since they require the evaluator to have more control over implementation.

Randomization may not always be feasible or ethical. In such circumstances, a nonrandomized evaluation design may be a better fit. Participants in nonrandomized evaluations are not randomly allocated to different groups. Instead, patients, providers, organizations, or communities are assigned or self-select into implementation or non-implementation groups. Thus, compared to randomized evaluations, these designs have more threats to internal validity. However, since nonrandomized designs are often implemented in more "real-world" settings without as much evaluator control, they typically exhibit higher external validity. To address concerns with lower internal validity, nonrandomized evaluations often enhance rigor by employing one or more of the following approaches to strengthen the counterfactual: (a) increasing the number of observed pre- and post-implementation time points; (b) adding comparison groups or comparison outcomes; or (c) matching across implementation and comparison groups. For programs that have a distinct launch date, increasing the number of time points observed before or after the beginning of implementation can be used to establish a counterfactual. Because this approach compares outcomes before and after implementation, they are called *pre–post designs*. Including a larger number of time points in a pre–post design helps increase confidence that the changes observed are indeed due to implementation itself. Additionally, comparisons can be created by evaluating whether there are differences after implementation between targeted outcomes versus other outcomes one would not expect to change due to implementation. Finally, *matching* refers to any method that aims to equate (or "balance") the distribution of observed characteristics of participants in the implementation and comparison groups. This approach attempts to eliminate baseline differences in participants without resorting to randomization. All three approaches can be used in combination in nonrandomized designs to strengthen the counterfactual and improve internal validity.

WHICH EVALUATION DESIGNS CAN BE USED FOR DIFFERENT IMPLEMENTATION QUESTIONS?

In this section, four common implementation evaluation questions are presented, along with potential study designs and research methods that can be used to address them.

Question 1: How Can Implementation Be Improved at a Local Level?

Evaluators working in health facilities or other local contexts may wish to evaluate how service delivery operates and iteratively improves. Many evaluation tools suitable for this environment arise from the manufacturing industry. For example, the field of *operations research* (related to systems engineering, management sciences, industrial engineering) emerged to optimize service delivery, typically using modeling (Monks 2016; Wagner et al., 2019). Models can be simple, such as process or flow maps that illustrate a specific step or set of steps needed for implementation. Models can also be complex, such as computer-based models that answer questions and guide decisions about resource allocation or staffing. The advantages of using models are that they are typically faster and less expensive than launching an implementation study and accompanying evaluation. However, the degree to which models can reflect what implementation might look like in the real world depends greatly on the data sources and assumptions used to create them. Thus, models may be particularly useful in brainstorming and prioritizing strategies to test in real life.

Similarly, **continuous quality improvement (CQI, or quality improvement [QI])** is an implementation strategy used at a local level to test iterative small changes to determine what changes improve targeted process or implementation outcomes. CQI may use qualitative or quantitative data to evaluate the small changes, often testing adaptations of the small changes in iterative cycles. For example, if a school district seeks to evaluate and optimize social support services for students, they might ask for qualitative feedback from a small number of school counselors who provide these services. Based on this feedback, evaluators could use quantitative measures to test if small changes to social support programming, such as introducing a service screening tool, increases the adoption of social support services in schools. Various additional operations research tools are often combined with CQI to brainstorm and prioritize ideas that should be tested in the local context; this process is similar to choosing implementation strategies to address a particular barrier in a particular context.

Question 2: Evaluators Would Like to Test a New Implementation Strategy and Have Received Grant Funding to Do So. What is the Effectiveness of This Implementation Strategy, Relative to Standard Practice?

The goal of this evaluation is to determine if a new implementation strategy is more effective than another strategy, such as the existing standard of care. Randomized evaluation designs are often used to determine the comparative effectiveness of various implementation strategies. This section describes how individually **randomized controlled trials**

(RCTs), cluster RCTs, and variants of these, such as the stepped wedge RCT, can be used to evaluate an implementation strategy.

In *an individual RCT*, the unit of randomization is an individual. Individual RCTs are less frequently used in implementation evaluations because implementation strategies are not often differentially applied at the level of the individual, but rather are rolled out at the group level in clinics or in communities. Individual RCTs are useful to evaluate the effectiveness of strategies in which it is unlikely that individuals randomized to the control arm would inadvertently get exposed to the strategy. It is additionally appropriate in instances where the effect of the strategy is not expected to be higher or lower based on what proportion of participants receive it (Brown et al., 2017). By controlling patient-level factors, individual RCTs have high internal validity, but potentially lower external validity due to restrictive enrollment criteria.

Unlike individual RCTs, the unit of randomization in *cluster RCTs* is groups such as health facilities, communities, districts, or schools. Cluster RCTs are more commonly used in implementation evaluations because many strategies are administered to groups of individuals or units that then deliver services to individual patients or clients, also referred to as nesting. For example, a cluster RCT could be used to evaluate the effectiveness of a teacher incentive program to improve teacher adoption of a stress-management program to effectively support their students and reduce stress at a student level. As the focus of implementation is at the school level, implementers would randomize some schools to participate in the incentive program and some not to. By engaging diverse schools in a cluster RCT, evaluators can increase external validity by reflecting a wider range of real-world settings.

The *stepped wedge RCT* is a variant of a cluster RCT where the implementation strategy is introduced sequentially to clusters over time. The order in which the clusters receive the strategy is randomized and occurs in a phased approach until all clusters have received it. A stepped wedge RCT is particularly helpful in scenarios where rolling out a strategy broadly all at once is logistically challenging, or when there is an ethical imperative to offer it to all clusters. The ethical advantage of this study design is that all clusters ultimately benefit from the implementation strategy. It is important to note that a stepped wedge RCT may take longer to conduct than a standard cluster RCT where intervention clusters receive the implementation strategy at the same time. Given that outcomes must be measured at each phase, the stepped wedge RCT also involves more frequent data collection than a standard cluster RCT, and it is best suited to outcomes that can be measured rapidly.

In summary, RCTs provide strong evidence of the comparative effectiveness of implementation strategies. The design of the RCT will depend on the unit of randomization and, as a result, the evaluator's comfort with balancing internal and external validity (see Table 9.2).

Question 3: A New Public Health Program Was Introduced. Evaluators Would Like to Understand the Effectiveness of This New Program.

Randomized designs are not always ethical or feasible to implement when new interventions, policies, and programs are introduced. In this case, nonrandomized study designs provide the opportunity to evaluate program effectiveness. The **difference-in-difference (DID)** design is a nonrandomized design that extends the simple pre–post design to strengthen internal validity (Handley et al., 2018). This design is used when there is only one, or a few, observations before and after implementation, such as when surveys are

TABLE 9.2 Study Design Features

CATEGORY	DESIGN	COMPARISON/ COUNTERFACTUAL SOURCE	TYPICAL INTERNAL VALIDITY	COMMON THREATS TO INTERNAL VALIDITY	TYPICAL EXTERNAL VALIDITY	COMMON THREATS TO EXTERNAL VALIDITY	TYPICAL COST
Randomized	Individual-level randomized controlled trial	Comparison individuals	+++	Few; most related to execution of design, not inherent in design	+	Population included may not reflect broader general population due to highly selective selection criteria	+++
	Cluster randomized controlled trial	Comparison clusters	+++	Clusters receiving intervention may differ from comparison clusters by chance	++	Clusters selected may not reflect other areas	+++ Less costly using program data
	Stepped wedge randomized trial	Comparison periods within clusters	+++	Clusters receiving intervention may differ from comparison clusters by chance; history (external events differ between intervention and comparison periods, time trends)	++	Clusters selected may not reflect other areas	+++ Less costly using program data
Non-randomized	Interrupted time series (no comparison sites)	Pre-intervention period and modeled time trend	+	History (external events differ between intervention and comparison periods, seasonality) Routine program data may define outcomes or populations differently than intended for evaluation	+++	Few; most related to execution of design, not inherent in design	+ More costly using primary data

(*continued*)

TABLE 9.2 Study Design Features (*continued*)

CATEGORY	DESIGN	COMPARISON/ COUNTERFACTUAL SOURCE	TYPICAL INTERNAL VALIDITY	COMMON THREATS TO INTERNAL VALIDITY	TYPICAL EXTERNAL VALIDITY	COMMON THREATS TO EXTERNAL VALIDITY	TYPICAL COST
	Interrupted time series (with comparison sites)	Concurrent comparison sites and pre-intervention period and modeled time trend	++	Selection of groups receiving intervention may be biased Routine program data may define outcomes or populations differently than intended for evaluation	+++	Few; most related to execution of design, not inherent in design	+ More costly using primary data
	Difference in differences	Concurrent comparison sites and pre-intervention period	+	Selection of groups receiving intervention may be biased Routine program data may define outcomes or populations differently than intended for evaluation	+++	Few; most related to execution of design, not inherent in design	+ More costly using primary data
	Regression discontinuity	Individuals or sites not qualifying for intervention based on cutoff value	++ Higher if cutoff value is only factor determining intervention	Invalid if selection of groups to receive intervention can be modified	+++	Few; most related to execution of design, not inherent in design	+ More costly using primary data
	Pre–post	Preintervention period	Poor	History (external events differ between intervention and comparison periods, time trends)	++	Few; most related to execution of design, not inherent in design	+

conducted every year or less frequently. The most common DID design measures changes in key evaluation outcomes before and after implementation in both an implementation group and a comparison group. In DID designs, evaluators measure if evaluation outcomes change more before versus after implementation in the implementation group (first difference) compared to the changes in the comparison group (second difference). The addition of a comparison group makes this design more robust to threats to internal validity compared to a simple pre–post design, as the comparison group "differences out" or removes the effect of other changes over time that occur at the same time as the new intervention, policy, or program. Thus, for example, for a new intervention to increase coverage of social support services in schools, it is important to ensure that the comparison schools are representative of the implementation schools; comparison schools could be selected from nearby districts with similar per-capita income levels. Changes in coverage of social support services before and after the intervention, in both the implementation and the comparison school districts, could be measured over time. If trends in service coverage are similar in implementation and comparison school districts before the program begins, evaluators may be more confident that they have identified an appropriate comparator.

Another nonrandomized design that can be used to evaluate public health programs is the **regression discontinuity (RD)** design. The RD design can be applied when there is a natural "cutoff score," such as socio-economic status of a community or size of a hospital, that dictates if the group has access to an intervention, program, or implementation strategy. The RD design compares individuals or groups who received the intervention and were just below the cutoff (eligible) to those who did not receive the intervention and were just above the cutoff (ineligible). The groups right above and right below the cutoff score should be similar on all factors except for access to the intervention. For example, if a school mental health program is only introduced in school districts meeting a specific per-capita income eligibility criteria, evaluators could compare coverage of mental health services in school districts just above and just below the cutoff. Thus, like the DID design, the RD design can be used to evaluate public health programs when there are a small number of outcome measurements over time. A flowchart for considering different design decisions, including determining the feasibility of randomization and availability of comparison groups, is presented in Figure 9.2.

Question 4: A New National Policy Has Been Implemented. How Can Evaluators Assess if It Is Effective?

When a new policy is implemented, evaluators rarely have control to randomize policy rollout. In such circumstances, there are a variety of approaches that can be used to evaluate effective implementation of the policy. **Interrupted time series (ITS)** designs are nonrandomized designs often used in implementation evaluations, and which can be used to evaluate policy implementation (Bernal et al., 2017). ITS considers the same group (people, regions, or other groups) at numerous time points before and after a strategy is introduced. Evaluators observe how a particular outcome changes in this group prior to implementation, then compare these measures to changes in the outcomes immediately after the strategy is introduced and over time after implementation. The visual representation of this analysis can be especially compelling and intuitive for stakeholders. For example, students' unmet social support needs were increasing gradually at a school during the 2-year period before a new social services policy was introduced; after the policy was introduced, there was no immediate impact, but over the next 2-year period there was a substantially faster reduction in unmet social support needs among students than in the prior 2 years.

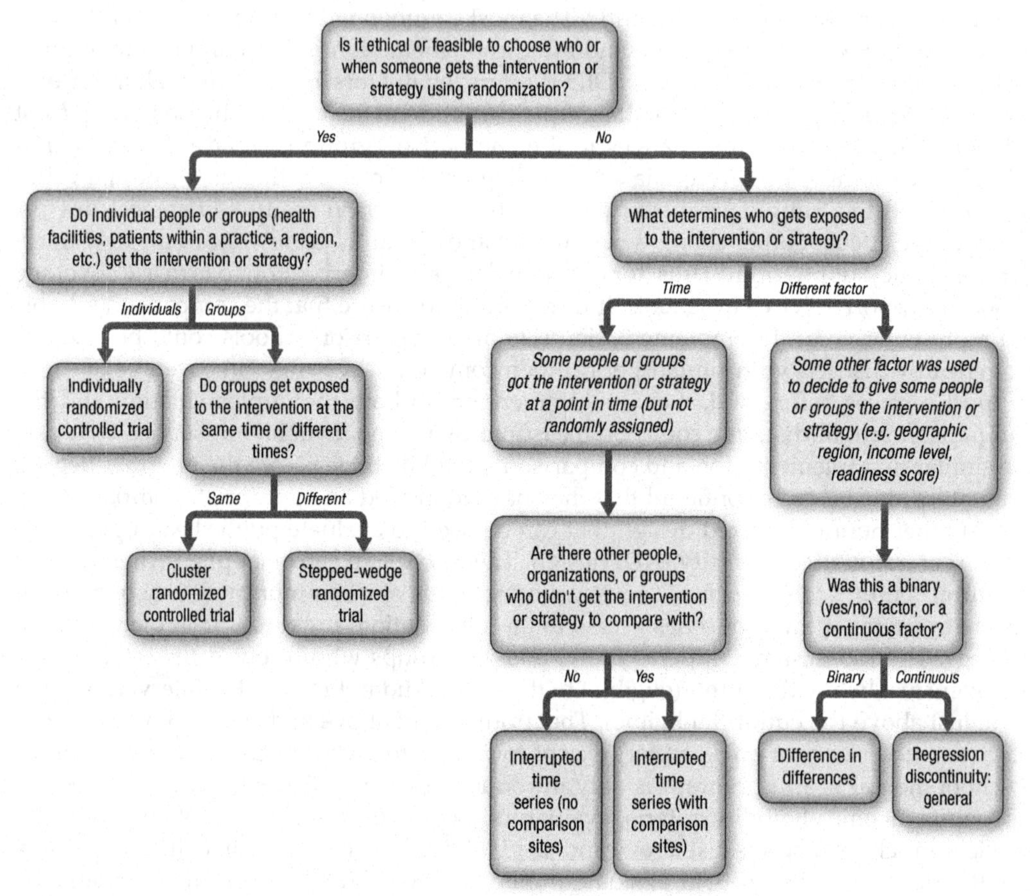

FIGURE 9.2 Flowchart of study design decisions.

The difference between the gradual increase in the "before" period and the substantial decrease in the "after" period can be interpreted as the impact of the policy. However, this is only internally valid if no other changes have happened during that period that could have caused the change.

The major weakness of the ITS design is that other events might happen over time that also affect the outcome. For example, if a teachers' strike takes place while a new school social support policy is introduced, it may not be possible to distinguish which caused the observed change in social service coverage outcomes. Adding comparison groups (e.g., groups of people or geographic regions) that have not received the strategy or adding a different outcome that is not affected by the strategy can help evaluators strengthen their counterfactual to overcome this challenge. This is known as ITS with comparison groups or comparison outcomes (Table 9.2). For example, if a new policy is introduced in one school district at the same time as a teachers' strike across several districts, including comparison districts in the ITS design can reveal if observed changes in outcomes are due to the policy, or the strikes that are taking place throughout the area. Importantly, evaluators should use the same data source and outcome definitions throughout the ITS and measure outcomes with sufficient (typically at least seven) data points before and after the strategy or policy is introduced.

Case study 9.2D highlights a case study of how to apply concepts learned in this chapter, including designing an implementation evaluation, choosing a study design, applying an evaluation framework, and measuring appropriate evaluation outcomes to answer the implementation question.

CASE STUDY 9.2D EVALUATING THE IMPLEMENTATION OF TEXT MESSAGE REMINDERS TO IMPROVE ADHERENCE TO TUBERCULOSIS PREVENTIVE TREATMENT IN KENYA

In this fictional case study, the Kenyan national government plans to roll out a short-course fixed dose combination drug regimen for TB preventive treatment also known as "3HP." This is a WHO-endorsed EBI that combines two drugs in a once-weekly dose for people at high risk of acquiring TB. The national government is interested in testing an implementation strategy that uses text messages to send weekly reminders to patients to take their 3HP dose. *Evaluation aim:* The Kenyan government hypothesizes that the text message reminders will facilitate smooth implementation and roll out of 3HP. Accordingly, evaluators aim to determine if these reminders increase the acceptability of 3HP to patients who receive them and, ultimately, their drug adherence. *Study design:* In a cluster RCT, evaluators randomize 10 health facilities to participate in the text message reminder strategy and another 10 facilities to launch 3HP without reminders. The evaluation is designed as a hybrid effectiveness-implementation design, meaning the evaluators are interested in both implementation outcomes (acceptability of the EBI) and clinical outcomes (adherence to the EBI). *Framework*: Evaluators will use the Implementation Outcomes Framework to structure the evaluation, with *acceptability* of 3HP being the primary implementation outcome. *Data collection:* The evaluators use a mixed methods design for data collection where quantitative data were collected first, followed by qualitative data collection to help explain the quantitative evaluation findings. Patient surveys were conducted in all facilities 1 month after starting 3HP to determine the acceptability of 3HP. Based upon quantitative findings, patients were invited to participate in focus group discussions, with focus groups conducted among patients who find 3HP to be acceptable and those who find 3HP to not be acceptable, in both implementation and comparator facilities. Health workers also participated in focus groups to discuss their observations of factors influencing acceptability and adherence to 3HP. This cluster randomized, mixed methods evaluation provided the opportunity to maximize both internal validity and external validity, while also understanding key implementation outcomes from provider and patient perspectives.

SUMMARY

The design of an implementation evaluation requires defining the evaluation question, identifying the appropriate evaluation framework for the design (if one will be used), delineating the quantitative and qualitative components of the evaluation, deciding if clinical outcomes must be incorporated using a hybrid effectiveness-implementation design, and establishing priorities related to internal and external validity. After these decisions have been made, evaluators can select study designs that are most fit for purpose. These designs might include randomized designs (individual, cluster, or stepped wedge RCTs) or nonrandomized designs (DID, RD, and ITS). Whether an evaluation examines a small pilot study or widescale roll out of a new policy, it is imperative that evaluators share and disseminate their methodology and findings widely. Transparently sharing research methodology is important for ensuring that other public health practitioners and evaluators can assess the rigor of the evaluation, adapt the methodology, or compare their findings when implementing the same implementation strategy in other settings.

KEY POINTS FOR PRACTICE

1. Evaluation questions vary based upon the stage of implementation (pre-implementation, early or mid-implementation, and late implementation). A formative pre-implementation evaluation can help evaluators understand the implementation context and what barriers exist to implementation in the context, prior to roll out. A mid-implementation process evaluation helps determine if implementation is delivered as intended, and if any adjustments or adaptations should be made to the implementation process.
2. Evaluation frameworks can help evaluators structure their evaluation and define the outcomes that they would like to measure. Common evaluation frameworks include RE-AIM and the Implementation Outcomes Framework.
3. Many designs rely on quantitative statistical evaluations to answer the question, "Does implementation work?" However, qualitative and quantitative data can be used together to increase the depth of learning.
4. There is no one "ideal" or "best" evaluation design. An evaluator should choose the design that helps answer the evaluation question with strong evidence given practical considerations such as the time and resources needed to conduct the evaluation.
5. Randomized evaluation designs to test the effectiveness of an implementation strategy typically have the highest internal validity. On the other hand, they often lack external validity. It may not always be feasible or ethical to randomize individual or groups to a strategy, and in these cases nonrandomized designs may be better suited.
6. Nonrandomized evaluation designs are commonly used when strategies cannot feasibly be allocated randomly to groups or individuals. Compared to randomized designs, nonrandomized designs tend to have lower internal validity, but are more generalizable to real-world implementation settings.
7. DID and RD designs are both good choices for evaluation designs when there are fewer measurements of the outcome of interest over time. ITS is a good choice for a nonrandomized design when there are many measurements of the outcome of interest over time; they can be strengthened by adding comparison groups.

COMMON PITFALLS IN PRACTICE

1. Failing to carefully develop an evaluation question that is specific and appropriate to the stage of implementation.
2. Forgetting that quantitative and qualitative data can be intentionally integrated to validate, expand upon, or explain observed findings.
3. Ignoring the tradeoffs between internal and external validity when selecting an evaluation design or determining the generalizability of findings.
4. Assuming that a randomized evaluation design is the only, or the most rigorous, study design available.

DISCUSSION QUESTIONS

1. You are working with a local government and are in the very early stages of understanding the local context, and the barriers and facilitators to implementing a new school-based strategy to improve student mental health. What implementation outcomes do you think might be most important to consider at this stage?

2. You decide to use mixed methods to evaluate a new school-based strategy to improve student mental health. You want to first understand broadly teacher perceptions of, and preferences for, the tools that they use to support student mental health, and then follow-up with a small group of teachers to learn more in-depth information about how to adapt a new implementation strategy prior to rollout. What are the advantages or disadvantages of using this approach during the preimplementation period?
3. A colleague proposes a pre–post design with no comparison group as the evaluation design for the rollout of a new school-based implementation strategy. They say it is really the only option since you only have one measurement before implementation and one measurement after implementation. How would you describe to this colleague your concerns around internal validity that this design might pose? What are creative solutions to strengthen the internal validity of your colleague's design?
4. You are leading an evaluation team to evaluate the impact of a new policy influencing school mental health services. How would you go about choosing between a cluster randomized trial or a nonrandomized evaluation design such as a DID design for this evaluation? How would you communicate with your supervisor, in practical terms, the benefits and drawbacks of each design? What would shape your recommendations of which design to choose?

REFERENCES

Bernal, J. L., Cummins, S., & Gasparrini, A. (2017). Interrupted time series regression for the evaluation of public health interventions: A tutorial. *International Journal of Epidemiology, 46*(1), 348–355. https://doi.org/10.1093/ije/dyw098

Brown, C. H., Curran, G., Palinkas, L. A., Aarons, G. A., Wells, K. B., Jones, L., Collins, L. M., Duan, N., Mittman, B. S., Wallace, A., Tabak, R. G., Ducharme, L., Chambers, D. A., Neta, G., Wiley, T., Landsverk, J., Cheung, K., & Cruden, G. (2017). An overview of research and evaluation designs for dissemination and implementation. *Annual Review of Public Health, 38*, 1–22. https://doi.org/10.1146/annurev-publhealth-031816-044215

Chamberlain, P., Brown, C. H., & Saldana, L. (2011). Observational measure of implementation progress in community based settings: The Stages of Implementation Completion (SIC). *Implementation Science: IS, 6*, 116. https://doi.org/10.1186/1748-5908-6-116

Creswell, J. W., & Clark, V. L. P. (2017). *Designing and conducting mixed methods research*. Sage Publications.

Curran, G. M., Bauer, M., Mittman, B., Pyne, J. M., & Stetler, C. (2012). Effectiveness-implementation hybrid designs: Combining elements of clinical effectiveness and implementation research to enhance public health impact. *Medical Care, 50*(3), 217–226. https://doi.org/10.1097/MLR.0b013e3182408812

Enos, M., Sitienei, J., Ong'ang'o, J., Mungai, B., Kamene, M., Wambugu, J., Kipruto, H., Manduku, V., Mburu, J., Nyaboke, D., Ngari, F., Omesa, E., Omale, N., Mwirigi, N., Okallo, G., Njoroge, J., Githiomi, M., Mwangi, M., Kirathe, D., … Weyenga, H. (2018). Kenya tuberculosis prevalence survey 2016: Challenges and opportunities of ending TB in Kenya. *PLoS One, 13*(12), e0209098. https://doi.org/10.1371/journal.pone.0209098

Glasgow, R. E., Harden, S. M., Gaglio, B., Rabin, B., Smith, M. L., Porter, G. C., Ory, M. G., & Estabrooks, P. A. (2019). RE-AIM planning and evaluation framework: Adapting to new science and practice with a 20-year review. *Frontiers in Public Health, 7*, 64. https://doi.org/10.3389/fpubh.2019.00064

Glasgow, R. E., Vogt, T. M., & Boles, S. M. (1999). Evaluating the public health impact of health promotion interventions: The RE-AIM framework. *American Journal of Public Health, 89*(9), 1322–1327. https://doi.org/10.2105/ajph.89.9.1322

Handley, M. A., Lyles, C. R., McCulloch, C., & Cattamanchi, A. (2018). Selecting and improving quasi-experimental designs in effectiveness and implementation research. *Annual Review of Public Health, 39*, 5–25. https://doi.org/10.1146/annurev-publhealth-040617-014128

Hendricks-Brown, C., Curran, G., Palinkas, L. A., Aarons, G. A., Wells, K. B., Jones, L., Collins, L. M., Duan, N., Mittman, B. S., Wallace, A., Tabak, R. G., Ducharme, L., Chambers, D. A., Neta, G., Wiley, T., Landsverk, J., Cheung, K., & Cruden, G. (2017). An overview of research and evaluation designs for dissemination and implementation. *Annual Review of Public Health, 38*(March), 1–22. https://doi.org/10.1146/annurev-publhealth-031816-044215

Kadota, J. L., Musinguzi, A., Nabunje, J., Welishe, F., Ssemata, J. L., Bishop, O., Berger, C. A., Patel, D., Sammann, A., Katahoire, A., Nahid, P., Belknap, R., Phillips, P., Namusobya, J., Kamya, M., Handley, M. A., Kiwanuka, N.,

Katamba, A., Dowdy, D., ... Cattamanchi, A. (2020). Protocol for the 3HP Options Trial: A hybrid type 3 implementation-effectiveness randomized trial of delivery strategies for short-course tuberculosis preventive therapy among people living with HIV in Uganda. *Implementation Science: IS, 15*(1), 65. https://doi.org/10.1186/s13012-020-01025-8

Lewis, C. C., Mettert, K. D., Dorsey, C. N., Martinez, R. G., Weiner, B. J., Nolen, E., Stanick, C., Halko, H., & Powell, B. J. (2018). An updated protocol for a systematic review of implementation-related measures. *Systematic Reviews, 7*(1), 66. https://doi.org/10.1186/s13643-018-0728-3

Monks, T. (2016). Operational research as implementation science: Definitions, challenges and research priorities. *Implementation Science: IS,* 11(1), 81. https://doi.org/10.1186/s13012-016-0444-0

Nilsen, P. (2015). Making sense of implementation theories, models and frameworks. *Implementation Science: IS, 10,* 53. https://doi.org/10.1186/s13012-015-0242-0

Peters, D. H., Tran, N. T., & Adam, T. (2013). *Implementation research in health: A practical guide*. World Health Organization.

Pluye, P., & Hong, Q. N. (2014). Combining the power of stories and the power of numbers: Mixed methods research and mixed studies reviews. *Annual Review of Public Health, 35,* 29–45. https://doi.org/10.1146/annurev-publhealth-032013-182440

Proctor, E., Silmere, H., Raghavan, R., Hovmand, P., Aarons, G., Bunger, A., Griffey, R., & Hensley, M. (2011). Outcomes for implementation research: Conceptual distinctions, measurement challenges, and research agenda. *Administration and Policy in Mental Health, 38*(2), 65–76. https://doi.org/10.1007/s10488-010-0319-7

Turley, R., Gamoran, A., McCarty, A. T., & Fish, R. (2017). Reducing children's behavior problems through social capital: A causal assessment. *Social Science Research, 61,* 206–217. https://doi.org/10.1016/j.ssresearch.2016.06.015

Wagner, A. D., Crocker, J., Liu, S., Cherutich, P., Gimbel, S., Fernandes, Q., Mugambi, M., Ásbjörnsdóttir, K., Masyuko, S., Wagenaar, B. H., Nduati, R., & Sherr, K. (2019). Making smarter decisions faster: Systems engineering to improve the global public health response to HIV. *Current HIV/AIDS Reports, 16*(4), 279–291. https://doi.org/10.1007/s11904-019-00449-2

10

Dissemination Information About Evidence-Based Interventions

Jonathan Purtle, Margaret E. Crane, Katherine L. Nelson, and Ross C. Brownson

Learning Objectives

By the end of this chapter, readers will be able to:

- Describe how dissemination is distinct from, and related to, implementation, diffusion, health communication, and advertising
- Apply theories and dissemination strategies to change a target audience's knowledge, attitudes, intentions, and behaviors related to an evidence-based intervention (EBI)
- Identify the importance of audience segmentation and tailoring in dissemination campaigns
- Describe the process of evaluating a dissemination campaign

CASE STUDY 10.1 *FOR THE SAKE OF ALL*: COMMUNITY-PARTNERED DISSEMINATION TO IMPROVE KNOWLEDGE AND SUPPORT POLICIES THAT PROMOTE HEALTH EQUITY

Despite large and persistent health disparities in the United States, the U.S. general public and policy makers have limited knowledge about the existence of disparities and inequities in the social determinants of health that produce them. With the goal of addressing these knowledge deficits and cultivating public demand and political will for policies that promote health equity, the *For the Sake of All* dissemination and civic engagement campaign was developed and launched by researchers and community partners in St. Louis, Missouri (Purnell et al., 2018). The campaign first engaged a wide range of community, government, philanthropic, and media partners to develop and refine the goals of the project. Strategic messages and images were then developed and disseminated in partnership with mass media outlets in St. Louis. Local data were analyzed to create policy briefs that were tailored for the local context and disseminated to both the public and policy makers in the city. Discussion guides and toolkits—including elements such as sample social media posts and guidance for writing an op-ed for a newspaper—were developed and disseminated to provide the public with guidance about how to engage in advocacy and dissemination activities related to health disparities. Evaluation occurred continuously during the campaign, with website visits, social and news media attention, policy action, and survey data providing metrics of success.

INTRODUCTION

In many ways, dissemination is just another word for communication. **Dissemination** involves the strategic communication of information about evidence-based interventions (EBIs) to audiences who affect the population health impact of these interventions. The communication is *strategic* because the content of messages, the sources from which they are distributed, and the channels through which they are delivered are intentionally selected to influence specific knowledge, attitudes, intentions, and ultimately behaviors related to the EBI among target audiences. These target *audiences* can range from policy makers who make regulatory and funding decisions related to an EBI, to practitioners who deliver it in clinical and community settings, to patients who would benefit from seeking out the EBI, and to the broader general public who can influence policymaking related to the EBI. At the center of any dissemination effort is an **actor** (e.g., a professional organization, a government agency, a passionate researcher, a concerned citizen) that is making deliberate decisions and taking purposeful actions to communicate information about an EBI to target audiences. In the absence of an active dissemination effort, information about an EBI is simply left to passively diffuse. Although diffusion can affect dissemination outcomes, diffusion in isolation (i.e., in the absence of dissemination) can exacerbate health inequities. When the evidence supporting an EBI is left to passively diffuse, key information about an EBI is less likely to reach historically and currently socially disadvantaged populations and the practice audiences who serve them, particularly in the form of messages that are clear and compelling.

In this chapter, we first contextualize dissemination within the broader context of strategic communication. Specifically, we highlight how dissemination is distinct from, and related to, implementation, diffusion, health communication, advertising, and applied political science. Understanding key ideas from these different disciplines can help maximize the impact of dissemination campaigns. Second, we summarize theories from different disciplines that can be useful to informing the design and execution of dissemination campaigns. We then illustrate how direct-to-consumer (DTC) marketing principles can be applied to disseminate information about EBIs to the general public. Next, we summarize information about four broad types of dissemination strategies that can be used in dissemination campaigns. Finally, we conclude by detailing steps to design, execute, and evaluate a dissemination campaign.

D → I > D & I

"D & I" is the ubiquitous acronym for "dissemination and implementation" research and practice. This expression is commonly used as shorthand for the enterprise of implementation science, but it is not critically examined. The exercise of questioning this acronym, however, can shed light on the relationship between dissemination and implementation. There are several key questions to consider. Why are "D" and "I" separated by an ampersand? The separation suggests that dissemination and implementation are conceptually distinct, but what are the key attributes of dissemination that differentiate it from implementation? Second, the ampersand suggests that the dissemination and implementation are complementary concepts, but how are they complementary? Is the ampersand really the most appropriate symbol to express the relationship between dissemination and implementation? Below we provide clarification and insights about why D → I is a more practical way think about the relationship between dissemination and implementation than D & I.

The U.S. National Institutes of Health (NIH, n.d.) defines dissemination research as "the scientific study of *targeted distribution of information and intervention materials* to a specific public health or clinical practice audience" In contrast, the NIH defines implementation research as "the scientific study of the use of *strategies to adopt and integrate evidence-based health interventions* into clinical and community settings," (NIH, n.d.). Leeman and colleagues (2017) define **dissemination strategies** as those that target knowledge, attitudes, and intentions to adopt an EBI; and implementation strategies as those that target the execution of behaviors related to an EBI.

According to these definitions, the defining attribute of dissemination is that it relates to the spread of information to influence what practice audiences think and know, whereas the defining attribute of implementation is that it relates to strategies that directly influence what practice audiences do. However, we feel it is important to offer two amendments to this definition of dissemination that have implications from a dissemination practice perspective. First, we contend that members of the general public who are not practitioners can also be the target audience of dissemination campaigns that spread information about EBIs. The NIH recognizes this in describing knowledge gaps related to dissemination (NIH, n.d.). Dissemination campaigns targeting the general public can foster patient demand for EBIs and also cultivate a sociopolitical context that is supportive of policies that are aligned with EBIs. Second, we believe that behavior change can be conceptualized as a dissemination outcome. This is because persuasive communication can sometimes be sufficient to change behavior related to an EBI (e.g., Doctor et al., 2018; Sacarny et al., 2018). Furthermore, additional constructs can be considered dissemination outcomes (e.g., skills, self-efficacy) if they align with the specific goals of the dissemination campaign (Purtle, Marzalik, et al., 2020; Purtle, Nelson, et al., 2020).

The preceding definitions shed some light on the relationship between "D & I": dissemination and implementation are complementary concepts because changes in knowledge, attitudes, and intentions related to an EBI are often necessary, even if not sufficient, to subsequently change behaviors related to an EBI (implementation costumes). Given that changes in knowledge, attitudes, and intentions typically *precede* and can causally contribute to changes in behaviors, an arrow may be a more appropriate symbol than an ampersand (D → I). In other words, effective dissemination can foster readiness for implementation among a target audience and cultivate a context that supports implementation. While dissemination and implementation are distinct concepts, the distinction is often blurry—and that is okay. Whether language of "dissemination" or "implementation" is used to describe strategies is somewhat arbitrary. What really matters is a clear conceptualization of how strategies can be used to achieve goals related to the EBI.

Actively Disseminating Information Is Different Than Letting It Diffuse, and That Matters for Health Equity

Another area of confusion lies in the use of the terms *dissemination* and *diffusion*. These terms are often used interchangeably, but we believe they are not synonymous concepts. In a foundational 1993 paper on terminology related to knowledge translation, Lomas contended that dissemination was distinct from diffusion because dissemination entails active and strategic efforts to spread information while diffusion relates to the passive and "haphazard" spread of information (p. 263). However, Everett Rogers—creator of the Diffusion of Innovations (DOI) theory (detailed in the following)—and other diffusion scholars do view dissemination and diffusion as being synonymous (Rogers, 2010). We agree with Lomas and believe that there is practical utility in thinking about dissemination as a distinct concept. Dissemination activities, as opposed to diffusion activities, should be strategically planned and carried out by an actor for the purpose of spreading information about an EBI. Although information about an EBI can spontaneously spread through a population and affect dissemination outcomes (e.g., influence knowledge and attitudes), the intentional nature of dissemination differentiates it from diffusion.

As previously noted, diffusion without dissemination is often problematic from a health equity perspective. Exclusively relying on spontaneous diffusion to spread information about EBIs is analogous to a laissez-faire approach to the economy—in which government regulation is limited and market forces drive outcomes. Although diffusion does result in information spreading throughout a social system, people with more power and privilege are more likely to receive the information, receive it sooner, and receive it in the form of messages that are clear and compelling. This dynamic contributes to inequities in information about EBIs and subsequent disparities in their reach and health benefits, similar to the way that the dynamics of laissez-faire economic approaches contribute to income disparities. In contrast, the active dissemination of information about an EBI *can* be analogous to an interventionism approach to the economy in which government regulation corrects market failures and promotes the equitable spread of information about EBIs. The emphasis is on "can" because a necessary criterion for success is for the actor or actors leading the dissemination campaign to be cognizant of issues of inequity and purposefully strategize to address them in dissemination decisions.

Fields of Research and Practice That Are Relevant to Dissemination

Dissemination, with its focus on the strategic communication of information, is relevant to many other fields of research and practice that are focused on persuasive communication. Although a detailed review of these fields is beyond the scope of this chapter, Table 10.1 highlights three of these fields and notes how they relate to dissemination. We believe that this information is useful to dissemination practice because it highlights the breadth of fields that contain tools and ideas that can be applied to enhance the impact of dissemination campaigns.

Advertising is one field that is highly relevant to dissemination. Informed by theories of consumer psychology, the advertising industry uses sophisticated and data-driven messaging techniques and has been extremely effective at persuading consumers and influencing their purchasing behavior (Haugtvedt et al., 2018; Liu-Thompkins, 2019). Another relevant field is health communication. Heath communication campaigns have been tremendously successful at persuading individuals to engage in health promoting behaviors (e.g., stop smoking, eat healthier; Snyder, 2007). Health communication principles (e.g., framing, detailed in the following) have also been effective at cultivating support for evidence-supported health policies (Gollust et al., 2017; McGinty et al., 2013, 2018; Niederdeppe et al., 2015). Health communication and advertising are considered dissemination strategies when research evidence related to the EBI is the focus of the information being communicated. Finally, the field of applied political science is relevant to dissemination campaigns that target policy maker audiences. Studies and practice initiatives in this area have strategically communicated information to policy makers to influence their behaviors in ways that benefit democratic processes and the public (Butler & Nickerson, 2011; Jason & Rose, 1984; Nyhan & Reifler, 2015).

TABLE 10.1 Fields Relevant to Dissemination: Key Similarities and Differences

FIELD	TARGET OF CHANGE	AUDIENCE THAT IS TARGETED WITH INFORMATION
Dissemination	Knowledge, attitudes, intentions, and behaviors related to EBI	People working in their professional capacity, and members of the general public who would benefit from accessing the EBI
Implementation	Behavior related to an EBI	People working in their professional capacity
Health communication	Personal health behavior	General public
Advertising	Purchasing behavior	General public
Applied political science	Political behavior	Policy makers

THEORIES AND PRACTICE APPROACHES USEFUL TO DISSEMINATION

Theories from the fields described in the previous section, and many others, can be useful to dissemination practice (Glanz & Bishop, 2010). In the following we provide high-level summaries of four of these theories and approaches and offer examples of their application to dissemination practice.

Diffusion of Innovations

The theory of the DOI, developed by Everett Rogers and originated in the fields of agricultural and rural sociology, focuses on the processes through which ideas and technologies that are perceived as new (i.e., innovations) are adopted by members of a social system over time (Dearing & Kee, 2012; Rogers, 2010). DOI is a macro-level theory and can be helpful in conceptualizing how the dissemination of information about EBIs might fit within the broader social context in which a target audience operates. Broadly, DOI focuses on how both attributes of adopters (i.e., people in a social system) and attributes of the innovation affect diffusion. In terms of attributes of adopters, a fundamental premise of DOI is that early adoption among key opinion leaders is integral to the spread of an innovation.

DOI constructs related to the attributes of innovations can be helpful in crafting messages and dissemination materials related to an EBI. DOI posits that these constructs have major influence on the speed with which an innovation spreads, if it spreads at all. Table 10.2 defines Rogers's attributes of innovations constructs, notes how they affect diffusion, and provides examples of how the constructs can be applied to inform dissemination planning and practice. It is important to emphasize that all the constructs relate to an audience's *perceptions of the EBI*, not "objective realities" of the EBI as defined by intervention developers, researchers, advocates, or any actor that might disseminate information about an EBI. In other words, the attributes of innovations are in the eye of the beholder.

Elaboration Likelihood Model

The Elaboration Likelihood Model (ELM) is from the field of social psychology and was developed to illuminate how persuasive communication can change attitudes and behaviors (Petty & Cacioppo, 1986; Petty & Krosnick, 2014). A key difference between ELM and DOI theory is that ELM is more focused on cognitive and emotional processes at the individual level. In short, ELM proposes that messages are processed through two routes: a *central route* and a *peripheral route.* The central route is cognitive and analytic, and the peripheral route is more emotional and reliant on heuristics (i.e., cognitive shortcuts) that are used to process information (Petty & Cacioppo, 1986). According to ELM, a message can change attitudes via the central route if a person is *motivated* and *able* to process a message. Perceived relevance of the message is a key factor that affects this motivation. If a person does not have the motivation or ability to process a message, the message can still change attitudes if a *peripheral cue* is perceived in the message. A peripheral cue could be a specific word, metaphor, story, or image that elicits a strong emotional response or the source from which the message was sent (e.g., a source that is perceived as a trusted expert). Although messages can change attitudes via central or peripheral routes, changes that occur via the central route generally result in more long-lasting attitude changes and subsequent changes in behavior (Haugtvedt & Kasmer, 2008).

TABLE 10.2 Applying Attributes of Innovations Constructs From the Diffusion of Innovations Theory to Dissemination Planning and Practice

DOI ATTRIBUTES OF INNOVATIONS CONSTRUCT	DEFINITION OF CONSTRUCT	IMPLICATION OF CONSTRUCT FOR SPEED OF DIFFUSION OF THE INNOVATION	APPLICATION OF CONSTRUCT FOR DISSEMINATION PLANNING AND PRACTICE
Relative advantage	The extent to which an EBI is perceived as superior to the alternative	Greater perceived advantage = faster diffusion	Consider what the alternatives are to the EBI for the audience (e.g., engage in another practice that is more familiar or less costly, doing nothing to address the issue that the EBI is focused on)
Compatibility	The extent to which an EBI is perceived as consistent with the experiences, values, and needs	Greater perceived compatibility = faster diffusion	Consider how the EBI might be perceived as consistent with and in conflict with the day-to-day practice realities of the audience, their needs, values, and social norms
Complexity	The extent to which an EBI is perceived as being complicated	Greater perceived complexity = slower diffusion	Consider how complex to adopt the audience might perceive the EBI and how dissemination materials could make the EBI seem less complex
Trialability	The extent to which an EBI can be tried and abandoned if desired	Greater perceived trialability = faster diffusion	Consider how to communicate about the costs (e.g., time, money) needed to adopt the EBI and how the audience could revert back to the status quo with limited costs if the EBI is perceived as undesirable after adoption
Observability	The extent to which the benefits of an EBI are observable to others	Greater perceived observability = faster diffusion	Consider how to communicate about what the benefits of adopting an EBI might look like to an adopter and their peers, especially in the short term, and how the benefits can be easily measured

Source: Adapted from Rogers, E. M. (2010). *Diffusion of innovations*. Simon & Schuster.

ELM can be useful to dissemination practice because it can guide decisions about the content of messages for different target audiences. For example, imagine that the primary goal of a dissemination campaign is to increase the reach and fidelity of trauma-focused cognitive behavioral therapy (CBT) for youth in foster care. For an audience of therapists working in child welfare systems, it can be assumed that many will perceive issues related to childhood trauma and CBT as being relevant to their work (motivation is criterion satisfied) and will be able to understand technical information about the clinical dynamics of trauma focused-CBT (TF-CBT; ability criterion satisfied). Thus, to spur information processing via the central route, dissemination materials for this clinical audience might emphasize the evidence base for TF-CBT, the prevalence of trauma exposure among youth in foster care, and technical practice guidelines related to the delivery of TF-CBT. In contrast, for an audience of state legislators who make funding decisions about child welfare systems, it is unlikely that many will perceive such information as relevant or comprehendible. Thus, dissemination materials for this policy maker audience might emphasize peripheral cues—such as a story about a child in their legislative district who benefited from TF-CBT in foster care—to prompt message processing via the peripheral route.

Theory of Planned Behavior

The theory of planned behavior (TPB), also rooted in social psychology, has utility in dissemination practice as well. In contrast to ELM theory, which is focused on the processes through which messages influence attitudes, TPB is focused on processes through which attitudes (along with social norms and beliefs about how difficult it would be to perform a behavior) influence behavior (Ajzen, 1991). TPB can be useful to dissemination because the goal of campaigns is to ultimately affect a behavior related to an EBI (Breslin et al., 2001; Casper, 2007; Yoong et al., 2015).

One specific way that TPB can inform dissemination decisions is by guiding the selection of the targets of dissemination strategies. For example, TPB constructs were used in a survey of addiction program counselors to assess the extent to which attitudes, subjective norms, and perceived behavioral control related to an EBI were associated with the intention to adopt the EBI at baseline and actual adoption of EBI at 6-month follow-up (Breslin et al., 2001). The survey found that subjective norms were significant predictors of intention to adopt the EBI, which was a predictor of actual adoption. The implication for dissemination is that strategies which target these norms, as opposed to attitudes about the EBI, might have the most impact. Similarly, a survey of youth in Australia found that attitudes and intentions related to their delivery of psychological first aid practices prospectively predicted their use of these practices; the implication being that attitudes about psychological first aid practices might be the prime targets for dissemination strategies among this population of youth (Brownson et al., 2018; Yap & Jorm, 2012).

Direct-to-Consumer Social Marketing Approaches

DTC social marketing approaches are often well-suited to achieve dissemination goals when patients who would benefit from an EBI are the target audience. DTC social marketing provides consumers of EBIs with information to improve their understanding of the issue that the EBI could address (e.g., a behavioral or physical health problem) and to inform their treatment decision-making (Friedberg & Bayar, 2017). Unlike commercial marketing, which aims to increase company profit, social marketing aims to provide a benefit to consumers and society at large (Kotler & Zaltman, 1971).

DTC marketing campaigns differ from other dissemination campaigns because they directly target the consumers without intermediaries (e.g., clinicians, policy makers). The consumer is the user of the EBI, while the customer is the person who chooses and pays for a service. With EBIs for adults, the consumer and the customer are often the same person (i.e., the patient/client). With EBIs for youth, the consumer is typically the youth, and the customer is typically their caregiver (Becker, 2015). Both consumer and customer characteristics, needs, and preferences should be considered when designing DTC campaigns.

The "four Ps" of DTC marketing are used to design campaigns in accordance with considerations related to *product, price, place,* and *promotion channel* (Becker, 2015). The four Ps framework is often referred to as the "marketing mix" because each of these Ps are considered at the same time, rather than sequentially (Zeithaml et al., 2012). The marketer must determine how to describe the *product* (i.e., the EBI) that they are promoting. Consumer perceptions of the "attributes of the innovation" (i.e., the EBI) are important to consider in this regard. Related to the *price* of the EBI, DTC marketing initiatives should consider both financial and practical barriers to service seeking. *Place* refers to both the physical location where the EBI is provided as well as where and from whom consumers receive information.

Promotion integrates information gathered about the product, price, and place to create a promotional campaign. This includes the key message of the campaign, as well as when, how, and where it will be marketed. Although it is useful for consumers to understand that some services have more research support than others, describing EBIs as "evidence-based" may be unhelpful. Research suggests that consumers are unfamiliar with the term "evidence-based" and may even dislike the concept of "evidence-based" treatment (Becker et al., 2016; Carman et al., 2010; Meyer et al., 2019). Lay language, such as "treatments that work" or "effective therapy," is likely more appealing to consumers (Becker et al., 2018; Crane et al., 2021). See the Dissemination Strategies section for details on specific strategies that can be used to tailor DTC marketing campaigns based on the marketing mix. Case Study 10.2 provides an example of how DTC marketing has been applied to EBIs.

CASE STUDY 10.2 USING DIRECT-TO-CONSUMER SOCIAL MARKETING TO DISSEMINATE INFORMATION ABOUT EVIDENCE-BASED INTERVENTIONS TO PARENTS OF ADOLESCENTS WITH SUBSTANCE USE ISSUES

The work of Becker et al. (2020) offers an example of how the marketing mix can be used to design dissemination materials to help parents of adolescents with substance use issues seek EBIs for their children. The team first used qualitative and quantitative surveys to assess parents' preferences for receiving information, then further assessed how those preferences varied by sociodemographic characteristics and the behavioral health issues of their children. For the product, many parents surveyed preferred an individualized approach to therapy that emphasized the therapeutic relationship. Further, parents with lower levels of education, with lower incomes, and identified as racial/ethnic minorities were more likely to incorrectly define "EBI" and dislike the principles and concepts of "EBIs." Parents with youth who had a history of juvenile justice system involvement believed the term "evidence-based" had a legal connotation. For the price, they found that parents were willing to commute an average of 38 minutes and were willing to pay an average of $42 for services; parents with higher incomes and with higher levels of education were willing to pay more. For the place, parents wanted to receive information about services from websites, brochures, and social media. They wanted to receive the therapy either in a "center focused on adolescents" or through their pediatrician. For the promotion strategy, the term that parents preferred for describing EBIs depended on their child's behavioral health history.

The team took this information from the marketing mix to design a user-informed infographic, which they compared to a standard description of EBI used by a national organization. An infographic was chosen because of parents' preference to receive information on social media. They used terms such as "effective therapy," "some therapies work better than others," and "every teen is different" given that many parents misunderstood or disliked the term "evidence-based" and because parents valued therapy that is customized to each client.

(*continued*)

CASE STUDY 10.2 USING DIRECT-TO-CONSUMER SOCIAL MARKETING TO DISSEMINATE INFORMATION ABOUT EVIDENCE-BASED INTERVENTIONS TO PARENTS OF ADOLESCENTS WITH SUBSTANCE USE ISSUES *(continued)*

Parents of adolescents with a history of legal problems were more likely to request additional information about EBIs after viewing the user-informed infographic, and parents of adolescents with a history of substance use issues preferred the user-informed infographic. Thus, this user-informed infographic, which was four times shorter and written at a lower reading level than standard educational materials, was a better DTC marketing strategy to encourage parents to see EBIs for their adolescent's substance use issues.

DISSEMINATION STRATEGIES

As noted, dissemination strategies are communication actions that seek to influence an audience's knowledge, attitudes, intentions, and behaviors related to an EBI through the distribution of strategic messages via intentionally selected sources and channels. Such communications include, but are not limited to, the development of evidence summaries (e.g., policy briefs, practice guidelines) distributed via email, social media, websites, podcasts, and presentations. Numerous reviews have synthesized information about dissemination strategies for specific audiences—such as healthcare providers (McCormack et al., 2013), public health practitioners (Brownson et al., 2018), policy makers (Ashcraft et al., 2020; Purtle, Marzalik, et al., 2020; Purtle, Nelson, et al., 2020), and members of the public who might seek out EBIs. Drawing from these literatures, this section highlights four broad types of dissemination strategies that can be applied to various communication actions.

Audience Segmentation

Audience segmentation is the process of identifying sub-groups within a population who have similar knowledge, attitudes, intentions, behaviors, demographics, or other characteristics relevant to the EBI that is the focus of a dissemination campaign (Kreuter & Bernhardt, 2009; Slater, 1996; Slater et al., 2006). The purpose of identifying these subgroups is to inform the development of different messages and dissemination campaigns for different types of people within a target population (see the following sections on adaptation tailoring and framing). The basic premise of audience segmentation is that disseminating different types of messages for different types of people is a more effective strategy than a "one-size-fits-all" dissemination approach (Dijkstra, 2008).

Audience segmentation can promote health equity by helping tailor dissemination materials about EBIs to reflect the practice realities of audiences who serve populations with varying degrees of social advantage (e.g., therapists in private practice versus community mental health centers) and populations of diverse cultural backgrounds (e.g., therapists in multilingual settings). There are two broad approaches to audience segmentation—demographic separation and empirical clustering (Smith, 2017). Here we describe both approaches and compare their strengths and weaknesses.

Demographic Separation: Creating Groups Based on Demographics

As the name suggests, **demographic separation approaches to audience segmentation** involve dividing an audience into segments based on demographic characteristics. "Demographic" has a broad meaning in this context. Segmenting demographics could include characteristics such as race/ethnicity, gender, age, as well as professional role (e.g., front-line clinician or administrative manager), type of organization (e.g., government versus non-government), or political ideology, as well as differences in knowledge, attitudes, intentions, and behaviors related to an EBI. In ideal circumstances, decisions about which demographic characteristics to segment upon are based on empirical data about the target population. However, such data are often not available and practical considerations drive segmentation decisions. Even without data to inform demographic separation segmentation decisions, such segmentation can still be effective if supported by theory about how audience members with specific demographic characteristics might respond differently to messages about an EBI. Case Study 10.3 provides an example of a data-driven demographic separation audience segmentation analysis of U.S. city mayoral officials.

CASE STUDY 10.3 DEMOGRAPHIC SEPARATION AUDIENCE SEGMENTATION TO DISSEMINATE EVIDENCE ABOUT HEALTH EQUITY TO CITY MAYORS IN THE UNITED STATES

A health-focused foundation has the goal of improving health equity in the United States. To help achieve this, they engage in dissemination activities targeting a range of audiences to increase knowledge about the existence of health disparities and to foster attitudes that are supportive of public policies that reduce disparities. Within this context, the foundation contracted with researchers to conduct a demographic separation audience segmentation analysis of U.S. city mayors and their mayoral officials (i.e., senior staff) in terms of their knowledge and attitudes about health disparities and health equity (Purtle, Henson, et al., 2018; Purtle et al., 2021).

The researchers worked with a survey firm to try and survey the mayors of all U.S. cities with a population of 50,000 or more. The survey was web-, post/mail-, and telephone-based and 230 mayoral officials responded (101 mayors, 129 mayoral senior staff; response rate = 30%). The survey assessed knowledge and attitudes related to health disparities, dissemination preferences (e.g., preferred sources and features of policy briefs), and collected demographic information about respondents. Key demographic variables of interest were social and fiscal ideology because prior research with the United States found ideological differences in knowledge and attitudes about health disparities.

The demographic separation analysis found large and statistically significant differences in knowledge about attitudes about health disparities between ideologically liberal and conservative mayoral officials. For example, socially liberal mayoral officials were much more likely than socially conservative officials to strongly agree that disparities existed in their city (61% versus 18%), believe that these disparities were very unfair (49% versus 10%), and believe that city policies affect health disparities (29% versus 8%). The demographic separation analysis also observed differences in the dissemination preferences of socially liberal and conservative mayoral officials. For example, a significantly larger proportion of liberal than conservative officials

(*continued*)

CASE STUDY 10.3 DEMOGRAPHIC SEPARATION AUDIENCE SEGMENTATION TO DISSEMINATE EVIDENCE ABOUT HEALTH EQUITY TO CITY MAYORS IN THE UNITED STATES *(continued)*

identified inclusion of information about the impacts of an issue on constituents as a very important feature of disseminated health evidence (88% versus 69%) and identified advocacy organizations as a very trustworthy source of research evidence (44% versus 17%). Conversely, industry sources were rated as among the least trustworthy sources of research among socially liberal mayoral officials while they were rated as among the most trustworthy sources among conservatives (22% versus 43%).

This demographic separation audience segmentation analysis has implications for dissemination practice. First, results indicate value in developing different dissemination materials, such as policy briefs, for liberal and conservative mayoral officials. For example, policy briefs tailored for liberal mayoral officials might use words that resonate with liberal worldviews (e.g., "equity") while those tailored for conservative mayoral officials might use words that typically resonate more strongly with conservative worldviews (e.g., "opportunity"). Furthermore, given differences in baseline knowledge and attitudes about health disparities, policy briefs for liberal mayoral officials might emphasize information about specific city policies that can address disparities, whereas those tailored for conservative officials might include more general information about the existence of health disparities in cities and their consequences. Second, the policy briefs might be sent from different sources to account for ideological differences in dissemination preferences. For example, partnerships with health equity advocacy organizations (e.g., National Association for the Advancement of Colored People) could be formed so that they can distribute policy briefs to liberal mayoral officials; partnerships could be developed with industry sources (e.g., American Medical Association) so that they can distribute the policy briefs to conservative mayoral officials.

Empirical Clustering: Creating Groups Based on Statistics

With **empirical clustering approaches to audience segmentation**, statistical techniques are used to identify relationships between multiple variables within a target population, rather than differences between groups based on single variables as is done in demographic clustering. Survey data are typically used to conduct empirical clustering audience segmentation analyses, but administrative data on the practice patterns of a dissemination audience could also be used for such analyses. The number of variables included in an empirical clustering audience segmentation analysis is determined by sample size and statistical power, but generally ranges from five to 15 variables. Latent class analysis (LCA) is a statistical technique typically used for these purposes, although *k*-means clustering can be used as well. LCA identifies latent "classes" (i.e., audience segments) that reflect relationships between variables and then members of the sample are assigned to the class to which they have the highest probability of belonging. After the quantitative process of identifying audience segments, a qualitative process is used to create names for the segments that reflect their most salient features.

For example, an empirical clustering audience segmentation analysis using LCA with survey data identified three audience segments of U.S. state legislators who vary in their knowledge, attitudes, and legislative behaviors related to behavioral health issues (Purtle, Lê-Scherban, et al., 2018). The largest audience segment (47% of the sample) was named "Budget-Oriented Skeptics With Stigma" because these legislators prioritized budget concerns over the strength of research evidence, were skeptical about the effectiveness of behavioral health treatments, and had high levels of stigma toward people with mental illness. An implication of this analysis for dissemination is that messages targeting this group should emphasize the cost-savings that can be produced by investments in mental health and should be cautious to not amplify stigma toward people experiencing mental illness (e.g., avoid use of frames which imply that people with mental illness can be dangerous; McGinty et al., 2018).

Empirical clustering audience segmentation also has utility with the public. While not a "practice population," the public is an important dissemination audience because public support is a key determinant of policy changes that increase the reach of EBIs (Purtle, 2020). For example, Bye and colleagues (2016) conducted a nationally representative survey of U.S. adults and used *k*-means clustering to identified audience segments related to attitudes about health disparities and the role of public policy in promoting health equity. Six audience segments were identified, ranging from "Committed Activists" to "Disinterested Skeptics."

Comparing Demographic Separation and Empirical Clustering Approaches

Demographic separation is the more pragmatic, although potentially less precise, approach to audience segmentation. As noted, while empirical data about a target audience are ideally used to inform segmentation decisions, appropriate use of theory can be sufficient when such data are not available. Another strength of demographic separation is that many segmenting variables are readily observable. This makes it possible to know to which segment a person belongs when disseminating materials to them. A weakness of demographic separation, however, is that it assumes that there is meaningful homogeneity within each segment in terms of knowledge, attitudes, and other factors that could influence the effectiveness of a dissemination campaign. Such homogeneity does not always exist within demographic segments, however, and as a result, demographic separation may not identify the most meaningful sub-groups within a population (Smith, 2017).

The main benefit of empirical clustering is that it can identify highly nuanced and meaningful sub-groups within a population because multiple variables are used to identify audience segments (Smith, 2017). By identifying these sub-groups, dissemination materials can be tailored with greater precision (described in the following) which can make them more effective at achieving dissemination goals. Further, well-funded for-profit advertising agencies often use this approach. The primary downside of empirical clustering approaches relates to the fact that primary data, such as survey data, are needed about a target population. These data are often difficult, and costly, to acquire.

Message Tailoring

As a dissemination strategy, **tailoring** involves the manipulation of dissemination materials and messages so that they are aligned with the personal attributes of individual message recipients. A large body of evidence from the fields of health communication and marketing indicate that tailored dissemination materials and messages are more effective than "one-size-fits-all" messages (Kreuter et al., 2013; Noar et al., 2007). Web-based communication (e.g., email, website content) has dramatically enhanced the efficiency and precision of tailoring (Kosinski et al., 2013). Drawing from a typology proposed by Dijkstra (2008), we provide an overview of three types of tailoring strategies that are relevant to the dissemination: *personalization*, *adaptation*, and *feedback*.

Personalization Tailoring

Personalization involves integrating recognizable aspects of message recipients (e.g., their name, professional title, organization) into messages. Taking simple and low-cost steps to personalize emails that disseminate information about EBIs for members of a target audience (e.g., using a mail merge or an email distribution program) can significantly increase engagement with dissemination materials. For example, an experiment found that including the message recipient's first name in the subject line increased the probability of opening the e-mail by 20% and reduced the probability of unsubscribing from future emails by 31% (Sahni et al., 2018).

Per the ELM, personalization might be an effective tailoring strategy because it signals that a message is relevant to the recipient, therein increasing the chances of them reading the message and processing the information through the central (i.e., cognitive) route (Hawkins et al., 2008; Petty et al., 1983). Personalization could also prompt information processing via the peripheral (i.e., emotional) route because people generally have positive attitudes toward salient features of themselves, such as their name (Munz et al., 2020). Although personalization is generally a recommended practice in dissemination, it can be counterproductive in certain circumstances. For example, personalization could have unintended consequences if it prompts information privacy concerns (e.g., a message recipient angrily asking: "How did you get this personal information about me to personalize this message?!).

Adaptation Tailoring

Adaptation entails modifying messages for different types of people within a target population to align the message with the characteristics of the recipient (Dijkstra, 2008). Messages can be adapted in terms of their content, the sources from which they are sent, and the modes through which they are delivered. Adaptation occurs after audience segmentation is conducted and is the reason why audience segmentation would be carried out in the first place. Adaptation is an effective tailoring strategy because it increases congruence between the message and the person receiving it, which in turn enhances engagement with and cognitive processing of the information (2008). Adaptation differs from personalization in that it involves tailoring messages, not simply offering cues (e.g., including a message recipient's name and professional title) to increase the likelihood of engagement with the information.

Message adaptation is a core strategy in advertising; and the rise of social media in which people leave "digital footprints" has accelerated the development, delivery, and precision of adapted messages (Kosinski et al., 2013). For example, adapting Facebook advertisements to reflect user personality traits, as predicted by their Facebook "likes," was found to result in 40% more advertising clicks and 50% more purchases (Matz et al., 2017). The notorious Facebook-Cambridge Analytica data scandal—in which social media data was (unethically and without appropriate permission) used to create complex psychological profiles of individuals and deliver messages based on these profiles to influence voting behavior in the 2016 U.S. election—is a prime example of message adaptation (Illing, 2018).

Feedback Tailoring

Feedback-tailored messages provide recipients with information about themselves as it relates to the EBI and their knowledge, attitudes, intentions, or behaviors that the dissemination campaign targets. For example, in health communication interventions focused on promoting healthy behaviors, a feedback-tailored message might include information about how many steps a person took in the current week compared to the prior week (using smartphone data to track this). A dissemination campaign focused on changing clinician prescribing behaviors might include information about how a clinician's prescribing behavior of a specific drug compares to that of their peers (using medical records or insurance claims data to track this). Such feedback-tailored dissemination strategies have demonstrated success changing clinician prescribing behaviors (Doctor et al., 2018; Sacarny et al., 2018).

Feedback-tailored messaging as a dissemination strategy is similar to the implementation strategy of audit and feedback. The key distinction is that, as a dissemination strategy, feedback tailoring is typically limited to the asynchronous and unidirectional provision of information, whereas audit and feedback often includes other components (e.g., training, facilitation). Feedback intervention theory (Kluger & DeNisi, 1996) posits that feedback which includes negative information coupled with feasible recommendations for improvement can increase motivation and positively change behavior. The following is an example of a tailored message for primary care physicians that reflects feedback intervention theory: "Electronic medical record (EMR) data show that you only screened 25% of patients over age 65 for depression last month. That is much lower than the health system average of 75%. Opting into the EMR reminder prompt for this screening has helped other doctors increase their screening rate."

Framing

Framing involves selectively emphasizing certain aspects of an EBI to influence specific knowledge, attitudes, intentions, and behaviors among a target audience (Druckman & Lupia, 2017; Milkman & Berger, 2014). Framing is similar to the tailoring strategy of adaptation (described earlier), but broader because information can be deliberately framed regardless of whether audience segmentation and message tailoring are conducted. For example, all members of a target audience might receive an identical message in which information about an EBI is strategically framed. Framing decisions can be deliberate, but all information is framed when communicated, whether done intentionally or not. For example, including information about cost-effectiveness in a policy brief frames the EBI in monetary terms; the inclusion of information about the EBI reducing disparities frames the EBI in terms of equity and justice. Framing can be a particularly useful strategy when disseminating evidence to audiences that have little prior knowledge about an EBI—as is often the case with elected policy makers (Vis, 2019). Framing is important with these audiences because they rely more heavily on heuristics (i.e., cognitive shortcuts) when processing information about a topic they have little prior knowledge.

Framing decisions are ideally informed by data about the target audience as well as theory about the mechanisms through which a specific frame would affect dissemination outcomes. When such data are lacking, as they often are, theory can be sufficient. Formal theories such as ELM and TPB, detailed earlier, can inform framing decisions as can more general, untested theoretical principles that are based on the synthesis of relevant evidence related to a topic. For example, Farrer and colleagues (2015) conducted a synthesis to develop guiding principles related to effective communication and advocacy about health equity. A dissemination campaign focused on increasing public awareness about the social determinants of health disparities was named *For the Sake of All*, which frames health disparities as an issue that has consequences for everyone (Purnell et al., 2018). Corrigan and Watson (2003) created a theoretical framework to inform the dissemination of research evidence about mental health issues to policy makers. The framework posits that policy makers' decisions about mental health issues are influenced by the extent to which they perceive people as being responsible for their mental health issues. Informed by this theory, a dissemination campaign might frame mental health issues as often having origins in childhood trauma, abuse, and neglect (factors beyond a person's control).

Identifying and Leveraging the Power of Opinion Leaders and Knowledge Brokers

DOI theory (Rogers, 2010) and other theories relevant to dissemination highlight the transformative role that influential individuals play in the spread of information about EBIs. Opinion leaders and knowledge brokers are two types of these individuals. Social network analysis—a methodological approach that focuses on relationships between individuals rather than relationships between characteristics of individuals (i.e., demographic characteristics)—supports the notion that opinion leaders and knowledge brokers can be integral to the success of dissemination campaigns (Valente & Davis, 1999).

Opinion Leaders

Opinion leaders are individuals who have a substantial interpersonal influence on others in their social network. They are often referred to as "change agents" in the literature (Miech et al., 2018). Opinion leaders can help successfully introduce new ideas, depict old ideas in newly positive light, and change the behavior of peers within their social networks (Green et al., 2009). For these reasons, identifying and partnering with opinion leaders is a widely used and often effective dissemination strategy (Miech et al., 2018; Valente & Pumpuang, 2007). In these instances, the entity disseminating information about the EBI partners with opinion leaders and then the opinion leaders disseminate the information to their peers. Effective techniques for identifying opinions leaders include asking members of a social network to identify who the opinion leaders are, in addition to asking opinion leaders to identify themselves (Valente & Pumpuang, 2007). Key attributes to consider when selecting opinion leaders include: their ability to influence the opinions of others in their network, their ability to communicate information persuasively to different audiences, the extent to which they understand the organizational and local context in which they work, and the extent to which they are respected, credible, and well-liked by peers (Bonawitz et al., 2020; Miech et al., 2018). To leverage opinion leaders as champions of an EBI, there likely will need to be an engagement process to gain opinion leader support of the EBI they are promoting.

Knowledge Brokers

Knowledge brokers can function similarly to opinion leaders in the dissemination process, but they are different in the sense that their primary job responsibilities relate to the spread of information about EBIs. Knowledge brokers facilitate, translate, and diffuse knowledge by developing positive relationships between knowledge producers (e.g., researchers) and knowledge users (e.g., clinicians, policy makers) to encourage the use of

EBIs (Bornbaum et al., 2015). Knowledge brokers work with members of different social networks and systems to exchange information and cultivate support for the EBI, filling structural gaps between clusters of individuals that do not necessarily interact (Burt, 2005). Knowledge brokers work to spread information about EBIs and influence dissemination outcomes through activities such as developing positive relationships between knowledge produces (e.g., researchers) and knowledge users (e.g., policy makers, clinicians), facilitating dialogue, and repackaging (i.e., adaption tailoring) information about an EBI for different audiences (Bornbaum et al., 2015; Dobbins et al., 2009).

DESIGNING, EXECUTING, AND EVALUATING A DISSEMINATION CAMPAIGN FOR PRACTICE AUDIENCES

Drawing from the precedingsections, we now summarize four steps to designing, executing, and evaluating a dissemination campaign. Across all these steps, engagement with key stakeholders (e.g., members of the population who are the primary audience of the dissemination campaign, members of the organization who are executing the campaign) are critical to success. Piloting campaign messages with key stakeholders can help increase the relevance and acceptability of the dissemination campaign.

Step 1. Define the Goals of Your Dissemination Campaign

What would success look like if the dissemination campaign were successful? In what ways would an audience change if dissemination strategies were effective? Such questions can help establish clear goals for a dissemination campaign. It is important to identify dissemination goals early in the planning process because they should drive decisions about the dissemination strategies that are used. It is often helpful to establish both proximal and distal dissemination goals. Proximal goals may relate to improvements in knowledge, attitudes, intentions to adopt an EBI among a practice audience, whereas distal goals may relate to behaviors related to adoption of the EBI and having the EPI reach a defined threshold (e.g., 65%) of the eligible population.

Step 2. Define and Characterize Your Audience

It is important to clearly define the target audience of the dissemination campaign early on in the goal-setting process. The size and specificity of target audiences can vary dramatically, and professional role and geography are two key dimensions that can help establish the boundaries of a target audience. For example, in a policymaker-focused dissemination campaign, professional roles could be limited to elected policy makers, administrative policy makers, or include both; and geography could range from those with policymaking authority at the national, state/provincial, and/or local level.

Understand the Audience's Baseline Knowledge, Attitudes, Intentions, and Behaviors Related to the Evidence-Based Intervention

As described in the previous sections about audience segmentation and adaptation tailoring, it is important to consider the baseline knowledge, attitudes, intentions, and behaviors related to the EBI among the target audience. This information is important to designing the dissemination campaign and can also be useful in developing its goals. Ideally, primary data are collected from a sample of the target audience (e.g., surveys or interviews) to characterize relevant knowledge, attitudes, intentions, and behaviors. However, in instances when such primary data collection is not possible, it is still important to consider these factors. Informal correspondence with members of the target audience paired with theory can be useful when primary data collection is not an option. Audience segmentation should also occur at this step in the planning process, using guidance related to audience segmentation detailed earlier in the chapter.

Understand the Audience's Preferred Channels and Modes for Receiving Information About the Evidence-Based Interventions

Identifying the preferred channels and modes for receiving information about the EBI can inform decisions about how information is delivered to the target audience. Examples of such challenges include interactive websites, static documents (e.g., policy briefs and practice guidelines in PDF format), synchronous or asynchronous webinars, in-person trainings, and podcasts. Again, primary data are ideally collected from a sample of the target audience to obtain information about these preferences. However, while baseline knowledge, attitudes, intentions, and behaviors often vary dramatically from one EBI to another, a target audience's preferences for specific channels and modes are likely similar for information about different EBIs.

Understand the Audience's Preferred Sources of Information About the Evidence-Based Interventions

Dissemination materials do not have impact unless they reach the target audience. Therefore, it is important to consider where the audience turns to for information and to disseminate information to that source, or better yet develop mutually beneficial partnerships with that source and co-create dissemination materials and a distribution plan. Examples of sources of information about EBIs include university researchers, advocacy organizations, professional trade associations, and government agencies. There is often substantial heterogeneity in the preferred sources of information within a target population (as noted in Case Study 10.3).

Step 3. Develop and Distribute Dissemination Materials

The development and distribution of dissemination materials is where the "rubber hits the road" in the dissemination campaign. The development and distribution process should be informed by theory, data if possible, and entails making decisions about audience segmentation and dissemination strategies (e.g., how dissemination materials will be tailored, framed, and the sources through which they will be distributed).

The "3-30-3" rule is useful to keep in mind when developing dissemination materials. The rule states that you have 3 seconds to capture a message recipient's attention, 30 seconds to persuade them that the dissemination materials are worth engaging with, and 3 minutes for them to engage with the actual dissemination materials. As an example, think of a policy brief about an EBI that is being emailed to policy makers. The subject line of the email should be compelling in 3 seconds or less, the body text should be compelling in 30 seconds or less, and the policy brief itself should be comprehendible in 3 minutes or less.

Visual elements such as maps and infographics can be effective elements in dissemination materials. With maps, such as those displaying the prevalence of a health condition, it is ideal to tailor the maps to align it with the geographies that are most relevant to the target audience (i.e., use state or local as opposed to national data if possible). PolicyMap (a free web-based mapping tool) and other data dashboards that map health issues can be useful in this regard. Taking screenshots of maps on these dashboards can be a more efficient approach then re-creating them in a mapping program. A variety of no-cost web-based design tools, such as Canva, can help facilitate the development of infographics and other dissemination materials, such as policy briefs. The *Getting Research Into Policy in Public Health* initiative (n.d.) has centralized tools to provide concrete guidance about developing and distributing policy briefs, with many of these resources focused on policy makers in low- and middle-income countries. Materials are enhanced by visual images that are appealing, use images relevant to the target audience, include adequate white space, and connect closely with the text.

The inclusion of narratives (i.e., brief stories about people, real or fictional) in dissemination materials can play a powerful role in framing an issue (Frank et al., 2015). Narratives contain elements such as a character, a setting, a plot, a conflict, and a resolution. Scales exist to assess how effective narratives are by assessing the extent to which they "transport the reader" (Green & Brock, 2000). Exhibit 10.1 provides an example of a narrative that was used to disseminate information about a clinical practice guideline for opioid prescribing to emergency medicine physicians (Meisel et al., 2016).

The distribution of dissemination materials can occur through "push" and "pull" approaches, both of which can be used simultaneously in a dissemination campaign (Lavis et al., 2006). Push approaches send information to target audiences such as through personalized tailored emails from trusted and/or credible sources, social media posts, post-mailings, podcasts, and presentations. Pull approaches enable and encourage target audiences to obtain information from websites, EBI clearinghouses, and other repositories. As an example of pull initiative, Lavis and colleagues (2011) curated a database of policy-relevant systematic reviews, complete with quality ratings and lay language summaries. The database was created for policy analysts and advisors in the Ontario Ministry of Health and Long-Term Care to access and review with the goal of these reviews informing policy decisions.

Step 4. Evaluate the Dissemination Campaign

Evaluation is essential to knowing the extent to which the goals of the dissemination campaign were achieved and to provide information for improving current and future efforts. Purtle and colleagues (2021) have detailed a research approach for data-driven dissemination that can be useful in thinking about evaluation. There is an important difference between dissemination outputs (e.g., number of social media posts, number of webinars provided) and dissemination outcomes. Table 10.3 provides examples of dissemination outcomes spanning a proximal-distal continuum across three domains: engagement with dissemination materials; knowledge, attitudes, and intentions; and behaviors. These outcomes can be assessed descriptively using cross-sectional designs, with quasi-experimental methods (Handley et al., 2018), or experimentally in a randomized controlled trial (RCT) approach in which messages, sources, or modes of dissemination are manipulated during the campaign.

While a full-fledged RCT might initially seem beyond the scope of dissemination campaigns that are focused on practice as opposed to research, dissemination RCTs can

Exhibit 10.1 Example of a Narrative Used to Disseminate Information About a Clinical Practice Guideline to Emergency Medicine Physicians

STORIES FROM THE EMERGENCY DEPARTMENT: MEDS AND MARRIAGE

My husband Bill and I used to argue about opioids. A lot. We are both emergency physicians and met during residency. After a few years, we found ourselves happily married by the end of training.

By all accounts, Bill and I have similar professional temperaments—I believe we are thoughtful, compassionate, and procedurally adept. But we used to have fundamentally different approached to treating pain. Bill felt that all patients with acute or chronic pain should be treated with as much analgesia as was required to get them completely comfortable. Sometimes that meant sending them home with prescriptions for large quantities of hydrocodone or dilaudid. "Pain is the fifth vital sign and if I don't fully treat it I am doing a lousy job as a doctor," he would say.

I would roll my eyes; I've seen patients come back to the ED addicted to opioids after therapeutic uses for acute pain. I was worried about the growing epidemic of prescription pill overdoses. "Where do you think all these pills are coming from?" I'd say, "Doctors like you."

Looking back, I think that we boxed ourselves into positions on treating patients with pain. We knew that both of our approaches were problematic. But we didn't have good tools to help us risk stratify our patients and optimize their care.

Evidence-based recommendation on opioid prescription helped us get out of our boxes. The American College of Emergency Physicians' (ACEP) clinical policy statement helped us negotiate the care of those "in between" patients where it wasn't clear what the best strategy was for pain management.

Click here to see the ACEP Clinical Policy on Opioid Prescribing

We started using the prescription drug monitoring program (PDMP) for our state. The database was filled with surprises—like the elderly grandparent that we discovered was a doctor shopping for Percocet—but it also made us feel more comfortable about prescribing opioids to other patients who were not flagged in the PDMP.

Click here to Get to Your State's PDMP

We now use the guidance to help explain to our patients, colleagues, and students whey we are making our clinical decisions.

For the most part, we have stopped arguing about prescribing opioids. Too bad there isn't a guideline about who should do the dishes.

Source: From Meisel, Z. F., Metlay, J. P., Sinnenberg, L., Kilaru, A. S., Grossestreuer, A., Barg, F. K., Shofer, F. S., Rhodes, K. V., & Perrone, J. (2016). A randomized trial testing the effect of narrative vignettes versus guideline summaries on provider response to a professional organization clinical policy for safe opioid prescribing. *Annals of Emergency Medicine, 68*(6), 719–728. Reprinted with permission.

TABLE 10.3 Outcomes to Evaluation Dissemination Campaigns

OUTCOMES	MODES OF MEASUREMENT
Engagement with dissemination materials	■ Email view rates ■ Link click rates ■ Social media views, likes, and re-tweets and other engagement metrics ■ Website visit volume
Knowledge, attitudes, and intentions	■ Surveys ■ Interviews
Behaviors	■ Surveys ■ Interviews ■ Analysis of administrative data/documents (e.g., health care claims, introduction of policy proposals)

be executed easily with little or no additional cost. For example, a target audience can be randomized to receive an email with information about an EBI with one of three different messages in the subject line—each of which frames the EBI a different way. Email open and link click rates can then be compared across the three study arms to determine which subject frames, if any, were more effective than others. Google Analytics Optimize is a free and useful tool for RCTs of dissemination campaigns because it can randomly assign website visitors to see versions of webpages. Link click behavior within the website can then be assessed as an outcome. This tool was recently used, for example, to assess the effect of altering the headings of a websites about a clinical practice guideline (Werntz et al., 2020).

SUMMARY

Dissemination is communication. It is communication about an EBI, and communication that is strategic as it reflects intentional decisions about the content of messages, the sources from which they are distributed, and the channels through which they are delivered to different audiences. Dissemination campaigns generally seek to influence knowledge, attitudes, intentions, and ultimately behaviors related to an EBI among a target audience. As such, dissemination campaigns can complement and set the stage for implementation strategies that are more squarely focused on behavior change related to an EBI. Dissemination is important from a health equity perspective because it can help reduce disparities in the spread of information about EBIs—disparities that are likely to occur if information is simply let to diffuse. Dissemination campaigns can be enhanced by using elements of theories (e.g., the ELM, theory of the DOI) and four broad types of strategies: audience segmentation, message tailoring, framing, and using opinion leaders and knowledge brokers.

The extent to which theory, data, and the full range of dissemination strategies are used in a dissemination is typically influenced by the resources available. It is better to use at least some of the strategies in the dissemination toolbox than to rely on diffusion to spread information about an EBI.

KEY POINTS FOR PRACTICE

1. Define and know your audience.
2. Segment your audience, even if adequate primary data are not available to drive segmentation decisions.
3. Partner with opinion leaders, knowledge brokers, and trusted intermediary organizations to spread dissemination materials and information about EBIs.
4. Thoughtfully develop messages, consider how messages are framing the EBI.
5. Tailor dissemination materials to the highest degree feasible, even if just by the message recipient's first name.
6. Identify clear goals and outcomes for a dissemination campaign and engage with key stakeholders through the dissemination planning, execution, and evaluation process.

COMMON PITFALLS IN PRACTICE

1. Assuming that the words and frames that are most common and accepted among researchers are those that are best suited for communicating with practitioners and consumers of EBIs.
2. Using a "one-size-fits-all" dissemination approach that does not account for different audience segments.
3. Not drawing from relevant theory about DOI and persuasive communication when developing dissemination materials.
4. Equating dissemination outputs (e.g., number of social media posts, number of webinars provided) with dissemination outcomes (e.g., changes in knowledge, attitudes, and intentions).

DISCUSSION QUESTIONS

1. Using data from a target audience to conduct audience segmentation analyses, and subsequently tailoring dissemination materials for audience members if different segments, is recognized as a best practice for dissemination. However, organizations that execute dissemination campaigns rarely have sufficient data and resources to conduct detailed audience segmentation analyses and tailoring. Given this, how can principles of audience segmentation and tailoring be applied to improve dissemination campaigns executed by organizations with limited resources?
2. Identify a specific EBI that is of interest to you. If information about the EBI is simply let to diffuse without active dissemination, what might the implications be from a health equity perspective?
3. Dissemination strategies can target practice audiences who affect the delivery of and access to EBIs, as well as members of the general public who are consumers of EBIs. For a specific EBI that you identify, how might a practice audience–focused

dissemination campaign and consumer-focused DTC marketing campaign work synergistically to increase the reach of the EBI?

4. Dissemination, as defined in the field of implementation science, is a relatively new concept. However, the study and practice of persuasive communication has existed for over a century. With its focus on EBIs, is dissemination truly distinct from other fields that focus on persuasive communication, such as advertising and health communication? How so?

REFERENCES

Ajzen, I. (1991). The theory of planned behavior. *Organizational Behavior and Human Decision Processes, 50*(2), 179–211. https://doi.org/10.1016/0749-5978(91)90020-T

Ashcraft, L. E., Quinn, D. A., & Brownson, R. C. (2020). Strategies for effective dissemination of research to United States policy makers: A systematic review. *Implementation Science, 15*(1), 1–17. https://doi.org/10.1186/s13012-020-01046-3

Becker, S. J. (2015). Direct-to-consumer marketing: A complementary approach to traditional dissemination and implementation efforts for mental health and substance abuse interventions. *Clinical Psychology: Science and Practice, 22*(1), 85 – 100. https://doi.org/10.1111/cpsp.12086.

Becker, S. J., Helseth, S. A., Tavares, T. L., Squires, D. D., Clark, M. A., Zeithaml, V. A., & Spirito, A. (2020). User-informed marketing versus standard description to drive demand for evidence-based therapy: A randomized controlled trial. *American Psychologist, 75*(8), 1038. https://doi.org/10.1037/amp0000635

Becker, S. J., Spirito, A., & Vanmali, R. (2016). Perceptions of 'evidence-based practice' among the consumers of adolescent substance use treatment. *Health Education Journal, 75*(3), 358–369. https://doi.org/10.1177/0017896915581061

Becker, S. J., Weeks, B. J., Escobar, K. I., Moreno, O., DeMarco, C. R., & Gresko, S. A. (2018). Impressions of "evidence-based practice": A direct-to-consumer survey of caregivers concerned about adolescent substance use. *Evidence-Based Practice in Child and Adolescent Mental Health, 3*(2), 70–80. https://doi.org/10.1080/23794925.2018.1429228

Bonawitz, K., Wetmore, M., Heisler, M., Dalton, V. K., Damschroder, L. J., Forman, J., Allan, K. R., & Moniz, M. H. (2020). Champions in context: Which attributes matter for change efforts in healthcare? *Implementation Science, 15*(1), 1–10. https://doi.org/10.1186/s13012-020-01024-9

Bornbaum, C. C., Kornas, K., Peirson, L., & Rosella, L. C. (2015). Exploring the function and effectiveness of knowledge brokers as facilitators of knowledge translation in health-related settings: A systematic review and thematic analysis. *Implementation Science, 10*(1), 1–12. https://doi.org/10.1186/s13012-015-0351-9

Breslin, C., Li, S., Tupker, E., & Sdao-Jarvie, K. (2001). Application of the theory of planned behavior to predict research dissemination: A prospective study among addiction counselors. *Science Communication, 22*(4), 423–437. https://doi.org/10.1177/1075547001022004004

Brownson, R. C., Eyler, A. A., Harris, J. K., Moore, J. B., & Tabak, R. G. (2018). Research full report: Getting the word out: New approaches for disseminating public health science. *Journal of Public Health Management and Practice, 24*(2), 102. https://doi.org/10.1097/PHH.0000000000000673

Burt, R. S. (2005). *Brokerage and closure: An introduction to social capital.* Oxford University Press.

Butler, D. M., & Nickerson, D. W. (2011). Can learning constituency opinion affect how legislators vote? Results from a field experiment. *Quarterly Journal of Political Science, 6*(1), 55–83. https://doi.org/10.1561/100.00011019

Bye, L., Ghirardelli, A., & Fontes, A. (2016). Promoting health equity and population health: How Americans' views differ. *Health Affairs, 35*(11), 1982–1990. https://doi.org/10.1377/hlthaff.2016.0730

Carman, K. L., Maurer, M., Yegian, J. M., Dardess, P., McGee, J., Evers, M., & Marlo, K. O. (2010). Evidence that consumers are skeptical about evidence-based health care. *Health Affairs, 29*(7), 1400–1406. https://doi.org/10.1377/hlthaff.2009.0296

Casper, E. S. (2007). The theory of planned behavior applied to continuing education for mental health professionals. *Psychiatric Services, 58*(10), 1324–1329. https://doi.org/10.1176/ps.2007.58.10.1324

Corrigan, P. W., & Watson, A. C. (2003). Factors that explain how policy makers distribute resources to mental health services. *Psychiatric Services, 54*(4), 501–507. https://doi.org/10.1176/appi.ps.54.4.501

Crane, M. E., Helseth, S. A., Scott, K., & Becker, S. J. (2021). Adolescent behavioral health problems are associated with parent perceptions of evidence-based therapy and preferences when seeking therapeutic support. *Professional Psychology: Research and Practice.* https://doi.org/10.1037/pro0000361

Dearing, J., & Kee, K. (2012). Historical roots of dissemination and implementation science. In R. Brownson, G. Colditz, & E. Proctor (Eds.), *Dissemination and implementation research in health: Translating science to practice* (pp. 55–71). Oxford University Press.

Dijkstra, A. (2008). The psychology of tailoring-ingredients in computer-tailored persuasion. *Social and Personality Psychology Compass*, *2*(2), 765–784. https://doi.org/10.1111/j.1751-9004.2008.00081.x

Dobbins, M., Robeson, P., Ciliska, D., Hanna, S., Cameron, R., O'Mara, L., DeCorby, K., & Mercer, S. (2009). A description of a knowledge broker role implemented as part of a randomized controlled trial evaluating three knowledge translation strategies. *Implementation Science*, *4*(1), 1–9. https://doi.org/10.1186/1748-5908-4-23

Doctor, J. N., Nguyen, A., Lev, R., Lucas, J., Knight, T., Zhao, H., & Menchine, M. (2018). Opioid prescribing decreases after learning of a patient's fatal overdose. *Science*, *361*(6402), 588–590. https://doi.org/10.1126/science.aat4595

Druckman, J. N., & Lupia, A. (2017). Using frames to make scientific communication more effective. In K. H. Jamieson, D. M. Kahan, & D. A. Scheufele (Eds.), *The Oxford handbook of the science of science communication* (pp. 243–252). Oxford University Press.

Farrer, L., Marinetti, C., Cavaco, Y. K., & Costongs, C. (2015). Advocacy for health equity: A synthesis review. *The Milbank Quarterly*, *93*(2), 392–437. https://doi.org/10.1111/1468-0009.12112

Frank, L. B., Murphy, S. T., Chatterjee, J. S., Moran, M. B., & Baezconde-Garbanati, L. (2015). Telling stories, saving lives: Creating narrative health messages. *Health Communication*, *30*(2), 154–163. https://doi.org/10.1080/10410236.2014.974126

Friedberg, R. D., & Bayar, H. (2017). If it works for pills, can it work for skills? Direct-to-consumer social marketing of evidence-based psychological treatments. *Psychiatric Services*, *68*(6), 621–623. https://doi.org/10.1176/appi.ps.201600153

Getting Research Into Policy in Public Health. (n.d.). https://blogs.lshtm.ac.uk/griphealth/

Glanz, K., & Bishop, D. B. (2010). The role of behavioral science theory in development and implementation of public health interventions. *Annual Review of Public Health*, *31*, 399–418. https://doi.org/10.1146/annurev.publhealth.012809.103604

Gollust, S. E., Barry, C. L., & Niederdeppe, J. (2017). Partisan responses to public health messages: Motivated reasoning and sugary drink taxes. *Journal of Health Politics, Policy and Law*, *42*(6), 1005–1037. https://doi.org/10.1215/03616878-4193606

Green, L. W., Ottoson, J. M., Garcia, C., & Hiatt, R. A. (2009). Diffusion theory and knowledge dissemination, utilization, and integration in public health. *Annual Review of Public Health*, *30*. https://doi.org/10.1146/annurev.publhealth.031308.100049

Green, M. C., & Brock, T. C. (2000). The role of transportation in the persuasiveness of public narratives. *Journal of Personality and Social Psychology*, *79*(5), 701. https://doi.org/10.1037/0022-3514.79.5.701

Handley, M. A., Lyles, C. R., McCulloch, C., & Cattamanchi, A. (2018). Selecting and improving quasi-experimental designs in effectiveness and implementation research. *Annual Review of Public Health*, *39*, 5–25. https://doi.org/10.1146/annurev-publhealth-040617-014128

Haugtvedt, C. P., Herr, P. M., & Kardes, F. R. (2018). *Handbook of consumer psychology*. Routledge.

Haugtvedt, C. P., & Kasmer, J. A. (2008). Attitude change and persuasion. In C. P. Haugtvedt, P. M. Herr, & F. R. Kardes (Eds.), *Handbook of consumer psychology* (pp. 419–435). Taylor & Francis Group/Lawrence Erlbaum Associates.

Hawkins, R. P., Kreuter, M., Resnicow, K., Fishbein, M., & Dijkstra, A. (2008). Understanding tailoring in communicating about health. *Health Education Research*, *23*(3), 454–466. https://doi.org/10.1093/her/cyn004

Illing, D. (2018). *Cambridge Analytica, the shady data firm that might be a key Trump-Russia link, explained*. VOX. https://www.vox.com/policy-and-politics/2017/10/16/15657512/cambridge-analytica-facebook-alexander-nix-christopher-wylie.

Jason, L. A., & Rose, T. (1984). Influencing the passage of child passenger restraint legislation. *American Journal of Community Psychology*, *12*(4), 485–494. https://doi.org/10.1007/BF00896507

Kluger, A. N., & DeNisi, A. (1996). The effects of feedback interventions on performance: A historical review, a meta-analysis, and a preliminary feedback intervention theory. *Psychological Bulletin*, *119*(2), 254. https://doi.org/10.1037/0033-2909.119.2.254

Kosinski, M., Stillwell, D., & Graepel, T. (2013). Private traits and attributes are predictable from digital records of human behavior. *Proceedings of the National Academy of Sciences*, *110*(15), 5802–5805. https://doi.org/10.1073/pnas.1218772110

Kotler, P., & Zaltman, G. (1971). Social marketing: An approach to planned social change. *Journal of Marketing*, *35*(3), 3–12. https://doi.org/10.1177/002224297103500302

Kreuter, M. W., & Bernhardt, J. M. (2009). Reframing the dissemination challenge: A marketing and distribution perspective. *American Journal of Public Health*, *99*(12), 2123–2127. https://doi.org/10.2105/AJPH.2008.155218

Kreuter, M. W., Farrell, D. W., Olevitch, L. R., & Brennan, L. K. (2013). *Tailoring health messages: Customizing communication with computer technology*. Routledge.

Lavis, J. N., Lomas, J., Hamid, M., & Sewankambo, N. K. (2006). Assessing country-level efforts to link research to action. *Bulletin of the World Health Organization*, *84*(8), 620–628. https://doi.org/10.2471/blt.06.030312

Lavis, J. N., Wilson, M. G., Grimshaw, J. M., Haynes, R. B., Hanna, S., Raina, P., Gruen, R., & Ouimet, M. (2011). Effects of an evidence service on health-system policy makers' use of research evidence: A protocol for a randomised controlled trial. *Implementation Science*, 6(1), 1–8. https://doi.org/10.1186/1748-5908-6-51

Leeman, J., Birken, S. A., Powell, B. J., Rohweder, C., & Shea, C. M. (2017). Beyond "implementation strategies": Classifying the full range of strategies used in implementation science and practice. *Implementation Science*, *12*(1), 1–9. https://doi.org/10.1186/s13012-017-0657-x

Liu-Thompkins, Y. (2019). A decade of online advertising research: What we learned and what we need to know. *Journal of Advertising*, *48*(1), 1–13. https://doi.org/10.1080/00913367.2018.1556138

Lomas, J. (1993). Diffusion, dissemination, and implementation: Who should do what? *Annals of the New York Academy of Sciences*, *703*(1), 226–237. https://doi.org/10.1111/j.1749-6632.1993.tb26351.x

Matz, S. C., Kosinski, M., Nave, G., & Stillwell, D. J. (2017). Psychological targeting as an effective approach to digital mass persuasion. *Proceedings of the National Academy of Sciences*, *114*(48), 12714–12719. https://doi.org/10.1073/pnas.1710966114

McCormack, L., Sheridan, S., Lewis, M., Boudewyns, V., Melvin, C. L., Kistler, C., Lux, L. J., Cullen, K., & Lohr, K. N. (2013). Communication and dissemination strategies to facilitate the use of health-related evidence. In *Database of Abstracts of Reviews of Effects (DARE): Quality-assessed reviews [Internet]*. Centre for Reviews and Dissemination (UK).

McGinty, E., Pescosolido, B., & Goldman, H. (2018). Communicating about mental illness and violence: Balancing increased support for services and stigma. *Journal of Health Policy, Politics and Law*, *43*(2), 185–228. https://doi.org/10.1215/03616878-4303507

McGinty, E. E., Webster, D. W., & Barry, C. L. (2013). Effects of news media messages about mass shootings on attitudes toward persons with serious mental illness and public support for gun control policies. *American Journal of Psychiatry*, *170*(5), 494–501. https://doi.org/10.1176/appi.ajp.2013.13010014

Meisel, Z. F., Metlay, J. P., Sinnenberg, L., Kilaru, A. S., Grossestreuer, A., Barg, F. K., Shofer, F. S., Rhodes, K. V., & Perrone, J. (2016). A randomized trial testing the effect of narrative vignettes versus guideline summaries on provider response to a professional organization clinical policy for safe opioid prescribing. *Annals of Emergency Medicine*, *68*(6), 719–728. https://doi.org/10.1016/j.annemergmed.2016.03.007

Meyer, M. N., Heck, P. R., Holtzman, G. S., Anderson, S. M., Cai, W., Watts, D. J., & Chabris, C. F. (2019). Objecting to experiments that compare two unobjectionable policies or treatments. *Proceedings of the National Academy of Sciences*, *116*(22), 10723–10728. https://doi.org/10.1073/pnas.1820701116

Miech, E. J., Rattray, N. A., Flanagan, M. E., Damschroder, L., Schmid, A. A., & Damush, T. M. (2018). Inside help: An integrative review of champions in healthcare-related implementation. *SAGE Open Medicine*, *6*, 2050312118773261. https://doi.org/10.1177/2050312118773261

Milkman, K. L., & Berger, J. (2014). The science of sharing and the sharing of science. *Proceedings of the National Academy of Sciences*, *111*(Suppl 4), 13642–13649. https://doi.org/10.1073/pnas.1317511111

Munz, K. P., Jung, M. H., & Alter, A. L. (2020). Name similarity encourages generosity: A field experiment in email personalization. *Marketing Science*. https:doi.org/10.2139/ssrn.3244125

National Institutes of Health. (n.d.). *Department of Health and Human Services, Part 1: Overview information*. https://grants.nih.gov/grants/guide/pa-files/PAR-19-274.html

Niederdeppe, J., Roh, S., & Shapiro, M. A. (2015). Acknowledging individual responsibility while emphasizing social determinants in narratives to promote obesity-reducing public policy: A randomized experiment. *PLoS One*, *10*(2), e0117565. https:doi.org/10.1371/journal.pone.0117565

Noar, S. M., Benac, C. N., & Harris, M. S. (2007). Does tailoring matter? Meta-analytic review of tailored print health behavior change interventions. *Psychological Bulletin*, *133*(4), 673. https:doi.org/10.1037/0033-2909.133.4.673

Nyhan, B., & Reifler, J. (2015). The effect of fact-checking on elites: A field experiment on US state legislators. *American Journal of Political Science*, *59*(3), 628–640. https:doi.org/10.1111/ajps.12162

Petty, R. E., & Cacioppo, J. T. (1986). The elaboration likelihood model of persuasion. In *Communication and persuasion* (pp. 1–24). Springer.

Petty, R. E., Cacioppo, J. T., & Schumann, D. (1983). Central and peripheral routes to advertising effectiveness: The moderating role of involvement. *Journal of Consumer Research*, *10*(2), 135–146. https://doi.org/10.1086/208954

Petty, R. E., & Krosnick, J. A. (2014). *Attitude strength: Antecedents and consequences*. Psychology Press.

Purnell, J. Q., Goodman, M., Tate, W. F., Harris, K. M., Hudson, D. L., Jones, B. D., Fields, R., Camberos, G., Elder, K., Drake, B., & Gilbert, K. (2018). For the sake of all: Civic education on the social determinants of health and health disparities in St. Louis. *Urban Education*, *53*(6), 711–743. https://doi.org/10.1177/0042085916682574

Purtle, J. (2020). Public opinion about evidence-informed health policy development in US Congress. *Translational Behavioral Medicine*, *10*(6), 1549–1553. https://doi.org/10.1093/tbm/ibz083

Purtle, J., Henson, R. M., Carroll-Scott, A., Kolker, J., Joshi, R., & Diez Roux, A. V. (2018). US mayors' and health commissioners' opinions about health disparities in their cities. *American Journal of Public Health*, *108*(5), 634–641. https://doi.org/10.2105/AJPH.2017.304298

Purtle, J., Joshi, R., Lê-Scherban, F., Henson, R. M., & Diez Roux, A. V. (2021). Linking data on constituent health with elected officials' opinions: Associations between urban health disparities and mayoral officials' beliefs about health disparities in their cities. *The Milbank Quarterly, 99*(3), 794–827. https://doi.org/10.1111/1468-0009.12501

Purtle, J., Lê-Scherban, F., Wang, X., Shattuck, P. T., Proctor, E. K., & Brownson, R. C. (2018). Audience segmentation to disseminate behavioral health evidence to legislators: An empirical clustering analysis. *Implementation Science, 13*(1), 121. https://doi.org/10.1186/s13012-018-0816-8

Purtle, J., Marzalik, J. S., Halfond, R. W., Bufka, L. F., Teachman, B. A., & Aarons, G. A. (2020). Toward the data-driven dissemination of findings from psychological science. *American Psychologist, 75*(8), 1052. https://doi.org/10.1037/amp0000721

Purtle, J., Nelson, K. L., Bruns, E. J., & Hoagwood, K. E. (2020). Dissemination strategies to accelerate the policy impact of children's mental health services research. *Psychiatric Services, 71*(11), 1170–1178. https://doi.org/10.1176/appi.ps.201900527

Rogers, E. M. (2010). *Diffusion of innovations*. Simon and Schuster.

Sacarny, A., Barnett, M. L., Le, J., Tetkoski, F., Yokum, D., & Agrawal, S. (2018). Effect of peer comparison letters for high-volume primary care prescribers of quetiapine in older and disabled adults: A randomized clinical trial. *JAMA Psychiatry, 75*(10), 1003–1011. https://doi.org/10.1001/jamapsychiatry.2018.1867

Sahni, N. S., Wheeler, S. C., & Chintagunta, P. (2018). Personalization in email marketing: The role of noninformative advertising content. *Marketing Science, 37*(2), 236–258. https://doi.org/10.1287/mksc.2017.1066

Slater, M. D. (1996). Theory and method in health audience segmentation. *Journal of Health Communication, 1*(3), 267–284. https://doi.org/10.1080/108107396128059

Slater, M. D., Kelly, K. J., & Thackeray, R. (2006). Segmentation on a shoestring: Health audience segmentation in limited-budget and local social marketing interventions. *Health Promotion Practice, 7*(2), 170–173. https://doi.org/10.1177/1524839906286616

Smith, R. A. (2017). Audience segmentation techniques. In *Oxford Research Encyclopedia of Communication*. Oxford University Press.

Snyder, L. B. (2007). Health communication campaigns and their impact on behavior. *Journal of Nutrition Education and Behavior, 39*(2), S32–S40. https://doi.org/10.1016/j.jneb.2006.09.004

Valente, T. W., & Davis, R. L. (1999). Accelerating the diffusion of innovations using opinion leaders. *The Annals of the American Academy of Political and Social Science, 566*(1), 55–67. https://doi.org/10.1177/000271629956600105

Valente, T. W., & Pumpuang, P. (2007). Identifying opinion leaders to promote behavior change. *Health Education & Behavior, 34*(6), 881–896. https://doi.org/10.1177/1090198106297855

Vis, B. (2019). Heuristics and political elites' judgment and decision-making. *Political Studies Review, 17*(1), 41–52. https://doi.org/10.1177/1478929917750311

Werntz, A., Bufka, L., Adams, B. E., & Teachman, B. A. (2020). Improving the reach of clinical practice guidelines: An experimental investigation of message framing on user engagement. *Clinical Psychological Science, 8*(5), 825–838. https://doi.org/10.1177/2167702620920722

Yap, M. B. H., & Jorm, A. F. (2012). Young people's mental health first aid intentions and beliefs prospectively predict their actions: Findings from an Australian National Survey of Youth. *Psychiatry research, 196*(2–3), 315–319. https://doi.org/10.1016/j.psychres.2011.10.004

Yoong, S. L., Jones, J., Marshall, J., Wiggers, J., Seward, K., Finch, M., Fielding, A., & Wolfenden, L. (2015). A theory-based evaluation of a dissemination intervention to improve childcare cooks' intentions to implement nutritional guidelines on their menus. *Implementation Science, 11*(1), 105. https://doi.org/10.1186/s13012-016-0474-7

Zeithaml, V., Bitner, M. J., & Gremler, D. (2012). *Services marketing: Integrating customer focus across the firm* (6th ed.). McGraw-Hill Higher Education.

11

Scaling Up Evidence-Based Interventions

Ruth Simmons, Peter Fajans, and Laura Ghiron

Learning Objectives

By the end of this chapter, readers will be able to:

- Appreciate the importance of a focus on scale up in implementation science
- Understand concepts common to major scaling-up frameworks and approaches
- Be familiar with the ExpandNet/WHO scale-up framework, approach, and practical guidance tools, and understand how they can be used to support scale up of evidence-based interventions (EBIs)
- Be able to discuss key principles, lessons, and practices for sustainable scale up, as well as common challenges encountered

CASE STUDY 11.1 SCALING UP THE *STRONGER VOICES PROJECT* IN KYRGYZSTAN

The *Stronger Voices Project* was initially implemented in 10 villages across three districts in Kyrgyzstan by the national Ministry of Health (MoH), with support from the United Nations Population Fund (UNFPA). This project tested an innovation to develop community dialogues with different age and gender groups to address the sexual and reproductive health of youth, increase demand for family planning (FP), and promote the prevention of sexually transmitted infections (STIs). These interventions were based on the successful "Stepping Stones" model first tested in Uganda. In addition, the project intended to strengthen the provision of contraception and the management of STIs by staff of the village health centers.

Project interventions were designed following qualitative needs assessments using in-depth interviews with community members and health providers and observations of service delivery in each of the 10 villages. The assessments were conducted by senior MoH staff based in the capital city, Bishkek, together with senior staff from a national level non-governmental organization (NGO) experienced in community mobilization. The MoH officials then implemented trainings for service providers in each health center, while the NGO staff spent 2 weeks in each village conducting community mobilization exercises and training teachers at local schools to facilitate dialogues.

At the end of the first year of implementation, external evaluations demonstrated successful impact of the project on multiple indicators. The plan was to scale up activities to an additional 20 villages in the final 2 years of the project, using the same process of needs assessments and trainings conducted by the same senior staff, replicating the successful implementation process with a high degree of fidelity.

Do you think that this scale-up strategy could subsequently be used to achieve significant future impact in the 3,500 villages of Kyrgyzstan?

INTRODUCTION

Health and other development efforts of the last decades have relied on pilot, demonstration, or implementation research projects[1] to improve the lives of people throughout the world. Such projects have generally succeeded in demonstrating the value of evidence-based interventions (EBIs) for project participants or beneficiaries, but they have often not led to sustainable large-scale implementation. Since the early 2000s such small-scale efforts have come under increasing criticism for not leading to the larger impact that is needed to advance health and other development goals in low- and middle-income countries (LMICs; Simmons et al., 2007). A high-level official in the Democratic Republic of the Congo once remarked: "Projects kill programs" because they typically create conditions that are not replicable or sustainable and do not strengthen routine services provided by government programs (Mai et al., 2019). This problem must be addressed through efforts that may begin small, but which from the outset focus on both local relevance and feasibility, as well as the potential for large scale, lasting impact (ExpandNet & World Health Organization [WHO], 2009).

[1] The terms *pilot* and *demonstration projects* are used in the field of global health and development to refer to small-scale efforts to try out interventions in programmatic contexts, utilizing varying degrees of formal research methods.

The field of scale up has evolved to address these issues and has grown considerably in the last two decades. While differing in emphasis, various frameworks and approaches have emerged that share many common elements. These are discussed in this chapter, with special emphasis on the work of ExpandNet (www.expandnet.net), an informal network of individuals from international, bilateral and NGO organizations, academic institutions, and governmental ministries who seek to advance the science and practice of scaling up.

THE DEFINITION OF SCALING UP

A variety of definitions of scaling up have been used in the literature ranging from "doing more," to more complex descriptions that go beyond the expansion of ongoing implementation. These include other elements such as the importance of mobilizing human and financial resources, and adaptation of the interventions (Hartman & Linn, 2008; Mangham & Hanson, 2010).

The ExpandNet definition of scaling up, which has become widely cited in the literature and is used in this chapter, is as follows:

> *Deliberate efforts to increase the impact of successfully tested health innovations so as to benefit more people and to foster policy and program development on a lasting basis.* (ExpandNet & WHO, 2010, p. 2)

This definition emphasizes the following essential components:

- **"Deliberate efforts":** To succeed, scaling up typically requires carefully planned and guided efforts. It rarely happens spontaneously, and when it does the innovation tends to be only partially implemented and scaled up. Ad hoc approaches to scale up are often not successful.
- **"Successfully tested innovations":** ExpandNet uses the term *innovation* as introduced in the diffusion of innovation literature because the EBIs and related implementation strategies being expanded are new in the settings and for the people who are expected to benefit (Rogers, 2003). ExpandNet also emphasizes the need for testing the effectiveness and acceptability of innovations in the local health system and the social context.
- **"To benefit more people":** Here the emphasis is on expanding the innovation to more geographic areas, whether villages, districts, states, or to additional health facility catchment areas. This is referred to as expansion, roll-out, spread, or horizontal scale up and is what is most frequently meant when scale up is mentioned. However, one of the pitfalls of scaling up is a focus only on expansion, forgetting that it also requires embedding the innovation in policies and programs.
- **"Policy and program development":** This highlights the need to anchor innovations in their relevant institutional mechanisms; for example in policies, regulations, budgets, programmatic frameworks, and operational guidelines as part of ensuring sustainability. For example, a new policy may be needed that mandates that newborn umbilical cord stumps be treated with chlorhexidine, before expanding the innovation from pilot settings to additional areas. At the same time financial resources must be mobilized to train and supervise providers to ensure they can deliver such services with sufficient quality. A central point is that expansion and institutionalization are both required for successful scale up.
- **"On a lasting basis":** Given the importance of ensuring sustainability during scale up, the ExpandNet definition highlights this issue. Pilot or other small-scale implementation research projects often do not create conditions for sustainability. They typically benefit from special resources and attention and when these do not continue

to be available, the innovations disappear. Thus, scale-up initiatives, from the earliest stages of design, must focus on future sustainability. This means implementing the innovation under the conditions likely to be available in routine program contexts.

Common to most definitions is the key understanding that scale up is a policy, political, organizational development, and an implementation task rather than being tied to a particular technical health or development issue or intervention. Thus, various approaches to scale up draw heavily on the social sciences, particularly the diffusion of innovation literature and the management, political, and policy sciences.

WHY FOCUS ON SCALE UP

There are three key reasons why scale up is important for implementation science. First, a focus on scaling up the results of implementation research is essential for reaching global health and development goals. Relevant and effective innovations tested in a limited number of settings have the potential to contribute to achieving such goals, but only if they are sustainably scaled up. Attention to what will determine achieving future large-scale impact should therefore be part of initial planning and testing of innovations even at a small scale. Second, a failure to scale up promising innovations leads to wasted resources. Many projects begin with the goal that if successful, they will be scaled up to reach more people and become part of programs and policies. However, innovations conducted with special resources and leadership are often not scalable nor sustainable after the project ends. Equity imperatives are a third reason for the importance of a scale-up focus. Although difficult to achieve, the benefits of research and other successful health innovations should be extended to all who need them including the poor who are typically the hardest to reach (Zomahoun et al., 2019).

COMMON CHARACTERISTICS OF SCALE-UP APPROACHES

Over the last two decades many scale-up frameworks and approaches (sometimes combined with more practical guidance for implementors) have been published in the global development and implementation science literature. These various approaches differ considerably in their genesis, their fields of orientation, and their areas of emphasis. Many are based upon scale-up experiences from LMICs (Barker et al., 2015; Bradley et al., 2011; ExpandNet & WHO, 2009, 2010, 2011; Hartmann and Linn, 2008; Management Systems International [MSI], 2005, 2016, 2021; Massoud et al., 2006; Simmons et al., 2002, 2007; Spicer et al., 2014; Yamey, 2011). Others address scale up primarily in high-income countries (Ben Charif et al., 2017; Indig et al., 2017; Milat et al., 2014, 2016; Nguyen et al., 2020).

Zamboni et al. (2019) published tables reviewing some of these frameworks' theoretical bases and the various factors considered by each. Several of the frameworks have associated practical guidance tools to support scale-up efforts (ExpandNet & WHO, 2009, 2010, 2011; Milat et al., 2014, 2016; MSI, 2016, 2021). Although there are differences among these frameworks, they share the common goal of seeking to promote a systematic approach to scale up and have many of the following characteristics:

Evidence based: The systematic use of evidence is central to planning and implementing expansion and institutionalization, moving beyond more ad hoc approaches to scale up that have dominated the health and development fields in the past. The design and initial testing of a package of interventions for a particular context is often the first step. Documentation and stakeholder agreement about the evidence of effectiveness, feasibility, and acceptability of the intervention package is required before scaling up is considered. Although an intervention package may be acknowledged as an international best practice, local evidence is needed to demonstrate how the innovation can be implemented in the routine context where it is to be scaled up. As discussed in the following, this implementation research needs to begin with the end in mind by planning for scale up from the initial design of the innovation. If not, the model tested may not be feasible for future implementation and scale up.

Similarly, learning from the social sciences—and particularly the diffusion of innovation and knowledge utilization literatures—has contributed to the development of implementation frameworks and guidance to support scale up (Dearing & Cox, 2018; Glaser et al., 1983; Rogers, 2003). This literature has identified attributes of innovations that can facilitate scale up (Simmons & Shiffman, 2007).

An important step in applying an evidence-based approach to scale up is to identify the components of the innovation that are essential to attain the desired outcome and impact. The initial testing of EBIs in a new context frequently contains elements that are not required for success, and therefore can be eliminated to make scale up easier and more efficient. For example, to strengthen the demand for FP in urban communities, the Tupange project (Keyonzo et al., 2015) in Kenya first tested an innovation that included multiple sources of information about contraception for couples. These included print materials, radio spots, home visits by community health workers (CHWs) and community theater "edutainment." Following a mid-term evaluation that showed exposure to community theater was not related to contraceptive use it was subsequently dropped. It is important to note that when elements of the innovation are discontinued it is often necessary to test the simplified model during the first phase of expansion to confirm that nothing essential was omitted and that the expected outcomes are maintained.

Systems thinking: A key concept from the management sciences that should inform scaling efforts is the concept of *systems thinking* (Arnold & Wade, 2015). Expansion and institutionalization of innovations occurs within a complex network of interactions and influences. Changes in one element of a system tend to affect the others. Seeking an appropriate balance among all elements is a major task in designing and implementing a scaling-up strategy. When scaling up innovations in health services, it is important to consider the interactions between the package of interventions, the broader service delivery system and the intended target populations or communities, as well as how these interactions occur in a broader environmental context.

Lack of systems thinking typically occurs by planning to quickly expand a successfully tested innovation in settings that do not have the required organizational capacity or infrastructure to implement them. This is particularly true for the public sector in many low resource settings where capacities must be enhanced if scale up with sufficient quality of care is to succeed. Systems thinking often suggests a slower process that facilitates building the necessary implementation capacities as part of the process of scale up. For example, in Vietnam, the MoH initially thought that they could rapidly scale up the provision of depot medroxyprogesterone acetate (DMPA) an injectable contraceptive. However, after testing its provision in an implementation research project they learned that a slower and more systematic approach was necessary. Providers needed to be trained to inform women about the method's side effects and to counsel them with educational materials providing balanced information about all methods. Otherwise, women adopting the method quickly abandoned it and contraceptive choice was not increased (Fajans et al., 2007).

Context specific: The testing of innovations and subsequent development and implementation of scale-up strategies must be based on the understanding that one size does not fit all. There are not only major differences between LMIC and high-income settings, but also major differences among countries in both categories which substantially affect scaling up. The scaling-up process needs to be tailored to the local circumstances considering the various factors that determine whether implementation will succeed. Such tailoring requires deep understanding of the social context of the beneficiaries or target communities, as well as the institutional capacities of the implementing organization(s). This makes it possible to develop approaches that are feasible to implement and are acceptable to both service providers and target populations. As will be discussed, the context is not static, and strategies need to adjust to changes over time.

A phased process of learning and adaptation: A phased process is recommended by key scale-up frameworks and tools. It typically begins with an in-depth assessment of needs and the potential feasibility of the planned EBI and its implementation strategies, followed by the design of implementation research to test, on a limited scale, the effectiveness and acceptability of the innovation, and to learn of any unanticipated outcomes. This is followed by the development of a scale-up strategy to guide the initial scale up of the innovation. Early implementation of the strategy ideally takes place in a limited number of settings, testing the outcomes of the EBIs under the conditions of routine implementation, to learn about the adaptations needed to support continued and more rapid expansion and institutionalization of the innovations. As scale up continues, an iterative process using monitoring, learning, and feedback loops is necessary to ensure that scale up is proceeding appropriately, and the intended results continue to be achieved. This is further discussed in the following under the heading Phase 3: Managing the Implementation of Scale Up.

Stakeholder involvement throughout: The design of EBIs and their implementation strategies, as well as the testing and scale-up process, should be participatory, involving a full range of stakeholders including representatives of beneficiaries. Ownership and leadership should be in the hands of those who will be responsible for future full-scale implementation, even if initially the process will be supported by NGOs. This means that government involvement and preferably their leadership from the beginning are required for future scale up when strengthening public-sector services. Even pluralistic and private health systems typically depend on public-sector rules, regulations, and oversight. If government plays only a minor role, it is important to identify and involve in a central role the other institutions that are responsible for both implementation and regulatory oversight.

Focus on sustainability: A focus on sustainability of the innovation is required. In the past this has often been considered primarily in terms of continued financial support. However, it is now acknowledged that sustainability also includes maintaining activities, outcomes, and impacts (Lee, 2017; Shelton et al., 2018). Critical to this is the sustained capacity of responsible institutions and organizations to manage continued implementation of activities in the face of internal change, as well as changes occurring in the larger context. This requires institutionalized budgetary support, training capacity, the provision of necessary infrastructure and equipment, the health management information system (HMIS), and so forth. Thus, as mentioned earlier, scale up must address not only expansion, but also promote embedding innovations into policies, norms, programmatic frameworks, and operational guidelines to help create the conditions for sustainability.

Achieving sustainability may require hard choices such as the recognition that a simpler intervention package should be adopted because of its potential for sustainability, even though a more complex package might yield greater impact.

Values oriented: Scale up must be grounded in the values of equity, human rights, and gender perspectives, and guided by participatory and client-centered approaches that promote equitable access for all to quality services. These values are often adhered to as part of the initial implementation research. However, as innovations are expanded in large-scale public or private-sector settings without the special supports typically provided to initial trials, such values are difficult to maintain. Therefore, a focus on equity, human rights, and gender perspectives requires consistent emphasis throughout the process of scale up. If not, existing inequities in access to services based on gender or socio-economic status may be exacerbated.

The following sections outline the ExpandNet/WHO framework and approach, providing a detailed example of how proceeding systematically can serve to facilitate successful and sustainable scale up of health or other development innovations.

THE EXPANDNET/WHO FRAMEWORK

In the early 2000s, ExpandNet/WHO developed a systems framework (Simmons et al., 2002, 2007) to help implementors plan for and guide scaling-up processes. This framework, illustrated in Figure 11.1, was based on diverse literature reviews and members' practical experiences with scale-up initiatives. In this process multiple determinants of successful scale up were identified, pinpointing attributes of success whose relative presence or absence strongly affect outcomes. The scaling-up framework—which is discussed in more detail in ExpandNet/WHO guidance tools (2009, 2010, 2011)—consists of five elements inside the oval with the scaling-up strategy as the centerpiece and five strategic choice areas.

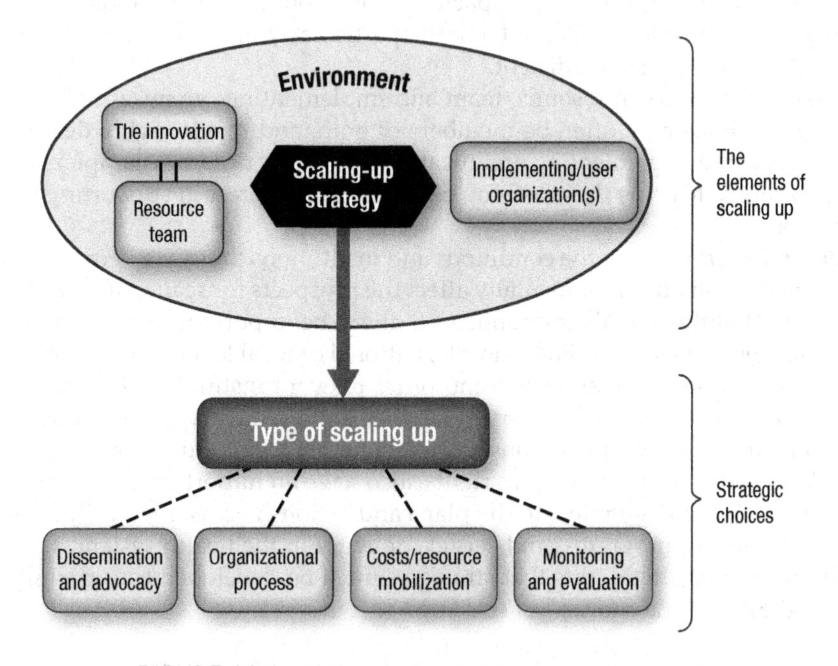

FIGURE 11.1 The ExpandNet/WHO scaling-up framework.

The Elements of Scaling Up

The innovation is the EBI and its associated implementation strategies–in other words, what is being scaled up. The innovation is typically a package of interventions, consisting of several components. These could be the introduction of new health technologies and activities necessary to provide them. In each case it is necessary to consider the technology or approach, as well as the multiple actions needed to implement them. In practice, the innovation often consists of at least one or more EBIs and activities necessary for their implementation. For example, introduction of a new health technology usually requires (a) training providers; (b) developing job aids and behavior change materials for clients; (c) strengthening supervision, logistics, and supply chains; (d) adapting (HMIS); and (e) ensuring ongoing budgetary commitments.

The resource team refers to the individuals and organizations that are promoting and facilitating wider use of the innovation. A resource team may be formally responsible for promoting the innovation or may act informally in this role. It should include members with the skills necessary to provide strong support to the scale-up process including advocacy, resource mobilization, management interventions, and technical skills related to the innovation. The resource team may be composed of program managers, researchers, technical experts including health policy and program analysts, service providers, policy makers from relevant ministries or other government organizations, representatives of national and international NGOs, as well as representatives of the beneficiaries or target populations. Resource teams benefit when some members hold senior, decision-making roles within institutions responsible for the scale-up process and have sufficient time to devote to the tasks of being a member.

The implementing organization(s), also known as the adopting or user organization(s), refers to the institution(s) or organization(s) that seek to or are expected to adopt and implement the innovation on a large scale. This could be the MoH or Education at national, sub-national, or local levels; an NGO or community-based organization; a network of private providers; or a combination of such institutions. As noted earlier, scaling up innovations typically involves building the capacity of the adopting organizations to implement the package of interventions on a wider scale, particularly in settings where the required implementation capacity is insufficient.

The distinction between resource team and implementing organization can be subtle and fluid. Individuals may often be members of both, and this is highly desirable. Over time, members of the implementing organization frequently become champions and members of the resource team as they develop expertise and interest in supporting scale up of the innovation.

The environment refers to the conditions and institutions that are external to the implementing organization but fundamentally affect the prospects for scaling up. There are multiple dimensions of the overall environment that can be important to address in planning for and implementing scale up. For example, national or local level politics and policies, in addition to government bureaucracies and other relevant institutions beyond the implementing organization (e.g., the Ministry of Finance or the Ministry of Education) can influence the scale up of health innovations. Socio-economic and cultural conditions, together with people's needs, perspectives, and rights, also have an important influence.

The scaling-up strategy refers to the plans and actions necessary to fully establish the innovation in policies, programs, and service delivery in the health system. The ExpandNet/WHO framework highlights that strategies must be developed considering the "elements" and the "strategic choices" of scale up.

Strategic Choices of Scale Up

A critical choice in developing a scaling-up strategy relates to the types of scale up to pursue. There are three types of deliberate or guided scale up: (a) institutional or vertical scale up, which refers to institutionalization through policy, political, legal, budgetary, or other health systems change; (b) expansion or horizontal scale up, which is also referred to as replication or spread to new geographic areas; and (c) diversification, which means adding new components to a tested innovation. In addition, there is a fourth type, spontaneous scale up, which occurs without deliberate guidance.

As is reflected in the ExpandNet/WHO framework, when developing a strategy there are strategic choices that must be made for each type of scaling up. These choices are related to: (a) dissemination and advocacy through policy briefs or other publications, policy dialogues, and technical assistance to ensure that the information about the innovations and plans for scale up are widely available and supported; (b) the organizational processes involved regarding the extent of geographic expansion, the number of institutions involved, and the degree to which the process is participatory; (c) costs and resource mobilization, which include linking scale up to funding mechanisms and ensuring adequate and sustainable budgetary allocations; and (d) monitoring and evaluation through a combination of collecting appropriate indicators, local assessments, special studies, and/or service statistics. For further detail see the section that follows on scaling-up strategy development and the guide titled *Nine steps for developing a scaling-up strategy* (ExpandNet & WHO, 2010).

THE THREE PHASES OF SCALE UP

Scale up involves a continuum of activities. As shown in Figure 11.2, ExpandNet conceptualizes a trajectory with three major phases beginning with (a) designing and implementing research or other projects to test promising packages of interventions, (b) developing a scaling-up strategy for the implementation of successfully tested EBIs, and (c) managing the process of scale up until implementation reaches the desired level of scale.

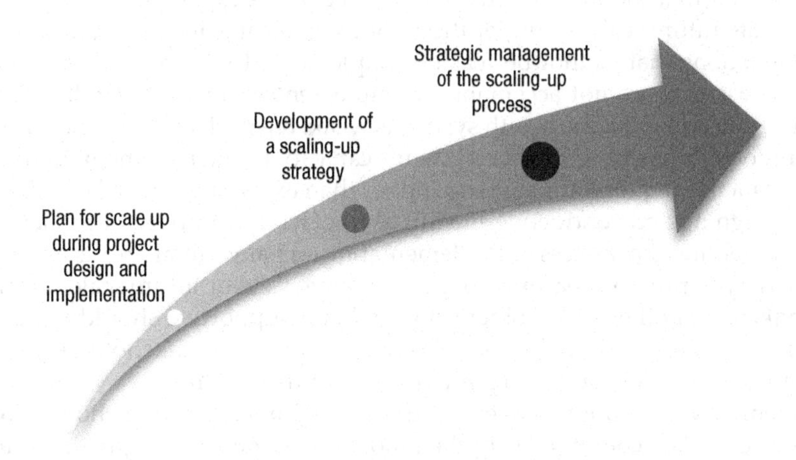

FIGURE 11.2 Three phases of scale up.

Phase 1: Planning Implementation Research for Scale-Up Success

ExpandNet has long called attention to the need for designing pilot and demonstration projects, as well as implementation research in ways that facilitate their potential for future scale up (ExpandNet & WHO, 2009, 2011; Simmons et al., 2002, 2007). The importance of designing projects for future scalability has now become widely accepted and numerous publications endorse key principles that enhance an innovation's suitability for scale up. ExpandNet/WHO published guidance entitled *Beginning with the end in mind: Planning pilot projects and other programmatic research for successful scale up* (BWEIM; ExpandNet & WHO, 2011). It discusses 12 recommendations for how to design and conduct projects in ways that increase the scalability of the innovation while simultaneously helping to ensure sustainability. Although each of the principles may appear on the surface to be common sense, they are often not followed when projects are designed and implemented. In summary, the recommendations are as follows.

The project team must have a clear vision of potential future scale up and build consensus on this vision with key stakeholders. Broad participation of key stakeholders, including representatives of the institutions that will be responsible for future implementation at scale up and of the intended beneficiaries, in the design and implementation process helps to create ownership of the activities. This is important for sustained implementation and scale up once the research or pilot phase has been completed.

The package of interventions must be relevant and evidenced based, acceptable to the intended beneficiaries or communities, and should be feasible for implementation within the routine institutional and resource constraints of the health system. It should also be tailored to the sociocultural and institutional settings where it will be implemented. In other words it needs to be designed using a systems perspective that takes into account how the innovation, implementing institutions, intended beneficiaries, and broader environment interact as a system.

Researchers should test innovations as much as possible under the conditions of routine program implementation, as well as in the variety of institutional settings where they will be scaled up. Sound evidence of effectiveness and acceptability must be generated in a range of settings representative of where scale up will take place to understand the outcomes of implementation in varied contexts, as well as to generate the political will and confidence of stakeholders to support and invest in a broader scale-up effort.

It is also vital that the innovation should be kept as simple and inexpensive as possible to facilitate future scale up under the resource and capacity constraints of the health system. Innovations that cannot be feasibly implemented within routine programmatic contexts or those that are not acceptable to implementers, or the intended beneficiaries should not be considered. If the health system is weak, the package of interventions should include components to strengthen the system's capacity for management, training, supervision, and data use required for scale up, rather than expecting this to be added later.

When designing and conducting the initial research it is important to plan on assessing and documenting the process of implementation and any initial results as they emerge. This is necessary to promote learning to facilitate advocacy for future scale up and to keep decision-makers and other stakeholders engaged and supportive should the final results warrant scale up. Early dissemination of results helps build stakeholders' commitment and willingness to provide budgetary support for future expansion.

Implementers should undertake early advocacy with relevant stakeholders for institutionalization of the key components of the innovation in policies, regulations, and guidelines, once results appear favorable. This helps prepare the ground for future scale up of the innovation. Likewise, advocacy with donors and other sources of funding for financial support beyond the research stage should start early and not wait for the completion of the project. At the same time, implementers also need to be cautious about initiating scale up before sufficient evidence of feasibility and effectiveness is available.

Finally, teams should not wait until the end of an externally funded project to begin planning for an appropriate end-of-project transition that will facilitate sustainable scale up. This is not solely an issue of ensuring funding, but also determining who will be responsible for providing strong leadership for the planning and implementation of the next phase of scale-up.

The ExpandNet/WHO BWEIM guide is intended for use by project implementers, researchers, policy makers, planners, program managers, technical-assistance providers, donors, and others who seek to ensure that programmatic or other implementation research tests innovations that are designed to facilitate scale up and lead to substantial and lasting impact. It can be used during the process of proposal development, throughout implementation, or to support evaluations to examine whether the project was appropriately designed for future scale up.

One project that used the BWEIM guidance from design throughout implementation was the multisectoral, integrated Health of People and Environment in the Lake Victoria Basin Project (HoPE-LVB) that ran from 2012 to 2018 (Ghiron et al., 2014; Omimo et al., 2018). The project had planned to implement several EBIs across the following sectors: maternal and child health, FP, water and sanitation, education, sustainable fisheries, agriculture, and environmental conservation. With support from ExpandNet, the Kenya and Uganda project teams used the ExpandNet/WHO BWEIM recommendations and the guide's scalability checklist to assess the proposed innovations. In the process they realized how the interventions could be adapted to improve the potential for future sustainability and scale up. For example, the project team had initially planned to independently train community members in project sites on agro-forestry innovations. However, when considering the BWEIM recommendations to tailor and test the innovation under the routine operating conditions and in the institutional settings where they will be implemented, they realized that Ugandan districts and subcounty administrative structures had personnel well suited to conduct these trainings. District-level natural resource officers and local village environmental committees had responsibility to conduct such trainings for communities, but lacked the resources and capacity to do so. Thus the project team involved them in the trainings, first as learners and then as trainers, thereby helping them gain the necessary skills and confidence. In this way the project built sustainable capacity to continue scaling up the innovations. The HoPE-LVB team conducted regular project reviews of all the EBIs using the BWEIM guide to ensure that the groundwork for future scale-up success continued to be laid.

When any implementation research project has been or is nearing completion with demonstrated success, the next step is to decide whether to proceed to scale up and develop a scaling-up strategy. Not all projects are capable of being sustained, or of being scaled up in a sustainable manner, particularly if they were not designed with scaling up in mind. Thus, a necessary step is to assess whether the innovations are in fact sustainable and scalable. In addition to the BWEIM checklist, there are several other recent publications that can be useful to retrospectively assess a project's potential future scalability (MSI, 2016, 2021; Milat et al., 2020; Zamboni et al., 2019).

Phase 2: Developing a Scale-Up Strategy for Successfully Tested Innovations

Once evidence exists that an innovation works within the local context and is considered relevant and feasible to implement in the wider health system, it is appropriate to develop a scaling-up strategy. Few development projects are designed using the principles presented in the BWEIM guide and as a result may not be easily scalable or sustainable. This does not mean they cannot be expanded to benefit more people and institutionalized in policies, plans, budgets, regulations, or laws. However, the scale-up strategy will need to address the fact that the innovation was designed and tested without thinking ahead to future scale up.

As previously mentioned, there are different frameworks, approaches, and practical tools to support scale up, including several for the development of scaling-up strategies. In the following, the ExpandNet/WHO approach is described in greater detail. This framework has been widely used in Africa, Asia, and Latin America for scaling-up innovations in the fields of health, education, gender and normative change, environmental conservation, and water and sanitation.

The practical guide entitled *Nine steps for developing a scaling-up strategy* (ExpandNet & WHO, 2010) is a tool to help design strategies for scaling up successfully tested innovations. It is organized around the ExpandNet/WHO framework discussed earlier. The first four steps focus on the elements of scaling up and elaborate how the strategy could potentially work:

- Step 1: Increase the scalability of the innovation
- Step 2: Strengthen the implementing (user) organization(s)
- Step 3: Enhance the fit of the EBI within the environment
- Step 4: Increase the capacity of the resource team to support scale up

The subsequent four steps analyze the strategic choices required to support the four different types of scale up:

- Step 5: Actions to support institutionalization
- Step 6: Actions to support expansion
- Step 7: Determining whether there is a need for diversification
- Step 8: Planning to address spontaneous scale up

In Step 9 the strategy is finalized by consolidating the recommended actions and identifying the next steps for its implementation.

Strategy development is ideally undertaken in a participatory, multi-stakeholder exercise where input from the local, sub-national, and the national levels contribute insight and recommendations for how the process should proceed. However, the exercise can also be undertaken by a smaller group of only project team members. When strategy development is undertaken with a broad range of stakeholders, the end results are often richer as they benefit from a wider range of insights. The HoPE-LVB project did both, starting with an internal strategy-development exercise with the project team, followed by a broader, more participatory process with stakeholders representing the various sectors that would implement the interventions.

During a strategy-development exercise, participants proceed sequentially through the nine steps, identifying recommendations for necessary actions which, when taken together, become the scaling-up strategy. For example, when participants address Step 1, which focuses on the EBI(s) and their implementation strategies, they consider actions to increase scalability, utilizing insights and lessons from the diffusion of innovation and knowledge utilization literatures. Past research has demonstrated that attributes of the innovation, such as its credibility, observability, and relevance, are associated with ease of scaling (Dearing & Cox, 2018; Glaser et al., 1983). To increase the credibility of the innovation, participants might recommend that summary results of the research or project evaluation be disseminated to key decision-makers. Observability of the EBIs and their outcomes might be enhanced by organizing opportunities for stakeholders to visit implementation sites and speak with providers and community members. Experience has shown that this contributes to increasing political will to support continued scale up of the innovation. Similarly, in the second step participants discuss what actions should be taken to increase the capacity of the implementing or user organization to manage and implement the package at multiple levels of the service delivery system. Recommended actions might include the need to strengthen district or regional training centers, develop job aids for providers, or improve the functioning of the HMIS.

Step 3 in turn requires identifying the various environmental sectors that are relevant for scale up and what can be done to maximize opportunities and minimize constraints. For example, an innovation tested in densely populated urban areas will have to be adapted when expanded to rural areas to better suit local conditions. Likewise, some implementation strategies tested in a predominantly Islamic region may need to be adapted when scaled to mainly Christian regions. Having a strong resource team to support scaling up of EBIs is essential. Step 4 therefore requires identifying at least some members who hold senior, decision-making roles in the implementing organizations and seeking their participation in the scale-up process.

Step 5, vertical scale up, addresses the policy, political, legal, regulatory, budgetary, or other health systems changes needed to institutionalize the innovation at the national or subnational level. If the government has not been involved in testing of the innovation, Step 5 must address strategic choices concerning advocacy for adopting the innovations within the national program. When innovations are to be scaled up within the NGO sector, some interactions with government will also be needed because of its policy and regulatory function. Other strategic choices address issues such as who will take responsibility for these activities, how necessary funding will be mobilized, and how progress toward institutionalization will be monitored.

Step 6 addresses the strategic choices to support expansion or horizontal scaling up to additional health centers, districts, or higher administrative levels. It requires deciding how the innovation will be disseminated to new areas or different population groups, how providers will be trained to implement the EBIs, how expansion will be organized, especially in terms of the pace and how widely it will be implemented, how resources will be mobilized and how the process, outcome, and impact will be monitored. When addressing resource mobilization, participants should discuss potential means of generating resources to support expansion. These could include linkages to health sectoral reforms, efforts to implement cost sharing with other ongoing activities, or advocacy with Ministry of Finance officials.

Step 7, diversification, consists of adding an additional innovation to one that is in the process of being scaled up; for example, adding a special component for adolescents in the process of scaling up an innovation that strengthens services for women. It requires proceeding through Steps 1 to 6 for this added component to determine whether diversification is feasible and if so, how best to integrate it into the package.

Step 8, spontaneous scale up, deals with the possibility that innovations spread without deliberate guidance. Such spontaneous scaling up is desirable if the intended results continue to be obtained. However, it may result in the innovation being incompletely replicated or the quality of the implementation may not be adequate. It is necessary to monitor spontaneous scale up to ensure that if needed, guidance is provided to ensure that results remain acceptable.

Discussion of Steps 1 to 8 is likely to lead to a long list of important recommendations. Collating these, prioritizing next steps, and identifying who will be responsible for implementing them is required, as is vetting the draft strategy with stakeholders who participated in the process. These activities constitute the final ninth step of strategy development. Presenting the strategy in a written document is required to provide a record and allow it to be widely shared.

Lessons Learned About Developing a Scaling-Up Strategy

Several lessons have been learned about applying the nine-step strategy development process in the field. The first lesson concerns the role of a participatory process. What is true for initial research or pilot project development also holds for developing a scale-up strategy: It should be a participatory process involving relevant stakeholders. If appropriate stakeholders have been involved from the beginning of project design, they should continue to be engaged throughout implementation and scale up. However, it is often necessary to include additional stakeholders throughout the process because strategy development and subsequent scale up will require new perspectives, skillsets, and champions among the resource team. The HoPE-LVB project demonstrated that involving new stakeholders in a second, more participatory strategy-development exercise opened windows of opportunity to embed the innovations in the work of additional stakeholders. For example, when government leaders from Kenya's Homa Bay County, where HoPE-LVB was initially implemented, shared their learning with their counterparts from the new scale up county, Siaya, the new leaders quickly understood how to institutionalize the innovations within their County Development Plan. Furthermore, the two counties set up a mentoring relationship that facilitated much faster initial implementation and scale up in Siaya than had occurred in Homa Bay.

Another important lesson concerns the innovation. While issues related to the future scalability of the EBI(s) would ideally have been addressed in phase I, this question continues to be of central concern at the time of strategy development. Implementation research often tests an innovation's acceptability and effectiveness with complex inputs and under non-routine conditions that are difficult to replicate on a large scale. Therefore, simplification (i.e., identifying interventions that are essential for effectiveness and dropping those that are not) is an important step during strategy development.

The Tupange Project in Kenya illustrates this point. The initial phase tested a wide range of EBIs and implementation strategies to address FP supply and demand, HIV prevention and treatment, and other maternal and child health issues. Initial implementation took place in four cities. The project utilized the ExpandNet nine step approach to develop a scale-up strategy to expand within these cities as well as to two additional semi-urban districts. In doing so the team realized they would need to simplify the innovation to make it more scalable and sustainable. This led to dropping some of the more complex components of the innovation and simplifying others. They decreased the number of days required for the provider training curriculum, decreased special project reporting and recording requirements, and relied on district level training centers rather than project staff to train CHWs, and more.

Even when planning for future scale up has been part of the initial testing of the innovation in phase 1, it may still be necessary to further simplify the model. However, under real-world conditions it is often not evident how best to do so while retaining effectiveness. Thus, it may be necessary when developing the scale-up strategy to plan for additional testing of the simplified model to ensure that it remains effective as early scale up is proceeding. This is often referred to as a "proof of implementation," in contrast to the initial testing of the innovation which may have been more similar to a "proof of concept" (Keyonzo et al., 2015).

An important lesson about strategy development concerns strategic choices related to the type and pace of scale up. Expansion or horizontal scaling up alone is normally insufficient to ensure that an innovation is fully integrated within existing institutions. To be sustainable, scaling up needs to focus on both expansion of implementation to new geographies and on institutionalizing the innovations as policies, budgetary change, and operational guidelines. Moreover, the pace of expansion often may have to be slower than what would ideally be desirable because the pace must be in balance with the complexity of the

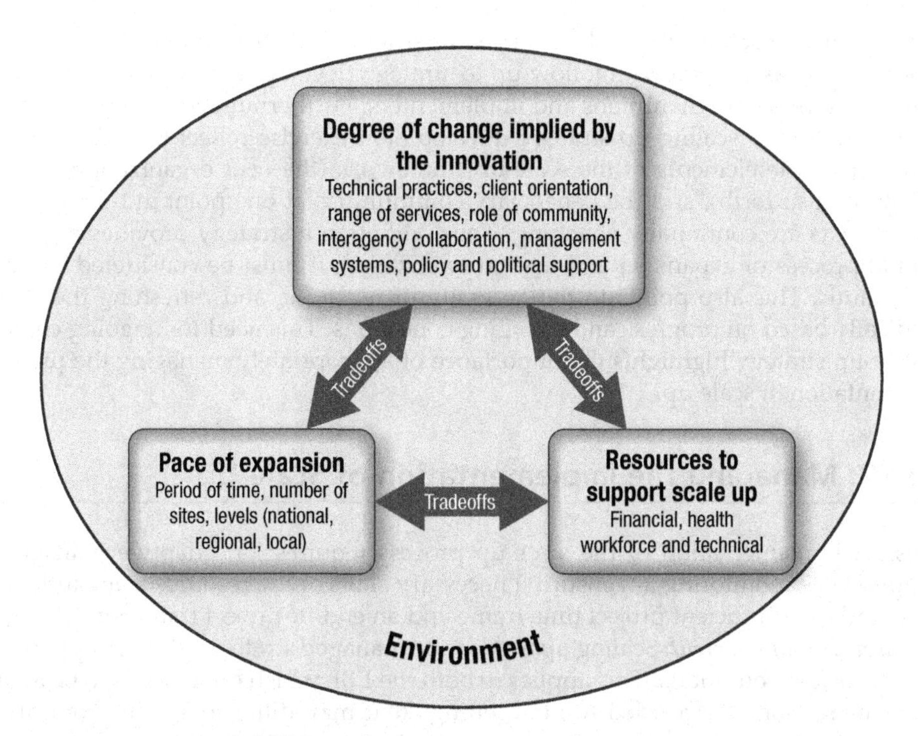

FIGURE 11.3 Strategic choices require tradeoffs.

innovation and the resources available to support the scale-up process (see Figure 11.3). Although it is often assumed that mainly financial resources are what are needed, it is clear from the literature and scale-up experience that extensive human and technical resources are also required. Here, human resources refer to the health workforce and their need for increased capacity to implement the innovation. The technical resources can be of two main types: those pertaining to infrastructure such as logistics, supplies, equipment, and facilities; and those related to technical skills including managerial expertise, leadership capacity, and to both external and internal technical support.

Figure 11.3 illustrates the potential tradeoffs involved. For example, if an EBI is of relatively low complexity and sufficient resources are available, then the pace of scaling can be faster. Conversely, if the EBI is more complex and/or resources are constrained, the pace of expansion must be slower. Overly rapid expansion can result in losing essential components of the innovation and typically these are the components most different from providers' current practices or those most difficult to implement. Actions to promote quality of care or values such as equity and gender perspectives are examples. A more gradual, phased process allows for learning about how sustainable expansion of all aspects of the innovation can be attained.

Strategy development requires facing the complexities and resource constraints of the real world. Implementers must ensure that the innovations being introduced are health system priorities and do not interfere with the provision of necessary existing services. This implies assessing EBIs and implementation strategies within the context of ongoing services within health systems and weighing the cost-effectiveness, efficiency, and impact of the interventions against that of alternative innovations (Zomahoun et al., 2019). Unfortunately, cost-related data are often not readily available.

Having a good scaling-up strategy does not ensure that an innovation will be sustainably scaled. A scaling-up strategy is likely to have components that must be implemented by a range of new actors who will need to endorse and implement the changes. Therefore, a major activity associated with follow up to strategy development is gaining buy-in and political will from new champions and implementers. Furthermore, the recommendations that emerge from a scaling-up strategy development exercise reflect the prevailing conditions across the elements of the scale-up framework (the user organization, the environment, and so forth), and the beneficiary communities at one point in time. However, these contexts are continually changing. Thus, although a strategy provides a guide for an initial process of expansion and institutionalization, it must be considered as flexible and dynamic. This also points to the necessity of revisiting and refreshing the strategy periodically based on progress and changing conditions. This need for ongoing change in the scale-up strategy highlights the importance of appropriately managing the process of implementation of scale up.

Phase 3: Managing the Implementation of Scale Up

Successful implementation of the scale-up process requires: (a) adaptive management, (b) appropriate monitoring, (c) ensuring necessary skills of the resource team and its continuity, and (d) a sufficient project time frame and an end-of-project transition strategy.

Adaptive management: Scaling up needs to be managed strategically to adapt to changing contexts and conditions. This applies to both the EBI, which often needs to be adapted as implementation is expanded to new settings that may differ markedly from original testing sites; and also, to the scaling-up process, which requires ongoing review, reflection, and learning about how it is proceeding and whether the intended outputs, outcomes, and impacts continue to be achieved over time. Adaptive management involves:

- Scaling up incrementally, building on success, and learning from failures
- Using rapid feedback loops based on ongoing program monitoring and context analysis to adapt EBIs and implementation strategies
- Changing strategies, plans, and activities to meet the overall goal, in response to new information (adapted from Mercy Corps, 2015)

For further discussion of the concept of adaptive program management, see Mercy Corps (2015) and Valters et al. (2016).

ExpandNet and its partners have learned that reviewing the strategy periodically and repeating the strategy development process can be an important component of adaptive management of scale-up. Experience with adaptive management of scale up has demonstrated that fixed strategies, and an emphasis on fidelity to the original model, which was an early focus of the implementation science literature, tend to become less effective over time or in new contexts. Although there is a need to ensure fidelity to the outcomes and impact of the EBIs, it is now recognized that a continuous process of learning, the use of feedback loops, and adaptation of the activities as the process of scale up proceeds are required. Such adaptation is especially necessary when expanding to new regions with differing social, cultural, linguistic, economic, institutional, and geographic realities, as well as when changes occur in institutions and communities with the passage of time (Chambers & Norton, 2016; Escoffery et al., 2018; Power et al., 2019; Shelton et al., 2018; Stirman et al., 2013). For example, a FP innovation developed in Northern Ghana that depended on village chiefs for community mobilization needed to be substantially adapted when scaled to Southern Ghana where local chiefs did not play such a role (Nyonator et al., 2007). A further example has been the global necessity to dramatically adapt scaling-up strategies for many EBIs in response to the COVID-19 pandemic.

Adaptive management is also particularly important in facilitating sustainability. Successful institutionalization of the innovation facilitates sustainability, but this is often not well-monitored or managed. Greater attention is frequently given to the management of expansion. Yet expansion without institutionalization to ensure sustainability wastes resources and risks the achievement of long-term outcomes.

During the process of scale up, sometimes it becomes apparent that additional EBIs need to be added to the innovation that is being scaled. For example, while expanding a set of tested interventions to strengthen community-based health services, the MoH may have decided to implement a new task-shifting policy for nurses and midwives. This innovation would require integration with the ongoing community-based activities and illustrates the type of scale up known as "diversification." In such a case the strategy-development process needs to be repeated to consider implementation of the additional intervention(s) within the scale-up process.

As mentioned earlier, repeated use of the ExpandNet/WHO framework and nine-step strategy development process has proven over time to be very useful for refining and adapting the process of scale up. The framework can be used as a basis for discussing and documenting the emerging lessons. Considering the elements, the types of scale up and each of the other strategic choice areas provides a systematic means of reviewing key decisions and making necessary adaptions to the innovation, or the process of scale up, as expansion moves to new areas and the context changes over time.

Monitoring scale up: To practice adaptive management, decision makers at multiple levels need reliable data about the process and outcomes of scale up. Therefore, monitoring systems need to address more than inputs, outputs, and outcomes associated with expansion of the innovation. Other types of information are needed including process-oriented indicators such as budget availability, appropriate training and supervision performed, the functioning of supply chains and the consistency of record-keeping, and so forth. Likewise, indicators of progress toward institutionalization (e.g., embedding the EBI and implementation strategies in policies, budgets, operational guidelines, and pre- and in-service training) need to be monitored as they are not routinely available from existing management information systems. These data can inform implementers why the results are being achieved or not. Both qualitative and quantitative data and indicators are needed and collecting these often requires special efforts or studies that should be organized in collaboration with key stakeholders.

Assessing whether spontaneous expansion is taking place should also be part of the monitoring process. When it does occur, key elements of the innovation are often dropped. As mentioned earlier, these are typically the most difficult to implement or those most different from routine patterns of work, and often are related to "soft" aspects of the innovation such as community empowerment or attention to equity or gender. It is therefore important to ensure that the expected outcomes and impacts continue to be achieved. Furthermore, spontaneous adoption of the innovation also presents an opportunity for learning about ways in which the guided process of expansion can be promoted more rapidly and efficiently.

Importance of a strong resource team during scale up: Ensuring continued availability of a strong resource team to guide scaling up is critical. The resource team in this phase requires the skills and tools needed to guide adaptive management. Specific technical skills include being able to help strengthen and utilize data and information systems, as well as establishing and facilitating management activities to implement any needed adaptations of either the innovation or the process of scale up. It is important that adequate funding is available to not only support the scaling up of implementation but to maintain and expand the resource team during the process. If such funding is not available, the strategy should be adapted to include efforts to mobilize these resources.

The resource team should continue to involve some of the individuals who were leaders during the first two phases, as well as key members of the organization that is implementing the scale-up process and responsible for future sustainability. When EBIs are being scaled up in the public sector, participation in, and ideally government leadership of the resource team are needed. With dual roles as members of both the resource team and the implementing organization, they are uniquely situated to facilitate future sustainable scale up. Such leadership builds government ownership of implementation, even when efforts are being supported by technical assistance agencies. It also prevents the initiative from being perceived as NGO- or donor-led, which can negatively impact local ownership, institutionalization of the innovation, resource mobilization, and long-term sustainability.

Other major stakeholders, including representatives of providers and target community groups should also continue to be involved. As in the strategy development process, the continued participation of a wide range of stakeholders ensures that diverse perspectives and input are incorporated into ongoing learning and adaptive management of scale up. For example, a representative from the Vietnam National Women's Union was included on the resource team for a project to strengthen quality of care in the Vietnamese FP program. Her input provided important feedback to the MoH about women's experiences with the use of a new method of tubal sterilization.

Extended project time frames: Scaling up normally takes a long time. This is especially true when it involves a complex package of EBIs and their implementation strategies in large public-sector bureaucracies. Successful scale up normally takes place over a period of years—often more than a decade—and it is unlikely that any donor or development agency would provide funding for all three phases. Thus, additional resource mobilization, particularly from government sources, is important not only at the time of original strategy development but throughout the scale-up process.

Another major challenge is that over time government champions, as well as project staff, are likely to change. Such turnover can be a significant pitfall in the scale-up process. New leaders may not have the same credibility, influence, or personal investment in scaling up the innovation and may not be familiar with its complexities.

Transition strategies: A final challenge in managing scale up is the importance of having an end-of-project transition strategy addressing how implementation of the innovation will be sustained after project funding has ended. Planning for this transition needs to begin as early as feasible and not be left until the final year of a project. It is important throughout the scale-up process but especially when approaching the final period of an externally funded effort. Clear and comprehensive plans for how to ensure sustainable implementation of the innovation should be made, including plans for continued funding beyond the project phase and for continued institutionalization of the innovation in policies, budgets, and operational guidelines.

In the HoPE-LVB experience, challenges related to the continuity of the project team and the need for an appropriate transition strategy emerged in the final year. Although the piloting and initial scale-up work were primarily undertaken within government systems and with beneficiary communities, the project team members were from externally funded NGOs. Efforts to implement ExpandNet's BWEIM recommendation to "advocate with donors and other sources of funding for financial support beyond the pilot stage" were delayed until the final year of support. As a result, they were not successful in securing sufficient resources to ensure that the NGO team could continue supporting the scale up of HoPE-LVB innovations within Ugandan project districts and Kenyan counties as well as nationally and regionally. However, during implementation several members of the resource team had begun replicating HoPE-LVB approaches with other organizations and funders. Thus, while the NGO-led HoPE-LVB project officially ended, much of the momentum that was built around implementing an integrated, cross-sectoral set of best practices in districts/counties and at the national and East Africa regional levels continued. For example, the parastatal Lake Victoria Basin Commission continued supporting integration projects modeled on HoPE-LVB. It is likely that with a strong transition strategy, begun 12 to 18 months before the scheduled end date, the project EBIs would have been scaled up further. However, it is common for such efforts to come to an end with no such plans in place.

CASE STUDY 11.2 A NEW APPROACH TO SCALING UP THE *STRONGER VOICES* PROJECT IN KYRGYZSTAN

UNFPA became concerned about the micro-level approach to scale up described in the introductory vignette to this chapter. Having learned about the ExpandNet/WHO approach they requested that ExpandNet and WHO facilitate a scale-up strategy development workshop with relevant stakeholders near the end of the second year of the project. The ExpandNet/WHO team joined national and local stakeholders to visit project villages to learn in detail about project implementation and to gain an understanding of community needs and perspectives, as well as the health system's capacities. Together they held a participatory workshop using the ExpandNet/WHO nine-step guidance to develop a new scaling-up strategy for the project. The comprehensive strategy that emerged emphasized activities to integrate project interventions in existing institutions and to create conditions for their wider and more rapid expansion to new areas. Key recommended actions included:

1. Embedding a standardized provider training curriculum in the national health staff training center, so that training in FP and sexual and reproductive health (SRH) services could be given to providers across the country.
2. Linking funding of the innovations to ongoing health sector reform and the national health plan, enabling mobilization of resources for various project components from budgetary changes and global health funding mechanisms.
3. Moving from a village-by-village implementation approach to a district-level focus which depended on local government institutions for implementation, thereby allowing for more rapid expansion of activities to additional villages and districts, using local government and NGO staff/experts.

The project team adopted the new strategy and began implementing the recommendations in the final year of the project. The ExpandNet/WHO team returned at the end of the year and facilitated a repeat of the nine-step strategy development process to lay the foundation for continued expansion and institutionalization of the innovation in a follow-up project. This exercise led to many refinements and adaptations of the various intervention components and the strategy for scale up. A key recommendation was to focus on integrating activities with other ongoing community-based health projects that were not addressing SRH. For example, the MoH, together with the Swiss Red Cross (SRC)/Swiss Development Corporation (SDC) was implementing a large community-based health project in over 600 villages which did not address youth, FP, or reproductive health.

Unfortunately, this case also illustrates a major pitfall of scaling up: the loss of donor support following relatively short project periods. Although the *Stronger Voices* team developed a strategic vision for scaling up, UNFPA headquarters decided not to fund a continuation of the *Stronger Voices* project. As a result, while some elements of the strategy were institutionalized in the Kyrgyz national program, the comprehensive package was not fully expanded. This illustrates the lesson that having a good

(*continued*)

CASE STUDY 11.2 A NEW APPROACH TO SCALING UP THE *STRONGER VOICES* PROJECT IN KYRGYZSTAN *(continued)*

strategy is only a first step—if scaling up is to succeed there must be dedicated human, financial and technical resources, as well as the political will to continue moving forward.

Fortunately, the story did not end there. The involvement in and resulting ownership of the *Stronger Voices* interventions by government champions created the will to continue to promote the innovation and to seek funding for expansion and continued implementation. The MoH and the Ministry of Education advocated with SRC/SDC to integrate the innovations into their ongoing village health project. As a result, over the following years most of the initial EBIs tested in 10 villages by *Stronger Voices* were scaled up to a significant proportion of the rural villages of Kyrgyzstan.

SUMMARY

Scale up is an essential component of implementation science. Applying the knowledge and tools that have been developed over the last two decades to facilitate sustainable scale up makes it possible to achieve health and other development goals more effectively than has often been the case in the past.

Scale up requires deliberate efforts to increase the impact of successfully tested interventions through expansion to new geographic areas or different population groups, as well as by embedding innovations in relevant institutional mechanisms including policies, budgets, operational guidelines, and training programs.

Although there are differences among the various scale-up frameworks, approaches, and guidance tools, they tend to share an emphasis on (a) evidence-based approaches, (b) systems thinking, (c) the importance of context, (d) a phased process of learning and adaption, (e) involvement of key stakeholders throughout the process to build ownership of the interventions, (f) a focus on sustainability, and (g) the values of equity, human rights, and gender perspectives.

The chapter discusses the ExpandNet framework and three phases of scale up and argues that success and sustainability require planning and conducting implementation research with future scale up in mind. Such research should be followed by a participatory, systematic process of strategy development. In turn, implementation of the strategy requires adaptive management by a strong resource team, based on appropriate monitoring of the process, outcomes, and impact of the interventions. If scale up takes place within the context of an externally funded project then strategy development, as well as the management of its implementation, must address an end-of-project transition to routine program implementation.

KEY POINTS FOR PRACTICE

1. Consider future scale up when designing innovations for testing in an implementation research study.
2. Create ownership of the innovation by involving key stakeholders in all three phases of scale up. This facilitates future sustainability.

3. Undertake a participatory and systematic process of scale-up strategy development once local testing of the EBI and its implementation approach are complete.
4. Ensure that a strong resource team facilitates all three phases of scale up.
5. Practice adaptive management during the process of scale up to promote necessary adaptations of the innovation and future sustainability.

COMMON PITFALLS IN PRACTICE

1. Assuming that scale up can be quickly implemented once local pilot testing has been completed.
2. Ignoring the importance of government and other forms of stakeholder ownership from the outset of the implementation research and continuing through the process of scale up.
3. Not developing a systematic scale-up strategy prior to broader implementation.
4. Forgetting that the implementing organization(s) have many other priorities for implementation and that addressing the challenges associated with the scale up of the EBI may not be viewed as worthwhile.
5. Assuming that government or the responsible NGO will be able to adequately support scale up without support from a dedicated resource team.
6. Failing to understand that scale up requires not only expansion of an EBI and its implementing strategies, but also institutionalization in policies, regulations, budgets, and operational guidelines.
7. Emphasizing implementation fidelity and ignoring the need to adapt EBIs and implementation strategies to changing contexts as scale up proceeds.

DISCUSSION QUESTIONS

1. The scale-up literature is much more extensive for LMIC than for the United States. Why do you think this is so?
2. Why does scaling up EBIs often take so much time?
3. How would you involve government to ensure their ownership of the scaling-up process?
4. Ensuring quality implementation of EBIs in the process of scale up is often difficult. How can this be addressed as EBIs are being expanded?
5. Even if large-scale implementation of an EBI has occurred, long-term sustainability may not be ensured. What can be done to facilitate sustainability and lasting impact?

ACKNOWLEDGMENTS

The authors would like to acknowledge financial support for the development of this chapter from the Bill and Melinda Gates Foundation and the MacArthur Foundation. The views and opinions are the authors' own and do not represent those of the foundations. The authors also wish to recognize the many ExpandNet members and colleagues whose scaling-up learning and experience are reflected in this chapter.

REFERENCES

Arnold, R. S., & Wade, J. P. (2015). A definition of systems thinking: A systems approach. *Conference on Systems Engineering, Procedia Computer Science*, *44*, 669–678. https://doi.org/10.1016/j.procs.2015.03.050

Barker, P. M., Reid, A., & Schall, M. W. (2015). A framework for scaling up health interventions: Lessons from large-scale improvement initiatives in Africa. *Implementation Science, 11*(1). https://doi.org/10.1186/s13012-016-0374-x

Ben Charif, A., Zomahoun, H. T., LeBlanc, A., Langlois, L., Wolfenden, L., Yoong, S. L., Williams, C. M., Lépine, R., & Légaré, F. (2017). Effective strategies for scaling up evidence-based practices in primary care: A systematic review. *Implementation Science, 12*(1). https://doi.org/10.1186/s13012-017-0672-y

Bradley, E. H., Curry, L., Pérez-Escamilla, R., Berg, D., Bledsoe, S., Ciccone, D. K., Fox, A., Minhas, D., Pallas, S., Talbert-Slagle, K., Taylor, L., & Yuan, C. (2011). *Dissemination, diffusion and scale up of family health innovations in low-income countries*. Yale Global Health Leadership Institute.

Chambers, D. A., & Norton, W. E. (2016). The adaptome: Advancing the science of intervention adaptation. *American Journal of Preventive Medicine, 51*(4 Suppl. 2), S124–S131. http://doi.org/10.1016/j.amepre.2016.05.011

Dearing, J. W., & Cox, J. G. (2018). Diffusion of innovations theory, principles, and practice. *Health Affairs, 37*(2), 183–190. https://doi.org/10.1377/hlthaff.2017.1104

Escoffery, C., Lebow-Skelley, E., Haardoerfer, R., Boing, E., Udelson, H., Wood, R., Hartman, M., Fernandez, M. E., & Mullen, P. D. (2018). A systematic review of adaptations of evidence-based public health interventions globally. *Implementation Science, 13*(1). https://doi.org/10.1186/s13012-018-0815-9

ExpandNet & World Health Organization. (2009). *Practical guidance for scaling-up health service innovations.* World Health Organization. Retrieved April 3, 2020 from https://www.who.int/reproductivehealth/publications/strategic_approach/9789241598521/en/ and http://www.expandnet.net/tools.htm

ExpandNet & World Health Organization. (2010). *Nine steps for developing a scaling-up strategy.* World Health Organization. Retrieved April 3, 2020 from http://www.who.int/reproductivehealth/publications/strategic_approach/9789241500319/en/index.html and http://www.expandnet.net/tools.htm

ExpandNet & World Health Organization. (2011). *Beginning with the end in mind: Planning pilot projects and other programmatic research for successful scaling up.* World Health Organization. Retrieved April 3, 2020, from https://www.who.int/reproductivehealth/publications/strategic_approach/9789241502320/en/

Fajans, P., Thom, N. T., Whittaker, M., Satia, J., & Phuong Mai, T. T. (2007). Strategic choices in scaling up: Introducing injectable contraception and improving quality of care in Viet Nam. In R. Simmons, P. Fajans, & L. Ghiron (Eds.), *Scaling up health service delivery: From pilot innovations to policies and programmes* (pp. 31–51). World Health Organization. https://expandnet.net/PDFs/Scaling_Up_HS_Delivery_Chapter_2.pdf

Ghiron, L., Shillingi, L., Kabiswa, C., Ogonda, G., Omimo, A., Ntabona, A., Simmons, R., & Fajans, P. (2014). Beginning with sustainable scale up in mind: Initial results from a population, health and environment project in East Africa. *Reproductive Health Matters*, 22(43), 84–92. https://doi.org/10.1016/s0968-8080(14)43761-3

Glaser, E. M., Ableson, H. H., & Garrison, K. N. (1983). *Putting knowledge into use: Facilitating the use and implementation of planned change*. Jossey-Bass.

Hartmann, A., & Linn, J. F. (2008). Scaling up: A framework and lessons for development effectiveness from literature and practice. *SSRN Electronic Journal.* https://doi.org/10.2139/ssrn.1301625

Indig, D., Lee, K., Grunseit, A., Milat, A., & Bauman, A. (2017). Pathways for scaling up public health interventions. *BMC Public Health, 18*(1). https://doi.org/10.1186/s12889-017-4572-5

Keyonzo, N., Nyachae, P., Kagwe, P., Kilonzo, M., Mumba, F., Owino, K., Kichamu, G., Kigen, B., Fajans, P., Ghiron, L., & Simmons, R. (2015). From project to program: Tupange's experience with scaling up family planning interventions in urban Kenya. *Reproductive Health Matters, 23*(45), 103–113. https://doi.org/10.1016/j.rhm.2015.06.010

Lee, H. (2017). Sustainability in international aid programs: Identification of working concepts of sustainability and its contributing factors. *International Journal of Social Science Studies, 5*(1). https://doi.org/10.11114/ijsss.v5i1.2055

Mai, M., Hassen, E., Ntabona, A. B., Bapura, J., Sarathy, M., Yodi, R., & Mujani, Z. (2019). Government ownership and adaptation in scale-up: Experiences from community-based family planning programme in the Democratic Republic of the Congo. *African Journal of Reproductive Health, 23*(4), 35–45. https://pubmed.ncbi.nlm.nih.gov/32227738/

Management Systems International. (2005). *Scaling up—From vision to large-scale change: A management framework for practitioners.* Management Systems International.

Management Systems International. (2016). *Scaling up – From vision to large-scale change: Tools and techniques for practitioners, second edition.* Management Systems International. https://msiworldwide.com/sites/default/files/additional-resources/2018-11/ScalingUp_3rdEdition.pdf

Management Systems International. (2021). *Scaling up – From vision to large-scale change: a management framework for practitioners, third edition.* Management Systems International.

Mangham, L. J., & Hanson, K. (2010). Scaling up in international health: What are the key issues? *Health Policy and Planning, 25*(2), 85–96. https://doi.org/10.1093/heapol/czp066

Massoud, M. R., Nielsen, G. A., Nolan, K., Schall, M. W., & Sevin, C. (2006). *A framework for spread: From local improvements to system-wide change.* IHI Innovation Series white paper. Institute for Healthcare Improvement.

Mercy Corps. (2015). *Managing complexity: Adaptive management at Mercy Corps.* Mercy Corps. https://www.mercycorps.org/sites/default/files/2020-01/Adaptive%20management%20paper_external.pdf

Milat, A., Newson, R., King, L., Rissel, C., Wolfenden, L., Bauman, A., Redman, S., & Giffin, M. (2016). A guide to scaling up population health interventions. *Public Health Research & Practice, 26*(1). https://doi.org/10.17061/phrp2611604

Milat, A. J., Newson, R., & King, L. (2014). *Increasing the scale of population health interventions: A guide.* NSW Ministry of Health. http://www.health.nsw.gov.au/research/Publications/scalability-guide.pdf

Milat, A., Lee, K., Conte, K., Grunseit, A., Wolfenden, L., Van Nassau, F., Orr, N., Sreeram, P., & Bauman, A. (2020). Intervention scalability assessment tool: A decision support tool for health policy makers and implementers. *Health Research Policy and Systems, 18*(1). https://doi.org/10.1186/s12961-019-0494-2

Nguyen, D. T., McLaren, L., Oelke, N. D., & McIntyre, L. (2020). Developing a framework to inform scale-up success for population health interventions: A critical interpretive synthesis of the literature. *Global Health Research and Policy, 5*(1). https://doi.org/10.1186/s41256-020-00141-8

Nyonator, F. K., Akosa, A. B., Awoonor-Williams, J. K., Phillips, J. F., & Jones T. C. 2007. Scaling-up experimental project success with the Community-based Health Planning and Services initiative in Ghana. In R. Simmons, P. Fajans, & L. Ghiron (Eds.), *Scaling up health service delivery: from pilot innovations to policies and programmes* (pp. 89–111). World Health Organization. https://expandnet.net/PDFs/Scaling_Up_HS_Delivery_Chapter_5.pdf

Omimo, A., Taranta, D., Ghiron, L., Kabiswa, C., Aibe, S., Kodande, M., Nalwoga, C., Mugaya, S., & Onduso, P. (2018). Applying ExpandNet's systematic approach to scaling up in an integrated population, health and environment project in East Africa. *Social Sciences, 7*(2), 8. https://doi.org/10.3390/socsci7010008

Power, J., Gilmore, B., Vallières, F., Toomey, E., Mannan, H., & McAuliffe, E. (2019). Adapting health interventions for local fit when scaling-up: A realist review protocol. *BMJ Open, 9*(1), e022084. https://doi.org/10.1136/bmjopen-2018-022084

Rogers, E. M. (2003). *Diffusion of innovations* (5th ed.). The Free Press.

Shelton, R. C., Cooper, B. R., & Stirman, S. W. (2018). The sustainability of evidence-based interventions and practices in public health and health care. *Annual Review of Public Health, 39*(1), 55–76. https://doi.org/10.1146/annurev-publhealth-040617-014731

Simmons, R., Brown, J., & Diaz, M. (2002). Facilitating large-scale transitions to quality of care: An idea whose time has come. *Studies in Family Planning, 33*(1), 61–75. https://doi.org/10.1111/j.1728-4465.2002.00061.x

Simmons, R., Fajans, P., Ghiron, L., Eds. (2007). *Scaling up health service delivery: From pilot innovations to policies and programmes.* World Health Organization. Retrieved April 3, 2020, from http://www.who.int/reproductivehealth/publications/strategic_approach/9789241563512/en/index.html and http://www.expandnet.net/tools.htm

Simmons, R., & Shiffman, J. (2007). Scaling up health service innovations: A framework for action. In R. Simmons, P. Fajans, L. Ghiron (Eds.), *Scaling up health service delivery: From pilot innovations to policies and programmes* (pp. 1–30). World Health Organization. https://expandnet.net/PDFs/Scaling_Up_HS_Delivery_Chapter_1.pdf

Spicer, N., Bhattacharya, D., Dimka, R., Fanta, F., Mangham-Jefferies, L., Schellenberg, J., Tamire-Woldemariam, A., Walt, G., & Wickremasinghe, D. (2014). 'Scaling-up is a craft not a science': Catalysing scale-up of health innovations in Ethiopia, India and Nigeria. *Social Science & Medicine, 121*, 30–38. https://doi.org/10.1016/j.socscimed.2014.09.046

Stirman, S. W., Miller, C. J., Toder, K., & Calloway, A. (2013). Development of a framework and coding system for modifications and adaptations of evidence-based interventions. *Implementation Science, 8*(1). https://doi.org/10.1186/1748-5908-8-65

Valters, C., Cummings, C., & Nixon, H. (2016). Putting learning at the centre: Adaptive development programming in practice. Overseas Development Institute. https://odi.org/en/publications/putting-learning-at-the-centre-adaptive-development-programming-in-practice/

Yamey, G. (2011). Scaling up global health interventions: A proposed framework for success. *PLoS Medicine, 8*(6), e1001049. https://doi.org/10.1371/journal.pmed.1001049

Zamboni, K., Schellenberg, J., Hanson, C., Betran, A. P., & Dumont, A. (2019). Assessing scalability of an intervention: Why, how and who? *Health Policy and Planning, 34*(7), 544–552. https://doi.org/10.1093/heapol/czz068

Zomahoun, H. T., Ben Charif, A., Freitas, A., Garvelink, M. M., Menear, M., Dugas, M., Adekpedjou, R., & Légaré, F. (2019). The pitfalls of scaling up evidence-based interventions in health. *Global Health Action, 12*(1), 1670449. https://doi.org/10.1080/16549716.2019.1670449

12

Sustaining Evidence-Based Interventions

Rachel C. Shelton and Nicole Nathan

Learning Objectives

By the end of this chapter, readers will be able to:

- Define sustainability and how it is distinct from implementation
- Explain why sustainability is important from the perspective of key stakeholders
- Identify key multi-level factors that impact sustainability
- Discuss practical considerations for sustaining evidence-based interventions (EBIs)
- Apply criteria to monitor and evaluate sustainability
- Select one or more strategies, tools, or frameworks to actively plan for sustainability

CASE STUDY 12.1 PLANNING FOR THE SUSTAINABILITY OF A CESSATION SMOKING PROGRAM IN A COMMUNITY MENTAL HEALTH CENTER

A program manager working within a community mental health center has been tasked with implementing an evidence-based smoking model of care for their clients. In reviewing existing evidence-based interventions (EBIs) and considering potential fit with the clients they serve in this setting, the manager selects the "2As and R" model of care. The "2As and R" model of care requires clinicians to: Assess patients' smoking status, provide brief Advice about quitting, and Refer to an evidence-based telephone counseling support service. The project manager is deeply committed to seeing this model of care be implemented and sustained, as there is strong evidence to show that this EBI can support patients attending mental health services to have successful quit attempts.

The program manager is aware that the clinicians within the mental health service are reluctant to adopt this model of care given the extra time it may require and competing demands that the clinicians face. However, the manager does not have the time, resources, or staff with expertise to adequately investigate all the potential barriers to implementing the program. The community mental health center has very finite human and financial resources to support this program; therefore, the program manager is mindful that strategies to support the ongoing delivery of the EBI need to be effective and cost-effective but is unsure of how to identify such strategies. They do know that due to budgetary constraints, it is likely that funding for implementation of the program will cease at the end of year; as such, whatever strategies are selected cannot be resource intensive. However, they do not want to see all their efforts go to waste in 12 months and have the program stop when the funding ends. What could the program manager do to help support or facilitate clinicians in continuing to implement this model of care once funding is withdrawn at the end of the year?

This vignette highlights some of the common challenges and considerations that practitioners working within clinical or community settings face when trying to sustain EBIs over time, including: limited time and resources, competing priorities, uncertain funding situations, and/or staff that may not have the knowledge or experience to adequately plan for sustainability. *We make a distinction in this chapter between* implementation, *which relates to the initial delivery of EBIs and the process of integrating EBIs within settings, and* sustainability, *which focuses on the extent to which EBIs are delivered and have impact over time and have capacity to support their delivery within the organizations and settings in which they are embedded (Rabin et al., 2010). Throughout this chapter, various theories, frameworks, tools, approaches, and strategies will be presented that have practical application for policy makers, practitioners, and researchers working to sustain EBIs across a range of clinical or community settings.*

INTRODUCTION: WHY SUSTAINABILITY IS IMPORTANT

Globally, there has been tremendous investment in the development and implementation of evidence-based interventions (EBIs) that aim to prevent and address chronic disease in communities (Emmons & Colditz, 2017). Despite such investments, sustaining the routine and widespread delivery of public health and healthcare interventions is a common and persistent challenge that has been identified across a broad range of settings, organizations, and populations (e.g., healthcare settings, community settings, schools, low- and middle-income countries, churches; Braithwaite et al., 2020; Proctor et al., 2015; Shediac-Rizkallah & Bone, 1998; Shelton et al., 2018). Empirical research in this area suggests that only about half of EBIs are sustained. As one example, researcher and project director Dr. Mary Ann Scheirer reviewed 19 health promotion programs from a portfolio of funded programs and found that 1 to 6 years after adoption, only 40% to 60% of programs were continually delivered to some extent (e.g., delivering at least one of the original components over time; Scheirer, 2005). As most EBIs have multiple program components to deliver, this highlights what a substantial challenge it can be to implement public health and healthcare EBIs routinely in real-world settings.

Similarly, a systematic review by Wiltsey Stirman et al. (2012) further indicates what a widespread problem it is to successfully sustain EBIs. They reviewed 125 empirical studies on the sustainability of a range of public health and clinical interventions and found that partial sustainability of EBIs was more common than sustainability of the full intervention, with less than 50% of EBIs continuing at high levels of fidelity to the original intervention. Furthermore, a review by Herlitz et al. (2020) which examined the sustainability of school-based health promotion interventions found that among the 18 interventions reviewed, none were sustained in their entirety following the withdrawal of implementation support (e.g., cessation of funding or resources). In light of these documented challenges, sustainability has been identified by experts in the field of implementation science as "one of the most significant translational research problems of our time" (Proctor et al., 2015, p. 2).

We should care about the persistent challenge of sustaining EBIs for several key reasons. First, there is often a latency period for many public health interventions whereby the impact or benefits to the community or at the population level may not be seen until many years after the EBI is first implemented (Walugembe et al., 2019). As such, discontinuation of programs means that the potential public health benefits cannot be optimally achieved or will not be maximized to their fullest potential, and may not reach the populations and settings that would benefit from them the most (e.g., organizational settings and populations that have fewer resources or face numerous structural barriers to health). Second, there is warranted concern that discontinued programs can reflect a loss or waste of substantial investment of time and resources for initial implementation on the part of funders, delivery organizations, staff, and administrators, which may result in frustration among implementers and may make staff wary of future implementation efforts. This is important to consider given that most public health and healthcare settings often have limited resources to work with. Additionally, abandoning, abruptly stopping, or failing to continue programs in clinical or community settings may also bring disillusionment to participants, create or reinforce negative perceptions and mistrust of research among community stakeholders, and pose subsequent obstacles to community mobilization. Again, this distrust may be particularly striking in communities experiencing persistent social and health inequities that have historically been and are currently marginalized and have not typically received the benefits of public health or healthcare innovations or investments. Additionally, there are ethical considerations and questions raised by policy makers, funders, and the public regarding the value and impact of developing new EBIs if the existing ones we have are not being sustained.

It is important to recognize that discontinuation of EBIs and issues of health equity are closely linked. Lack of sustainability has important implications for exacerbating health inequities, especially if the discontinuation of EBIs occurs more often or disproportionately in organizations and settings that serve populations and communities that experience a greater burden of health inequities. Maximizing the population health impact of EBIs and addressing the research-to-practice gap requires that we prioritize, invest, and proactively plan for the continued delivery of EBIs, particularly in settings and populations experiencing health inequities.

HOW TO THINK ABOUT SUSTAINABILITY

In the literature, there have been changing conceptualizations and definitions of sustainability over the years; this can be confusing and challenging for practitioners looking for advice about how to think about sustainability in public health and healthcare settings. As one example, researchers have made a distinction between **sustainability** as a process (e.g., planning for sustainability) or a characteristic of an intervention (e.g., extent to which an EBI can continue to be delivered over time), and **sustainment** as a potential outcome (e.g., evaluating the impact of different implementation strategies on sustainment).

Additionally, a number of variable terms have been used to refer to sustainability. Such terms have included *routinization, institutionalization, sustainment, durability, maintenance,* and *long-term follow-up/implementation*, as well as terms related to discontinuing programs (e.g., *discontinuation, de-adoption*; Braithwaite et al., 2020; Scheirer & Dearing, 2011; Wiltsey Stirman et al., 2012). While related, these terms are not synonymous and they often capture different but important aspects of sustainability. For example, historically there was a focus on conceptualizing sustainability as **institutionalization or routinization** (e.g., maintaining organizational practices, procedures, and policies started during implementation or integration into existing organizational routines, policies, or budgets within an institution; Yin, 1981). In recent years, there has been consideration that institutionalization may not fully capture all important dimensions of sustainability and there has been more focus on dynamic conceptualizations of sustainability (e.g., as a dynamic process as opposed to a static end goal).

Other commonly used terms like **long-term implementation** relate to continued delivery of the EBI (e.g., the extent to which all components of the program continue to be delivered over time), whereas other terms like **discontinuation** and **de-adoption** relate to failure to sustain the EBI or cessation of the EBI over time (Wiltsey Stirman et al., 2012). **Maintenance** has often been used to conceptualize multiple dimensions of sustainability, including: (a) institutionalization at the setting/organizational level; and (b) continued impact on health behaviors or outcomes at the individual level (Shelton et al., 2020).

The variation in these terms and definitions reveals important factors and dimensions of sustainability and highlights key considerations for how sustainability is being conceptualized. Recent definitions of sustainability capture more dynamic and multi-dimensional conceptualizations of sustainability and recognize the importance of potential adaptations of the EBI over time. For example, a commonly applied definition by Moore et al. (2017) is comprehensive and helps reconcile some of the more divergent conceptualizations of sustainability that have been used historically. Specifically, Moore et al. (2017) define sustainability as:

> *(1) after a defined period of time, (2) the program, clinical intervention, and/or implementation strategies continue to be delivered and/or (3) individual behavior change (i.e., clinician, patient) is maintained; (4) the program and individual behavior change may evolve or adapt while (5) continuing to produce benefits for individuals/systems.* (p. 5)

What does this conceptualization mean from a practical standpoint? For one, it is important that practitioners determine what constitutes a meaningful period of time for sustainability that is distinct from the implementation period. This may differ based on the nature of the EBI and its implementation delivery, as well as when health behavior change(s) or outcomes might be meaningfully impacted. Second, it is critical that practitioners decide and identify "what" it is they are seeking to sustain (e.g., a program, its health benefits and impact at the individual/setting level, program infrastructure or capacity to deliver the EBI, implementation strategies, or some combination). Third, if they are seeking to sustain delivery of an EBI and its strategies, it is important that practitioners have a detailed sense of what the core components are that comprise them (i.e., the essential functions or key ingredients of the EBI that are necessary to produce the desired outcome, informed by theory or through empirical testing), so they have a clear understanding of how the EBI has evolved or adapted over time. Additionally, while it can be useful to use multiple indicators of sustainability to gain a more comprehensive understanding (Scheirer et al., 2017), it may not always be feasible in real-world settings, particularly considering some of the resources that may be involved in doing so. In deciding which to prioritize, it is important to actively engage with and involve key stakeholders in the setting where you are based (e.g., providers, implementers, leaders, patients, community members) to determine which sustainability outcomes are meaningful and valued, are pragmatic and feasible to assess, and that there is consensus around how sustainability is being assessed.

RECONCILING FIDELITY AND ADAPTATION IN RELATION TO SUSTAINABILITY

Practitioners face a dilemma or decision in how to maintain fidelity (the extent to which an EBI is delivered as originally intended by intervention developers) to core components of the EBI (the essential functions or key ingredients that are necessary to produce the desired outcome). Here, a key consideration is how can the EBI continue to deliver health benefits while also being adapted to fit changing circumstances and contexts? Practitioners may find that sustaining the core components of EBIs with high fidelity is challenging and unrealistic, particularly in settings such as non-government agencies or social service settings that have limited resources. In fact, some planned adaptations to EBIs may actually be beneficial and necessary in delivering and ultimately sustaining EBIs, in order to fit population and setting needs and organizational capacity or to reflect the sociocultural characteristics of communities that differ from the original setting or population in which the EBI was developed or evaluated (Barrera et al., 2013; Kumpfer et al., 2017). Not making such adaptations may exacerbate health disparities, particularly if EBIs are not adapted to fit new sociocultural contexts and have less reach and engagement for communities that face structural barriers to health and healthcare (e.g., if an EBI is not adapted to Spanish or to reflect patient literacy levels and sociocultural norms in a clinic that serves predominately Spanish-speaking Latino people).

The **Dynamic Sustainability Framework** (DSF) introduced by Chambers et al. (2013) offers a way of resolving this dilemma by rethinking the relationships among fidelity, adaptation, effectiveness, and sustainability. The DSF recognizes that it is not realistic to think about sustainability as a static end goal and reframes sustainability amid the dynamic, complex, real-world contexts in which intervention delivery and impact occur over time. This framework challenges traditional public health assumptions that voltage drop (the idea that EBIs will deliver fewer benefits over time as they are sustained) and program drift (the idea that benefits will decline when deviating from strict fidelity protocols) are inevitable. Instead, the DSF offers a way of thinking about fidelity and adaptation that is less as a tension and more like a dynamic process that allows for capacity-building and planned adaptations in response to the dynamism of contexts, as reflected in changing and evolving scientific evidence, shifting population needs, and evolving multi-level contexts over time.

Specifically, the DSF focuses on several key elements and their "fit" *over time*: (a) the EBI (e.g., a decision-aid to support informed decision-making for cancer); (b) the context in which the EBI is delivered (e.g., a health clinic); and (c) the widespread system within which the settings exist (e.g., broader healthcare system and policies/regulations/insurance reimbursement). The DSF frames the benefits of the EBI in terms of its "fit" within a practice setting in a clinical, public health, or community setting (e.g., clinic, school, workplace) and posits that multiple factors within this context (e.g., resources, information systems, organizational culture and infrastructure, processes for training/supervising staff) will influence the impact of the EBI in this setting. Additionally, the DSF identifies the broader ecological system (the policy and regulatory environment, broader practice settings, characteristics and needs of broader population) as shaping implementation and sustainability of an EBI. Central to DSF is focus on change being constant across each of these three levels, necessitating that for an EBI to be sustained, it is important to assess and refine the fit of an EBI within both the practice setting and larger ecological setting over time and use quality improvement processes to refine, optimize, improve, and ultimately sustain EBIs.

The DSF and its focus on practice-based evidence, continual improvement, and ongoing learning has a number of important implications for practitioners to consider, as described in the following:

1. Practitioners can conduct continuous assessment (data monitoring, tracking, evaluation) to better understand, refine, and manage the fit between EBIs and the local context; that is, infrastructure, resources, and needs within the setting (including obtaining feedback on how well the EBI does among diverse patient populations or communities, to minimize potential health inequities). Ideally this assessment uses practical and relevant measures that leverage existing resources (e.g., claims data, electronic health record [EHR] data). For example, practitioners could do an organizational assessment annually to identify if there are any organizational changes made or planned that may have implications for sustainability (e.g., loss of funding, change in staffing/role, incorporation of new EHR system), and which may require a planned adaptation to the EBI.
2. Practitioners can conduct a needs assessment of their community or the patients they are serving to assess if the EBIs they are delivering are actually addressing priority health needs for their clients; if not, adaptations may be needed to address changing community needs. Additionally, it is important for practitioners to regularly assess the nature of the scientific evidence; it may be appropriate to adapt, refine, de-implement or replace the EBI or certain components if there is no longer evidence over time to support sustaining the EBI or if those components are not needed for achieving health impacts.
3. Practitioners can also apply rapid learning and ongoing problem-solving grounded in the real-world experiences of stakeholders and learning health systems to inform understanding of which EBI works for whom and inform resource allocation decisions under tight budgets. Such an approach requires a commitment to organizational learning and stakeholder engagement at the setting level and suggests the importance of a long-term plan and investment to have resources and time for ongoing engagement, assessment, and improvement.

In summary, the DSF can be a helpful framework for practitioners to use for sustainability planning and application of real-time assessment to improve practice.

PRACTICAL CONSIDERATIONS AND CHALLENGES IN SUSTAINING EVIDENCE-BASED INTERVENTIONS

There are several reasons why it can be challenging to sustain EBIs in real-world settings. It is important to note that sustainability is commonly conceptualized as the last or final stage in the overall life cycle of an EBI, with stages often including: development of EBIs or exploration of existing EBIs, preparation (e.g., understanding context, planning for adaptations of EBIs), adoption of the EBI, implementation, and sustainability. As such, people don't often think about sustainability up front, but wait until later along the implementation continuum. Often the focus is on development and testing of the new intervention for its effectiveness and the immediate challenges of adoption of EBIs and initial implementation (typically the first 6 months or one year of initial delivery of the EBI and its implementation strategies). As a result, people rarely plan for sustainability from the outset.

Some of the practical considerations and challenges that arise in implementing EBIs also arise in sustaining them. For example, characteristics of the intervention that may have implications for implementation also likely matter for sustainability, including how costly and complex it is, how adaptable it is, and how well it "fits" with the organizational and cultural context (Damschroder et al., 2009). Similarly, at the organizational level, factors that may matter for both implementation and sustainability include competing organizational priorities, organizational readiness, presence of a program champion, lack of support from leadership, and lack of funding and organizational infrastructure (Damschroder et al., 2009; Shelton et al., 2018).

There are also several key challenges to sustainability that practitioners may face that are specific to sustainability. First, dynamic policy landscape and shifting organizational priorities can make it difficult for practitioners to focus on a particular EBI over time (Chambers et al., 2013; Shelton et al., 2018); this may particularly be the case if there are new policy or organizational priorities that have financial implications or if new initiatives are introduced that have implications for competing demands on time. Second, the nature of funding, financing, and organizational resources to support EBI delivery is often minimal and short term which limits continuity over the long term without additional investment, support, or evidence of possible return on investment (Scheirer, 2005). Additionally, the long-term impact or value of sustaining a program may be challenging for a practitioner to document, track, or assess with limited resources, which may have implications for leadership or administrative support of delivering the EBI or maintaining political will to sustain an EBI. Finally, provider, practitioner, and implementer turnover and attrition over time are inevitable but critical and common threats to sustainment, and indicate the importance of planning for ongoing recruitment, training, supervision, and support of the workforce (Scheirer, 2013; Shelton et al., 2016; Walkosz et al., 2015).

Some of these foundational issues that impact sustainability of EBIs also have important implications for health equity (Baumann & Cabassa, 2020). Many existing EBIs weren't developed or evaluated with equity in mind. As such, trying to sustain programs or practices in low-resource settings or among diverse racial/ethnic groups may be a challenge if the EBI is not a good fit from the start. This can happen if the EBI wasn't developed with that community in mind, isn't culturally appropriate, and/or isn't acceptable or feasible in this context. Additionally, in the effort to develop interventions that work, intervention developers may develop EBIs that are too costly or complex for many real-world settings where they are later implemented. It is also important to recognize that in many countries, funding agencies, governments and donors, and the broader policy or political context drive a lot of decision-making about what to sustain and what is perceived as "unsustainable" from a financial perspective. As described in the following, conducting a sustainability assessment may be useful in anticipating and planning for some of these challenges to sustainability.

PERFORMING A SUSTAINABILITY ASSESSMENT

In practice, it is important to conduct a sustainability assessment to better understand the multi-level factors that may influence the long-term delivery and impact of an EBI. There is value in using an existing conceptual framework in informing this assessment as an initial starting place, to help provide shared grounding and guidance for practitioners. Conceptual frameworks can help build an evidence base for what factors matter in real-world settings by using shared constructs and terminology, promoting transparency, and can greatly enhance planning for sustainability (Damschroder, 2020; Tabak et al., 2012). Practitioners can use these frameworks as an initial starting place to help guide formal qualitative data collection or more informal feedback from various stakeholders in their setting (e.g., administrators, patients or community members, practitioners, leaders), to learn more about which factors stakeholders perceive as being important and may need to be actively addressed early in the implementation period to plan for sustainability. These data or feedback can be used to tailor or refine conceptual frameworks for the specific settings in which they are being applied, to account for any important factors that may be missing.

There are several established conceptual frameworks in the field that can be useful to guide a sustainability assessment, to identify and understand multi-level factors that may impact sustainability (Birken et al., 2020; Herlitz et al., 2020; Scheirer & Dearing, 2011; Wiltsey Stirman et al., 2012). While there are several frameworks to choose from, many of them overlap in terms of the factors that they contain and several are informed by the growing empirical literature on determinants that matter for sustainability (Shelton et al., 2018; Wiltsey Stirman et al., 2012). Historically, there has been much focus on the role of funding as being the key influence on sustaining EBIs in real-world settings. While research suggests that funding and resources can be important in the sustainability of EBIs (Palinkas et al., 2020), it is also likely that funding alone is insufficient to facilitate sustainability and that other multi-level factors also matter for sustainability (and in some cases may even be able to compensate for lack of funding or resources). Broadly speaking, most conceptual frameworks in this area identify determinants of sustainability at multiple levels: (a) policy or outer contextual factors; (b) inner contextual or organizational factors; (c) implementation processes; (d) characteristics of the EBIs; and (e) characteristics of implementers and populations.

The **Integrated Sustainability Framework** is an example of an empirically informed framework that identifies multi-level factors that have been commonly associated with sustainability across different settings, contexts, and populations, and can be used as a starting place for identifying and refining understanding of factors that are important to consider within a certain setting (Shelton et al., 2018; Shoesmith et al., 2021). This framework considers dynamic interactions between outer contextual or policy-related factors (the broader sociopolitical context, existing policies, funding environment, external partnerships with organizations/stakeholders); inner contextual or organizational-level factors (resources and internal funding, leadership, presence of program champions, organizational readiness and support, staff stability, alignment of internal practices/policies, EBI culture); implementation processes (ongoing training, planning for sustainability, stakeholder engagement, coaching/feedback, capacity-building); characteristics of the EBIs (adaptability, benefits, fit with setting and population); characteristics of implementers (skills, attitudes, motivations, role clarity); and characteristics of populations (literacy, language, experiences of stigma, mistrust, discrimination and other social characteristics). Table 12.1 provides an example of questions that practitioners may want to consider as they conduct a sustainability assessment at each of these levels, informed by the Integrated Sustainability Framework.

TABLE 12.1 Conducting a Sustainability Assessment, Informed by the Integrated Sustainability Framework

DOMAIN	QUESTIONS TO CONSIDER
Outer/Policy Context	▪ What **policies, regulations, and social norms** are in place that may have implications for sustainability? ▪ What's the **broader funding environment** like and are there external funds that could help sustain the EBI? ▪ Are there **external partnerships (with government agencies, healthcare systems, community-based organizations)** that can help bring resources, support, and commitment to sustain the EBI? ▪ How does EBI align with **national, state, local priorities**?
Inner/Organizational Context	▪ Are there **program champions** (community and organizational) who can help influence sustained delivery of the EBI? ▪ Does the EBI have **support from organizational leadership**? ▪ Within the organization, is there **organizational infrastructure** (time, financial resources, space) to support the EBI? How "ready" is the organization? ▪ How are **stakeholders continually engaged** related to EBI delivery?
Implementation Processes	▪ Are there processes in place to support the **recruitment and retention** of staff involved with EBI delivery? ▪ Are there **supervision and training** processes in place to support EBI delivery among staff over time? ▪ Are there processes in place or that could be added to **track or monitor data** on health impact of EBI or its delivery? ▪ Is there **strategic planning** about sustaining the EBI (e.g., grant writing, communications)?
Implementer and Population Characteristics	▪ Do the implementers have the **self-efficacy** to deliver the EBI over time? ▪ What are some of the **benefits and challenges** that implementers might experience in delivering the program over time? ▪ What are the **attitudes** of the implementers toward the EBI? ▪ What **characteristics or experiences of the population** served might impede sustainability (e.g., stigma, mistrust, literacy, poverty, experiences of discrimination)?
EBI Characteristics	▪ How **adaptable** is the EBI? ▪ How **costly** is the EBI? Is there a return on investment? ▪ How well does the **EBI "fit"** within the organizational context? ▪ Does the EBI continue to **address a priority or need** in the community?

EBI, evidence-based intervention.

When conducting a sustainability assessment, Scheirer (2013) has suggested that it can be helpful to consider that some sustainability factors may matter more than others depending on the specific nature or type of EBI being delivered according to their structure. As one example, for interventions that are implemented by individual providers or practitioners essentially implementing alone (e.g., clinicians prescribing a new medication, teachers delivering a new health curriculum), sustainability may be strongly influenced by whether payment for delivery is provided within regular streams of financial infrastructure and by their motivation to continue the new practice. Relevant to practitioners, Scheirer (2013) posits that sustainability of this type of EBI may necessitate less external support after providing initial training and feedback. As another example, other considerations may be more relevant for public health or clinical interventions requiring coordination across staff within organizations (e.g., programs that involve coordinated delivery among a variety of staff and practitioners, including health educators, providers, community health workers, and nurses). For this type of intervention, organizational leadership and administrative support may be particularly critical given the importance of delineating job roles/tasks and provision of training, supervision, coordination, and communication in such efforts. Inner contextual factors such as the presence of organizational program champions, administrative and financial support, EBI fit with organizational mission and culture, and financial and administrative support may also be relevant. For managers and practitioners trying to sustain such coordinated types of EBIs, it can be useful for them to plan at least 1 year before funding expires and investigate the resources needed to continue supporting staff, how those costs might be institutionalized, if there are options for a fee-for-service arrangement, and what new sources of funding or partnerships might help support it.

While there is some overlap, it is also likely that factors that influence sustainability differ across settings and contexts, or that certain factors are particularly important within certain contexts. For example, a recent review of 41 studies across 26 countries in sub-Saharan Africa suggests that community engagement, community resources, and mobilization may be especially important to consider in this region, as well as leveraging existing resources, providing adaptable interventions that are flexible to local context, and recognizing the important role of broader societal and political context and upheavals (Iwelunmor et al., 2016). This evidence suggests that in low- and middle-income countries it may be essential to facilitate opportunities for meaningful community ownership to ensure that appropriate changes are made during the numerous adaptations needed to address the local social, cultural, political, and policy contexts, and often limited available resources amidst healthcare worker shortages and vulnerable health systems. Ultimately, different factors may be most important in shaping sustainability in a particular setting. For example, several recent reviews have examined the factors that influence the sustainment of health-related EBIs in schools (Cassar et al., 2019; Herlitz et al., 2020; Shoesmith et al., 2021) and identified that aligning and prioritizing EBIs in the context of valued educational outcomes/metrics of schools is critical, as is the continued commitment from senior leaders and staff that are trained, motivated, and supported. Central to sustainability in many settings like schools and clinics/hospitals that have a strong organizational infrastructure involved in continued EBI delivery are issues of staff and implementer turnover and attrition (Cassar et al., 2019; Herlitz et al., 2020; Shelton et al., 2018). Given this possible distinctiveness of sustainability by setting, an implication for practice that follows is that it may be useful to select a sustainability framework specific to your context if you can (e.g., schools), and if that's not possible, try to do some assessment to understand factors that are distinctive to your context.

CASE STUDY 12.2 SUSTAINABILITY OF LAY HEALTH ADVISOR PROGRAMS IN LOW-RESOURCE COMMUNITY SETTINGS

From an equity perspective, sustaining EBIs that reduce or eliminate health inequities and the structural determinants underlying them is a priority. Lay Health Advisor (LHA) interventions are programs led by peer leaders who share similar social, economic, and cultural contexts as the communities they are seeking to reach. LHA programs have been highly effective in promoting behavior change in several areas from cancer screening to HIV prevention to chronic disease management, in both the U.S. and global contexts. However, there are challenges in sustaining these programs given limited resources and funding to support them, and programs experience high levels of LHA attrition. Researchers have partnered with the National Witness Program (NWP) to better understand how to support LHAs and sustain LHA programs in communities experiencing significant health inequities. NWP is an evidence-based LHA program nationally disseminated and implemented in community settings in the United States, developed by and for Black women to address inequities in breast and cervical cancer screening and to help women navigate systems to access screening and care (Erwin et al., 2003). An important component of the program is that Black cancer survivors provide testimonials and powerful narratives about their experiences.

Using surveys and in-depth interviews, in partnership with community sites nationally, several barriers to sustainability were identified among key stakeholders (Shelton et al., 2016, 2017), including: limited funding and the nature of funding as short-term; variable organizational infrastructure and/or instability of infrastructure; limited resources to support ongoing training; and some LHA burnout and attrition. Facilitators of sustainability included: organizational and community partnerships that provided access to resources, space, and funding; project director leadership and role as internal champions; the personal, social and professional benefits experienced by LHAs (and cancer survivors in particular; e.g., social support, sense of empowerment); and the gap this program addresses among Black women in being culturally competent and addressing issues of mistrust, stigma, and discrimination that women have experienced. Research conducted with sites suggests that context is very important in both influencing sustainability of the program at sites and supporting the retention of LHAs in the program. LHAs who were based at sites that had a strong partnership with academic or cancer centers were much more likely to remain and be active in the program. This finding suggests that having a program champion at partnering academic sites might be an important strategy, to help facilitate resources and infrastructure to support the program over time (e.g., address funding gaps, provide access to space and technology, connect to free or low-cost cancer screening services). Additionally, research highlighted the critical importance of social, community, and financial recognition for LHAs in these roles, and the importance of providing not only initial training but ongoing training to provide feedback and support to LHAs over time. Ongoing research is examining which multi-level factors identified previously predict the long-term sustainability of the program across sites nationally, with the goal of informing the planning, development, and delivery of sustainability strategies across these settings.

PLANNING FOR SUSTAINABILITY AND SUSTAINABILITY STRATEGIES

Planning to Sustain Evidence-Based Interventions

Benjamin Franklin once said *"If you fail to plan, you are planning to fail,"* which those wishing to sustain public health EBIs in community or clinical settings should definitely take heed. While it may not always be possible to foresee changes in priorities or regulations that will impact the sustainability of an EBI, the selection of the EBI, as well as the strategies required to support its ongoing delivery, can be crucial to its sustainability.

The development or selection of EBIs for implementation that are not suitable or a good fit for the context to begin with is a major impediment to their sustainment. As outlined, the capacity of an EBI to be sustained may be impacted by a range of organizational and contextual factors (Herlitz et al., 2020; Scudder et al., 2017; Shelton et al., 2018). For example, an EBI is unlikely to be sustained if it is too costly, complex, or irrelevant to end-users (Committee on Public Health Strategies to Improve Health, 2012). Similarly, the use of inappropriate strategies to support delivery of a community or clinical setting in delivering the EBI can also influence its sustainability. For example, if the implementation of the EBI has solely relied on researchers to drive the delivery of the intervention, without thought as to who might take this on after the research project ends, it is unlikely to be sustained. Ensuring that such factors are considered in the planning phase of an intervention may help ensure that the most sustainable interventions are implemented, reducing the risk that the investment in achieving initial implementation is wasted once implementation support is removed.

Tools to Help Plan for Sustainability

There are several useful sustainability planning frameworks available to help support policy makers, practitioners, and researchers identify, develop, or adapt EBIs so that they are more suitable for sustainment. *The Capacity for Sustainability Framework* (Schell et al., 2013), which may be used within both clinical and public health settings, developed by the Center for Public Health Systems Science (CPHSS) at Washington University in St. Louis, has identified eight core domains that affect a program's capacity for sustainability, including; environmental support, funding stability, partnerships, organizational capacity, program evaluation, program adaptation, communications, and strategic planning. Identifying needs related to these domains can help build the capacity for maintaining an EBI. The framework, and related measures, including the 35-item Clinical Sustainability Assessment Tool (CSAT; Malone et al., 2021) and the 40-item Program Sustainability Assessment Tool (PSAT; Calhoun et al., 2014), are assessment tools that those working in the clinical or public health setting can complete with staff and stakeholders to evaluate the sustainability capacity of an EBI. Once complete, the planning team can review the summary report of the overall sustainability of the EBI that is generated, which may inform the recommended next steps of developing and implementing an action plan for identifying and prioritizing the components of the EBI that need to be maintained, removed, or adapted. This will involve developing an action plan with specific action steps that prioritize areas where it will be important to build program sustainability capacity. While a few studies have utilized the CSAT or PSAT (Stoll et al., 2015; Tabak et al., 2016), the validity of these tools is still to be determined, and work is ongoing to see how well they accurately assess the determinants of sustainment.

Some other useful sustainability planning guides or models that one may consider for application are listed in the following. Common to all these tools is that the assessment is undertaken in collaboration with stakeholders. A shared understanding of factors that impact sustainability by practitioners, end-users, decision-makers, funding agencies, and researchers is integral for planning for sustainability as it allows stakeholder priorities and needs to be identified earlier. This may help avoid future obstacles, enabling adaptations to be made to the EBI or support strategies which may improve program fit before the obstacles arise (Shelton et al., 2018; Walugembe et al., 2019).

- *The National Health Service (NHS) Sustainability Model (Maher et al., 2010).* This is a diagnostic tool to help predict the likelihood of sustainment of a specific project or initiative. The tool, which is very easy to complete, may be used by practitioners to help brainstorm factors impacting on the sustainability of programs. Practitioners are encouraged to engage as many team members as possible to complete the model, to ensure that a broad range of sustainability views may be identified. The model consists of 10 factors relating to process, staff, and organizational issues, that NHS staff and key stakeholders identified as important in sustaining change in clinical settings. Individuals score each of the 10 factors against set criteria, which when pooled will identify the key areas that may need to be addressed for the project to be sustained. The accompanying NHS Sustainability Guide provides practical advice on how practitioners might increase the likelihood of sustainability of their initiative within their specific context.
- *Gruen et al.'s Model for Health-Program Sustainability (Gruen et al., 2008).* Based upon theories of dynamic sustainability and empirical evidence of program sustainability, Gruen's model poses a series of questions related to the health concern (e.g., what is it, is it recognized as an issue by the program drivers); the proposed program (e.g., is it evidence based, how will it be implemented); and the contextual fit and drivers (e.g., how are stakeholders involved and engaged in decision-making). Practitioners may use this to guide their planning; however, unlike the Capacity for Sustainability Framework or the NHS model, this model does not provide a score or grade regarding the sustainability of the innovation.
- *Getting to Outcomes (Johnson et al., 2013).* This is a nine-step comprehensive strategy that organizations can systematically work through to develop a sustainability strategy. The process involves an initial assessment of sustainability capacity and sustainable innovation characteristics, then progresses through planning, implementation, evaluation, and continuous quality improvement to sustain interventions. This process has been used across a broad range of public health issues including substance abuse, teen pregnancy, and mental health.

Effectiveness of Strategies to Sustain Evidence-Based Interventions

While there is a significant body of evidence describing implementation strategies and their effectiveness in clinical and community settings (Kingsland et al., 2018; Lau et al., 2015; Nathan et al., 2016, 2019, 2020; Wolfenden et al., 2016, 2018; Wolfenden, Nathan, Janssen, et al., 2017; Wolfenden, Nathan, Sutherland, et al., 2017), identifying sustainability strategies is still an emerging area within the field (Shelton & Lee, 2019). A 2019 systematic review (Hailemariam et al., 2019) of strategies used within community-based settings to sustain public health interventions identified just 26 studies, of which only nine sustainability strategies were reported. The review found that the most frequently utilized strategies were funding for EBIs, continued use and maintenance of workforce skills through continued training, booster training sessions, supervision, and feedback. Other, less frequently used strategies included adapting the EBI to increase continued fit/compatibility within the organization, obtaining organizational leadership and stakeholder support for prioritizing the continued use of the EBI, accessing new or existing financial support to facilitate sustainment, and monitoring EBI effectiveness. As few of these studies have empirically tested the effectiveness of these strategies, there is insufficient evidence to say how well these strategies work in successfully sustaining EBIs, either on their own or in combination. Examples of some of these projects and the strategies that they used are presented in Table 12.2. For practitioners, rather than trying to decide if a strategy is an implementation strategy as opposed to a sustainability strategy, it may be easiest to consider what barrier the strategy is trying to overcome. For example, while staff training may be necessary during the initial implementation phase to overcome barriers related to staff knowledge or skills to get the EBI initially implemented, booster training may be needed during the sustainability phase to overcome barriers related to staff knowledge or motivation to keep implementing the EBI (see the section "Describing and Selecting Sustainability Strategies" for a more detailed description of how to select sustainability strategies).

TABLE 12.2 Examples of Sustainability Strategies Used Within Community Health Programs

PROJECT AIM	STRATEGIES UTILIZED/ RECOMMENDED	THE IMPACT OF THESE STRATEGIES
CBRHP (Ahluwalia et al., 2010)—Aimed to examine the components that were sustained of CBRHP implemented by CARE-Tanzania to address high maternal mortality in two rural districts	▪ Promote capacity-building and community empowerment ▪ Mobilize formal and informal systems in communities	After 5 years the two components of CBRHP in six villages continued. From 2001 to 2006, the CBRHP-trained health workers continued to provide education and referrals to women in their communities including prenatal and emergency obstetric care; six villages with emergency transport systems continued for more than 5 years providing free or low-cost transport to health facilities
HELP (Bradley et al., 2005)—Aimed to examine key factors that influence sustainability in the diffusion of HELP in the United States as an example of an evidence-based, multifaceted, innovative program to improve care for hospitalized older adults	▪ Presence of clinical leadership (sustained leadership) ▪ Ensuring sustained funding is acquired ▪ The ability and willingness to adapt the original HELP protocols to local hospital circumstances and constraints ▪ The ability to obtain longer-term resources and funding for HELP	After 3 years 10 of the 13 hospitals studied were sustaining HELP at the end of the study period; three terminated the program (after 24, 12, and 6 months)

(continued)

TABLE 12.2 Examples of Sustainability Strategies Used Within Community Health Programs (*continued*)

PROJECT AIM	STRATEGIES UTILIZED/ RECOMMENDED	THE IMPACT OF THESE STRATEGIES
"Som la Pera" intervention: Adolescent Community Reinforcement Approach (Llauradó et al., 2018)—Aimed to improve the sustainability capacity of effective "Som la Pera," a school-based, peer-led, social-marketing intervention that encourages healthy diet and physical activity in low socioeconomic adolescents from Spain	Planning sustainability before implementation by: ▪ Developing collaborative bonds with institutions and community elements ▪ Organizing the different elements of the implementation by considering the community ▪ Including the intervention in the community, based on local policy	After 6–12 months the sustainability capacity assessment of the "Som la Pera" intervention was enhanced but only significantly improved in the deficient domains detected at the end of the first year. The strategic planning and a specific item of funding stability were improved significantly, overcoming the five cut-off points established over seven total points at the end of the second year of the intervention. The sustainability capacity assessment during the intervention allows its improvement before the program expires, ensuring the long-term implementation of the "Som la Pera" intervention program to encourage healthy lifestyles in adolescents

CBRHP, Community-Based Reproductive Health Project; HELP, Hospital Elder Life Program.

A 2017 randomized controlled trial (RCT) undertaken in 188 Australian community football clubs examined the effectiveness of a web-based program in sustaining the implementation of evidence-based alcohol management practices (e.g., prohibiting intoxicated patrons from entering or remaining at sporting venues, selling low or non-alcoholic beverages, providing food when alcohol is served). The web-based program was comprised of multiple strategies (audit and feedback, prompts and reminders, tools and resources, recognition and awards) and resulted in no significant difference in the proportion of community football clubs implementing safe alcohol management practices over time (McFadyen et al., 2019). Additional work evaluating which sustainability strategies are effective is still needed and a number of published protocols suggest that some studies are already underway (Johnson et al., 2018; Kastner et al., 2017; Vitale et al., 2018; Wiltsey Stirman et al., 2017). There are a number of naturalistic studies in low- and middle-income countries that have reported on the sustainment of EBIs (Ahluwalia et al., 2010; Llauradó et al., 2018; Vamos et al., 2014), which have adopted similar strategies in their efforts to sustain programs including capacity-building and community empowerment, mobilization of formal and informal systems in communities, train-the-trainer models, and quality assurance checks and feedback. However, with limited robust evidence regarding the sustainment of EBIs in low- and middle-income countries, future work is still needed on testing the effectiveness of these strategies in these settings, including the costs and value of such strategies (Hailemariam et al., 2019).

Describing and Selecting Sustainability Strategies

Currently, there is no specific taxonomy for sustainability strategies. Therefore, until one is developed or adapted, researchers and practitioners who conduct work on sustainability are encouraged to describe their strategies in sufficient detail to enable replication by others. Utilizing existing taxonomies such as the *Cochrane Collaboration's Effective Practice and Organization of Care* (EPOC, 2015), the *Expert Recommendations for Implementing Change* (ERIC; Powell et al., 2015), or taxonomies of behavior change techniques such as Michie et al.'s (2013) behavior change technique taxonomy (v1) may be useful for interventionists to characterize which strategies are used.

Similarly, in the absence of definitive evidence, we recommend that when selecting which strategies to use, practitioners apply learnings from the development of implementation strategies and interventions (Michie et al., 2013; Powell et al., 2015). Specifically, strategies can be selected based on: (a) the extent to which the strategy addresses the key determinants to implementation and/or sustainability (barriers and facilitators) and (b) the context that the EBI is being delivered in. Therefore, as recommended by Chambers et al. (2013) the continuous assessment of the determinants, context (structure, climate, culture, resources), as well as the fit between the EBI and the context and the intervention, not just prior to implementation, but over time is essential for informing appropriate selection of sustainability strategies. For example, the study described earlier on improving alcohol management practices in community football clubs found that the primary barriers to sustained implementation, as perceived by key stakeholders, related to program adaptability, the effectiveness of organizational system supports, and the internal and external support for the program (McFadyen et al., 2019). Such findings were distinct from those identified by the research team to impede initial implementation (Kingsland et al., 2015), which included leadership support, organizational readiness, and intervention characteristics (e.g., cost, complexity). This finding is consistent with the idea that implementation and sustainability may have distinct determinants that influence them and may require distinct strategies to address them (Scheirer, 2005; Shelton et al., 2018).

As with implementation strategies, we suggest that all sustainability strategies be assessed against some established criteria, to ensure that no strategy will create or exacerbate inequities. For example the *Acceptability, Practicability, Effectiveness, Affordability, Side-effects, and Equity* (APEASE) criteria developed by Michie et al. (2014) is a systematic approach for considering contextual factors that may impact on the appropriateness of the strategy for where the intervention is occurring and with whom. This includes considering the strategy in terms of whether it is: (a) acceptable to stakeholders and end-users; (b) practical to deliver in terms of resources and time; (c) effective and cost-effective; (d) affordable to be delivered; (e) has any side effects/safety issues; and (f) if it is equitable and will not disadvantage any community or population sub-group. The use of an APEASE grid (see Table 12.3) may help practitioners co-design a sustainability intervention or strategy (West et al., 2019). For example, advisory group members or end-users may be asked to rate on a scale (e.g., 0–10 or low, medium, high) the acceptability, practicability, effectiveness, affordability, side effects, or equity of each of the potential strategies being considered. If advisory group members are unsure of any of these specific details, they could use question marks in that cell. If practitioners felt that a specific criterion is more important than others for their context (e.g., equity over cost), then different weighting may also be given to these factors. Once completed, practitioners may then collate this information and facilitate a group discussion with their advisory group to resolve any discrepancies and reach agreement on the strategies that may be taken.

TABLE 12.3 Hypothetical Example of a Completed APEASE Grid to Assess and Select Strategies That May Support the Sustainability of a Community Weight Management Program Run by Hospital-Based Physiotherapists

STRATEGY	ACCEPTABILITY	PRACTICABILITY	EFFECTIVENESS	AFFORDABILITY	SIDE EFFECTS	EQUITY
	Rate on a scale of 0–10 or low, medium, high					
Audit and provide feedback	Low	High	Unsure	High	Low	High
Conduct educational outreach visits	High	Low	Unsure	Low	Low	Low
Distribute educational materials	High	High	Unsure	High	Low	High

CASE STUDY 12.3 SUSTAINING AUSTRALIAN SCHOOLS' IMPLEMENTATION OF A MANDATORY PHYSICAL ACTIVITY POLICY

WHAT IS THE PROBLEM?

In an attempt to improve the physical activity levels of children, multiple governments have released guidelines or policies mandating the minimum daily or weekly time elementary schools are to schedule structured physical activity for children (Nathan et al., 2019). Systematic reviews demonstrate that such guidelines and policies are effective in increasing student physical activity (Barr-Anderson et al., 2011; Robertson-Wilson et al., 2012; Strong et al., 2005). In Australia, almost all states and territories have a policy regarding the minimum time required for planned physical activity for children each week. Specifically, within New South Wales (NSW) schools are required to implement 150 minutes of planned physical activity across the school week, which may include time in physical education (PE), sport, active lessons, or short activity breaks such as energizers (Nathan et al., 2019). Application of implementation science methods have identified strategies to achieve effective implementation of this policy. A model of implementation support, which was co-developed by a local health promotion unit and end-user partners, was found to be effective in a pilot RCT to improve policy implementation from 33% to 62% (Nathan et al., 2020). These findings were replicated in a large-scale RCT undertaken in 62 elementary schools, with over 550 teachers (Nathan et al., 2019, 2021). After 12 months, the implementation trial successfully increased the proportion of schools who were compliant

(continued)

CASE STUDY 12.3 SUSTAINING AUSTRALIAN SCHOOLS' IMPLEMENTATION OF A MANDATORY PHYSICAL ACTIVITY POLICY *(continued)*

with the policy from 20% to 65%. However, 6 months after the implementation support ended, the health promotion unit conducted an audit of continued delivery of the policy and found that compliance had slipped to 40%. Without sustained program implementation, the potential public health benefits of EBIs cannot be achieved. Therefore, the health promotion unit decided that a sustainability intervention was needed if they are to avoid further slippage, and thus waste the substantial time and resources invested in initial implementation efforts. However, they were conscious that they cannot continue to support implementation over the long term, nor do they have the resources to be delivering an intervention that is as intensive as the implementation support.

WHAT DID THE LOCAL HEALTH PROMOTION UNIT DO?

A sustainability intervention was co-developed with the key partners, including health and education policy makers, health promotion practitioners, principals, teachers, as well as researchers with expertise in physical activity, implementation science, behavioral science, education, and public health. The development process was guided by formative evaluation undertaken by the research team and the Integrated Sustainability Framework (Shelton et al., 2018), a multi-level framework developed to help identify factors that influence sustainability that has been applied in the field of public health. Specifically, it included: (a) reviews of the scientific literature, (b) a quantitative survey with 240 teachers assessing factors associated with local sustainability of the physical activity policy using the PSAT, and (c) school-based observation and interviews with school staff to identify barriers to sustainability and potential strategies to address them. Utilizing this evidence, barriers were mapped to the domains of the Integrated Sustainability Framework, and a suite of potential strategies to address these were selected. Strategies were further refined following consultation with partner agencies and consideration informed by the APEASE criteria. A summary of the sustainability strategies prioritized for delivery include:

- *Sustainability support:* Schools have access to a project officer that contacts school champions and principals each term to answer any questions and check on progress.
- *In-school champions:* Schools nominate one or two school champions as the key contacts, to motivate and lead the coordination of sustainability support strategies in schools.
- *Executive support:* Principals demonstrate support for the sustained implementation of the physical activity policy via their regular *communication processes with staff.*
- *Training for teachers:* Schools are supported to ensure all teaching staff, including new teachers, annually attend relevant workshops or complete online training.
- *Communities of practice in schools:* Project officers work with existing peer teacher networks ("communities of practice") focusing on strategies to support the sustainment of the policy.

(*continued*)

CASE STUDY 12.3 SUSTAINING AUSTRALIAN SCHOOLS' IMPLEMENTATION OF A MANDATORY PHYSICAL ACTIVITY POLICY (*continued*)

NEXT STEPS?

The strategy was developed to (a) be consistent with Department of Education philosophy and national teachers' professional accreditation requirements, (b) be feasible, acceptable, and within existing resource capacity of local health districts, and (c) not require substantial and ongoing support from partner agencies. As such, the strategies, if found to be effective, have been designed to be integrated and adopted by partnering local health districts and the Department of Education.

MONITORING AND EVALUATING SUSTAINABILITY EFFORTS AND OUTCOMES

Monitoring and evaluation of all public health initiatives, whether that be at a local, state, national, or global level, are essential if we are to determine which interventions are, and continue to be, effective and cost-effective. For example, routine monitoring of EBIs over time may help identify any adaptations that are being made to the EBI by end-users or highlight unexpected challenges to its implementation which could require modifications to support strategies, both of which may impact on the effectiveness or cost-effectiveness of the EBI. Policy makers and practitioners may then use these data to make informed decisions as to whether EBIs should continue, be adapted, or be de-implemented (removed or replaced).

What to Measure

Public health practitioners may face many challenges when considering what to measure to determine if the implementation of their EBI has been sustained. For example, when considering Moore et al.'s (2017) definition of sustainability, this could require assessing if the program, clinical intervention, and/or implementation strategies have continued to be delivered (and potentially adapted), and whether individual (i.e., clinician, patient) behavior change is maintained. Additionally, others have also highlighted the importance of measuring the extent to which community and organizational infrastructure, capacity, and partnerships to deliver the EBI are maintained (Shelton et al., 2018). However, identifying what, when, and how to measure these items will vary for every public health initiative and may depend on a number of factors including obligations to policy makers, funding agencies or key stakeholders, the feasibility and acceptability of data collection tools and methods, the budget and time to do so, and the time that individual or organizational changes may take to have an effect or attenuate. See Figure 12.1 for different dimensions of sustainability that practitioners may want to consider assessing and discuss with their stakeholders to determine which are feasible and important.

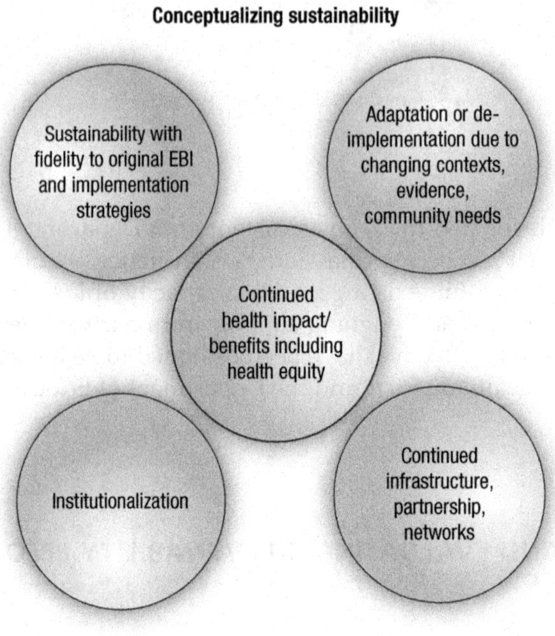

Conceptualizing sustainability

Sustainability with fidelity to original EBI and implementation strategies

Adaptation or de-implementation due to changing contexts, evidence, community needs

Continued health impact/ benefits including health equity

Institutionalization

Continued infrastructure, partnership, networks

FIGURE 12.1 Dimensions of sustainability practitioners may assess and discuss with stakeholders.

How to Measure

Despite the proliferation of sustainability theories and frameworks, few have developed valid and reliable tools for measuring sustainment or sustainability. For example, a 2014 study by Luke et al. (2014) reported that of the 17 sustainability frameworks identified within the public health literature, only two tools for measuring sustainability were available, neither of which was tested for reliability or validity. Findings from recent reviews (Mettert et al., 2020; Moullin et al., 2020) suggest that efforts are being made to overcome this problem in the field, with an increase in the development and psychometric evaluation of sustainment and sustainability determinants measures. For example, a 2015 review of implementation outcome measures within mental or behavioral health research identified just eight measures of sustainability (Lewis et al., 2015), which increased to 14 in the updated review in 2020 (Mettert et al., 2020). Unfortunately, the quality of these measures did not improve, with the review reporting that almost no measure could detect real change over time.

These findings are consistent with a review by Moullin et al. (2020) which used two large existing implementation science databases as well as supplemental searches to identify the most frequently used, comprehensive, and/or validated sustainability measures. Of the 11 measures included in the review, 10 measured constructs of sustainment as an outcome, and nine measured factors that influence sustainability (e.g., determinants). However, the authors reported that many of these tools were limited by several factors, including poorly reported psychometric properties, being too specific to context or intervention, being too long, and/or not pragmatic for use. The review does include a very useful summary of each of the tools which practitioners may find handy if trying to locate a relevant measure to use in their field.

For those wishing to measure sustainment, it is important to note that given the variability in clinical and public health initiatives and contexts, it may not be possible to have a "gold standard" measure for program sustainment. However, it is recommended that at a minimum the core components of a specific EBI (identified through theory or determined empirically) be measured. Furthermore, given programs may need to adapt over time in order to be sustained, measuring adaptations and the reasons for adaptations should be undertaken (Shelton et al., 2018). As a result, those wishing to measure sustainment of an EBI may need to utilize several tools to more accurately and comprehensively assess it. Similarly, for those with a particular interest in measuring the determinants of sustainability, the PSAT and CSAT may be useful; however, given that further work is needed to advance the psychometrics of these measures, researchers and practitioners are encouraged to use a range of data sources to identify determinants within the specific context in which the innovation is occurring and how this may change over time.

There are also existing frameworks and evaluation tools not specific to sustainability that can still be useful guides when planning for and measuring sustainability as an outcome. For example, the *Reach, Effectiveness, Adoption, Implementation, and Maintenance* (RE-AIM) framework is a widely used planning and evaluation framework, with an accompanying planning tool (Glasgow et al., 2019). RE-AIM has historically used the "maintenance" domain to capture long-term impact of the EBI and continued delivery of EBI program components after original implementation, which has typically been assessed at relatively short-term intervals (e.g., at least 6 months after EBI delivered or initially implemented). There has been a recent extension of RE-AIM to enhance sustainability, with a focus on dynamic context and health equity over time (Shelton et al., 2020). Specifically, this extension recommends: (a) extension of maintenance to include consideration of dynamic, longer-term sustainability across the life cycle of EBIs, which may include adaptation and even de-implementation due to changing evidence, context, and resources and emerging population needs over time; (b) iterative or periodic application of RE-AIM assessments to guide possible adaptations needed to plan for and/or enhance long-term sustainability; and (c) consideration of equity and cost as cross-cutting issues that have implications for sustainability and should be assessed and ideally addressed across RE-AIM dimensions. The RE-AIM framework also assists with pragmatic assessment of guiding questions and key elements for practitioners to consider as they are transitioning from initial implementation (typically the first 6–12 months of implementation) to longer-term sustainability for each of the RE-AIM dimensions and assessments. Example questions include: What sustainability strategies could be used to sustain the program beyond initial implementation or funding? Is the EBI being equitably sustained across populations and settings? How can we support, incorporate and institutionalize the EBI so its delivery is continued past initial implementation? What adaptations are needed to continue delivering the EBI long term and are there opportunities to build capacity at sites facing challenges to enhance sustainability?

Ideally, multiple indicators of sustainability as an outcome are measured first at 6 months post initial implementation and at least 12 months post EBI implementation and on an ongoing basis (e.g., annually). The time frame depends in part on the nature of the EBI and on what is relevant for the health issue/behavior studied. Qualitative data collection can be useful for comparing stakeholder insights within settings of interest regarding perceived historical and ongoing challenges with sustaining programs and to understand what strategies may be useful to plan for sustainability.

CASE STUDY 12.4 FACTORS TO CONSIDER WHEN MEASURING THE SUSTAINABILITY OF PUBLIC HEALTH PROGRAMS IN COMMUNITY SETTINGS

In order to improve the foods packed by parents and caregivers for their children to consume at school, the "SWAP IT" intervention used an existing school mobile communication app, already used by schools to communicate with parents, to provide healthy lunchbox information (Sutherland et al., 2019). Push notifications were sent to parents each week for 10 weeks to encourage them to "swap" discretionary foods from their child's lunchbox to healthier alternatives; for example, swapping out a pre-packaged cheese and biscuit snack which is high in fat and salt for wholegrain crackers and reduced fat cheese. Messages were designed to address parental barriers to packing a healthy lunchbox, identified using the *Behaviour Change Wheel*; for example, packing a lunchbox on a limited budget and food safety. The study, which was tested in a RCT in 12 schools in Australia with almost 1,400 students from kindergarten to grade 6, significantly impacted what was packed in children's lunchboxes and consequently on what children consumed. Furthermore, a large majority of parents opened the messages and found them to be useful. Based on these findings, "SWAP IT" has now been adopted as an EBI by the Department of Health to be delivered to all schools. Table 12.4 shows how the health promotion team that developed SWAP IT could measure the sustainability of SWAP IT and factors that need to be considered.

TABLE 12.4 Example of How an Evidence-Based Intervention Could Be Measured and Factors to Consider

MOORE'S DEFINITION OF SUSTAINABILITY	WHAT TO MEASURE?	HOW AND WHEN TO MEASURE THIS?	FACTORS TO CONSIDER IF MEASURING THIS?
The core components of the EBI continue to be delivered	SWAP IT (Sutherland et al., 2019) required schools to deliver the 10-week program at the start of each school year. Therefore, not only could the health promotion practitioners ensure that it is being delivered, they could measure the fidelity of its delivery (i.e., it is being delivered when it is supposed to, with all content, and for the full 10 weeks). They could also measure other factors as recommended by Proctor et al.'s (2011) core set of outcomes (i.e., acceptability, feasibility, uptake, penetration, and cost)	1. Surveys of schools who should have delivered the EBI to determine if they have implemented SWAP IT 2. Surveys of parents who should have received the EBI to determine if they have implemented SWAP IT Data could be collected once per year following the expected delivery of the program	Cost: This could be done at a relatively low cost if using online surveys Reliability/validity of the measure: This would be relying on self-report which is at risk of social desirability and recall bias Acceptability: It is unlikely that if this is collected once per year that this would cause participant burden Feasibility: The survey would be self-administered; therefore, there is no special training or skills required of data collectors

(continued)

TABLE 12.4 Example of How an Evidence-Based Intervention Could Be Measured and Factors to Consider (*continued*)

MOORE'S DEFINITION OF SUSTAINABILITY	WHAT TO MEASURE?	HOW AND WHEN TO MEASURE THIS?	FACTORS TO CONSIDER IF MEASURING THIS?
Strategies that support the implementation of the EBI are continued	To support schools to implement SWAP IT they were provided with prompts and reminders, resources for parents, and resources for teachers They could also measure other factors as recommended by Proctor et al.'s (2011) core set of outcomes (i.e., acceptability, feasibility, uptake, penetration, and cost)	1. The project records audits to determine if implementation support was provided to schools 2. Surveys of schools to determine if they have received the implementation support for SWAP IT Data could be collected once per year following the expected delivery of the program	Same as above.
Participant behavior change is maintained (e.g., the health behavior)	Parent/caregiver behavior of packing healthy lunchboxes is continued Student behavior of consuming healthy foods from their lunchbox continues	A valid and reliable lunchbox observational audit was undertaken whereby photographs were taken of children's lunchboxes prior to any food being consumed (i.e., at the start of the school day) and then again at the end of the school day following school meal breaks. Children placed all unconsumed or partially consumed items back into their lunchbox	Cost: This is incredibly time and labor intensive. The cost to collect such data across a large population would be substantial Reliability/validity of the measure: This is the gold standard measure for collecting such data Acceptability: This requires ethical approval and informed consent from schools, parents/caregivers, and children. While response rates were high (68%) it is not expected that routine observations would be acceptable to schools or parents. Feasibility: The collection of such data requires training of data collection staff and analysis by dietitians. If this measure is deemed essential it would only be feasible to conduct this in a sample of participating schools each year

EBI, evidence-based intervention.

Application of Learnings to Opening Case Study

At the start of this chapter, we presented a scenario where a program manager working within a community mental health center was aiming to implement and sustain the delivery of "2As and R," an evidence-based model of care to support their clients quit smoking. According to this model of care, clinicians: Assess patients' smoking status, provide brief Advice about quitting, and Refer them to an evidence-based telephone counseling support service. The funding for the project is time-limited, however, the manager wants to avoid the usual pitfalls of starting a project to support clinicians implementing the EBI which is not sustainable long term. What could the program manager do? Let's apply what we've learned:

1. *Undertake a sustainability assessment:* On the advice of a researcher from the local university, the manager reviews the Integrated Sustainability Framework and the DSF and uses them to identify the broad range of outer and inner contextual factors and processes that may influence the sustainability of clinician delivery of the EBI. Ideas generated from this assessment are discussed with members of the team who build upon it and inform planning of the next steps.
2. *Plan for sustainability:* The manager then uses the online CSAT tool to conduct a more formal assessment of their group's current capacity for sustaining the EBI. The assessment is rapid and helps provide additional information they use to guide their sustainability planning given in the following.
3. *Select sustainability strategies:* The community mental health center has no staff with the skills to conduct a rigorous literature review of potentially effective implementation and sustainability strategies. Given this potential barrier, the program manager:
   a. Conducts an anonymous paper survey with clinicians in the center to identify what their barriers are to implementing and sustaining the delivery of the EBI. They also include a list of strategies that they think are feasible to support clinicians' sustained delivery of the EBI. The clinicians are asked to select those that they think would be most helpful and acceptable. The list of barriers and potential strategies are those identified in steps 1 and 2.
   b. Forms an advisory group made up of relevant clinicians, consumer/patient representatives, and researchers from the local university who can provide advice on the implementation and sustainability strategies. Using the APEASE grid, advisory group members are asked, based on their knowledge and experience, to independently rate the Acceptability, Practicability, Effectiveness, Affordability, Side effects, and Equity of each of the potential strategies. The manager then compiles each of the advisory group member's ratings with the work undertaken in steps 1 and 2 and the clinician surveys to identify the most highly rated strategies. A group discussion with advisory group members is then held to resolve any discrepancies and reach agreement. These strategies are then presented back to the clinicians to gain their final agreement.
   c. Next, a sustainability plan is developed which identifies which components of the EBI need to be maintained or adapted, and the priority strategies needed to support and sustain the EBI, with specific detail of who is doing what, when, and how. This plan is then monitored and reported on during the managers meeting with clinicians.

4. *Developing a monitoring and evaluation plan*: As the community mental health center is part of a larger health network, there are already existing routine data collection processes that the manager realizes they could leverage to assess the sustained delivery of the EBI and the impact on clients' smoking status. The center uses a medical software program which all clinicians have to use to record each interaction with patients. As part of the strategy selection process (step 3), it was identified that this software could be modified to include a prompt for clinicians to Assess, Advise and Refer. The manager is therefore able to access the data collected by the software program to determine the proportion of clinicians that are delivering the EBI. They are aware, however, that the degree to which this is delivered with fidelity may vary significantly among the clinicians. Therefore, they have gained a commitment from the clinical supervisor to record the extent to which all three steps of the EBI are delivered during their monthly professional practice observations with all clinicians at the center. They will use the action plan developed in item 3c to monitor their implementation and fidelity of delivery. In addition, they have decided to ask clinicians to complete an anonymous survey every 3 to 6 months to assess their acceptability with the support provided to them.

SUMMARY

This chapter has described the most current evidence base in sustainability research and practice, while also providing practical methods, frameworks, and tools to use when planning for, or designing, sustainability interventions and strategies.

KEY POINTS FOR PRACTICE

1. Plan for sustainment from the outset. If we are to have an equitable impact on population health and make best use of public health funding and resources, we must invest in the most effective, cost-effective, and sustainable EBIs. To do this, we must proactively plan for the continued delivery of EBIs during the initial planning phase. This is particularly important for EBIs that take time (perhaps years or generations) to see public health impact for communities.
2. Adaptations for sustainment may be essential; however, it is important to ensure that if adaptations are made to the EBI or the support strategies, that the core components driving the intervention effect are not removed. Considering the dynamic real-world contexts in which EBIs are delivered, it is important to assess and refine the fit of an EBI to the practice setting over time and use quality improvement processes to refine, optimize, improve, and ultimately sustain EBIs.
3. Use an existing sustainability theory or framework to assess and plan your sustainability intervention. This is essential for identifying determinants important for intervention sustainment and will also contribute to the evidence base by informing the development and refinement of strategies that can support sustainability.

4. When selecting sustainment strategies, consider both the extent to which a strategy addresses the key determinants to implementation or sustainability and the context in which the EBI is being delivered. This may require a continuous assessment of the determinants, context, and EBI fit throughout the planning, implementation, and sustainability pipeline.

A summary of overarching key questions and points to consider for sustainability is presented in Table 12.5.

COMMON PITFALLS FOR PRACTICE

1. Selecting EBIs or support strategies that are not appropriate or not a good "fit." For example, the EBI may have originally been tested among a narrowly defined population or only ever tested in well-resourced academic settings. Alternatively, the EBI may not be conducive to sustainment; for example, it is too resource or time intensive to be delivered outside of a well-resourced trial.
2. Evaluating only initial intervention adoption and implementation. Long-term follow-up of EBIs and their effects are needed if we are to identify the most effective and cost-effective EBIs for sustainment.
3. Not planning for sustainability from the start among key stakeholders or thinking about sustainability during earlier stages of implementation.
4. Not recording adaptations to the EBI or strategies over time. Contextual factors (e.g., different populations, systems) may influence how the EBI needs to be implemented over time.
5. Only relying on quantitative data. Using mixed method designs with key stakeholders capturing the end-users as well as the implementer or practitioner experiences can provide insights that may help refine strategies to promote sustainment.

DISCUSSION QUESTIONS

Think about a public health initiative, program, or project that you have either delivered (or know of), but is no longer being implemented and consider the following questions:

1. Describe the initiative or project (i.e., what did the community, organization, system, or patient receive).
2. List the factors that may have impacted on the sustainment of the initiative or project. It may be useful to use a conceptual framework such as the Integrated Sustainability Framework to reflect on the range of sociopolitical, contextual/organizational, population, or intervention characteristics present at the time that may have impacted program sustainment.
3. What, if any, strategies could have been utilized to address these factors identified in question 2 above? When in the project timeline would they have been needed (i.e., project planning, project implementation, project sustainability)?
4. If the program is still being implemented in any capacity, what has changed since it was originally developed or implemented? Who decided to make these adaptations, how were they communicated, and were they tracked? How do you know if the program is still effective and delivering benefits?

TABLE 12.5 Overarching Questions to Consider Regarding Sustainability of Evidence-Based Interventions

Question	Considerations
1. Do I have a clear sense of the evidence-based practice/program and its core components and intended health impact?	■ Reach out to implementers (and possibly program developers) to access program materials and description
2. Have I worked with stakeholders to determine what "counts" as sustainability of the EBI?	■ Revisit conceptualizations of sustainability and discuss with stakeholders the advantages and disadvantages of various approaches (e.g., Sustained use of an EBI with fidelity? Maintenance of partnerships? Continued impact on health behaviors/outcomes?) ■ Consider the extent to which adaptations of EBIs are tracked, to understand their impact and how the EBI changes over time based on changing needs, evidence, and context. Consider tracking the extent to which such adaptations may reduce or exacerbate health inequities
3. Have I started to think about or plan for sustainability during the implementation phase or determine who will be involved in sustainability efforts?	■ Apply planning tools (e.g., Program Sustainability Assessment Tool [PSAT] or Clinical Sustainability Assessment Tool [CSAT]) or sustainability frameworks that help identify potential barriers and facilitators to consider and address specifically related to sustainability (e.g., Integrated Sustainability Framework)
4. Do I have a plan for measuring or assessing or monitoring sustainability over time?	■ Consider existing planning or evaluation tools (e.g., RE-AIM framework) and determine the time period when sustainability will be assessed (e.g., 6 months post implementation and annually over the next 5 years); if possible, assess using both qualitative and quantitative sources of information. Are there indicators of institutionalization that help inform understanding of sustainability (e.g., are staff roles and program costs included as part of annual budget)?
5. Have I considered delivering strategies to better support sustainability?	■ Think about linking identified barriers to sustainability with strategies that could address them ■ Provide opportunities to obtain feedback from stakeholders on how well they are working (are they feasible, acceptable, appropriate), so they can be iteratively refined as needed

EBI, evidence-based intervention; RE-AIM, reach, effectiveness, adoption, implementation, maintenance.

REFERENCES

Ahluwalia, I. B., Robinson, D., Vallely, L., Gieseker, K. E., & Kabakama, A. (2010). Sustainability of community-capacity to promote safer motherhood in northwestern Tanzania: What remains? *Global Health Promotion, 17*(1), 39–49. https://doi.org/10.1177/1757975909356627

Barr-Anderson, D. J., AuYoung, M., Whitt-Glover, M. C., Glenn, B. A., & Yancey, A. K. (2011). Integration of short bouts of physical activity into organizational routine: A systematic review of the literature. *American Journal of Preventive Medicine, 40*(1), 76–93. https://doi.org/10.1016/j.amepre.2010.09.033

Barrera, M., Jr., Castro, F. G., Strycker, L. A., & Toobert, D. J. (2013). Cultural adaptations of behavioral health interventions: A progress report. *Journal of Consulting and Clinical Psychology, 81*(2), 196–205. https://doi.org/10.1037/a0027085

Baumann, A. A., & Cabassa, L. J. (2020). Reframing implementation science to address inequities in healthcare delivery. *BMC Health Services Research, 20*, Article 190. https://doi.org/10.1186/s12913-020-4975-3

Birken, S. A., Haines, E. R., Hwang, S., Chambers, D. A., Bunger, A. C., & Nilsen, P. (2020). Advancing understanding and identifying strategies for sustaining evidence-based practices: A review of reviews. *Implementation Science, 15*, Article 88. https://doi.org/10.1186/s13012-020-01040-9

Bradley, E. H., Webster, T. R., Baker, D., Schlesinger, M., & Inouye, S. K. (2005). After adoption: Sustaining the innovation. A case study of disseminating the Hospital Elder Life Program. *Journal of the American Geriatrics Society, 53*(9), 1455–1461. https://doi.org/10.1111/j.1532-5415.2005.53451.x

Braithwaite, J., Ludlow, K., Testa, L., Herkes, J., Augustsson, H., Lamprell, G., McPherson, E., & Zurynski, Y. (2020). Built to last? The sustainability of healthcare system improvements, programmes and interventions: A systematic integrative review. *BMJ Open, 10*(6), e036453. https://doi.org/10.1136/bmjopen-2019-036453

Calhoun, A., Mainor, A., Moreland-Russell, S., Maier, R. C., Brossart, L., & Luke, D. A. (2014). Using the Program Sustainability Assessment Tool to assess and plan for sustainability. *Preventing Chronic Disease, 11*, 130185. https://doi.org/10.5888/pcd11.130185

Cassar, S., Salmon, J., Timperio, A., Naylor, P.-J., van Nassau, F., Contardo Ayala, A. M., & Koorts, H. (2019). Adoption, implementation and sustainability of school-based physical activity and sedentary behaviour interventions in real-world settings: A systematic review. *International Journal of Behavioral Nutrition and Physical Activity, 16*, Article 120. https://doi.org/10.1186/s12966-019-0876-4

Chambers, D. A., Glasgow, R. E., & Stange, K. C. (2013). The Dynamic Sustainability Framework: Addressing the paradox of sustainment amid ongoing change. *Implementation Science, 8*, Article 117. https://doi.org/10.1186/1748-5908-8-117

Committee on Public Health Strategies to Improve Health. (2012). Reforming public health and its financing. In Institute of Medicine (Ed.), *For the public's health: Investing in a healthier future*. National Academies Press. https://www.ncbi.nlm.nih.gov/books/NBK201015/

Damschroder, L. J. (2020). Clarity out of chaos: Use of theory in implementation research. *Psychiatry Research, 283*, 112461. https://doi.org/10.1016/j.psychres.2019.06.036

Damschroder, L. J., Aron, D. C., Keith, R. E., Kirsh, S. R., Alexander, J. A., & Lowery, J. C. (2009). Fostering implementation of health services research findings into practice: A consolidated framework for advancing implementation science. *Implementation Science, 4*, Article 50. https://doi.org/10.1186/1748-5908-4-50

Effective Practice and Organisation of Care. (2015). *EPOC Taxonomy*. Retrieved January 8, 2021 from epoc.cochrane.org/epoc-taxonomy

Emmons, K. M., & Colditz, G. A. (2017). Realizing the potential of cancer prevention — The role of implementation science. *New England Journal of Medicine, 376*(10), 986–990. https://doi.org/10.1056/NEJMsb1609101

Erwin, D.O., Ivory J., Stayton C., Willis, M., Jandorf, L., Thompson, H., Womack, S., & Hurd, T. C. (2003). Replication and dissemination of a cancer education model for African American Women. *Cancer Control, 10*(5_Suppl), 13–21. https://doi.org/10.1177/107327480301005s03

Glasgow, R. E., Harden, S. M., Gaglio, B., Rabin, B., Smith, M. L., Porter, G. C., Ory, M. G., & Estabrooks, P. A. (2019). RE-AIM planning and evaluation framework: Adapting to new science and practice with a 20-year review. *Frontiers in Public Health, 7*, 64. https://doi-org.ezproxy.cul.columbia.edu/10.3389/fpubh.2019.00064

Gruen, R. L., Elliott, J. H., Nolan, M. L., Lawton, P. D., Parkhill, A., McLaren, C. J., & Lavis, J. N. (2008). Sustainability science: An integrated approach for health-programme planning. *Lancet, 372*(9649), 1579–1589. https://doi.org/10.1016/s0140-6736(08)61659-1

Hailemariam, M., Bustos, T., Montgomery, B., Barajas, R., Evans, L. B., & Drahota, A. (2019). Evidence-based intervention sustainability strategies: A systematic review. *Implementation Science, 14*, Article 57. https://doi.org/10.1186/s13012-019-0910-6

Herlitz, L., MacIntyre, H., Osborn, T., & Bonell, C. (2020). The sustainability of public health interventions in schools: A systematic review. *Implementation Science, 15*, Article 4. https://doi.org/10.1186/s13012-019-0961-8

Iwelunmor, J., Blackstone, S., Veira, D., Nwaozuru, U., Airhihenbuwa, C., Munodawafa, D., Kalipeni, E., Jutal, A., Shelley, D., & Ogedegbe, G. (2016). Toward the sustainability of health interventions implemented in sub-Saharan Africa: A systematic review and conceptual framework. *Implementation Science, 11*, Article 43. https://doi.org/10.1186/s13012-016-0392-8

Johnson, J. E., Wiltsey-Stirman, S., Sikorskii, A., Miller, T., King, A., Blume, J. L., Pham, X., Moore Simas, T. A., Poleshuck, E., Weinberg, R., & Zlotnick, C. (2018). Protocol for the ROSE sustainment (ROSES) study, a sequential multiple assignment randomized trial to determine the minimum necessary intervention to maintain a postpartum depression prevention program in prenatal clinics serving low-income women. *Implementation Science, 13*, Article 115. https://doi.org/10.1186/s13012-018-0807-9

Johnson, K., Collins, D., & Wandersman, A. (2013). Sustaining innovations in community prevention systems: A data-informed sustainability strategy. *Journal of Community Psychology, 41*(3), 322–340. https://doi.org/10.1002/jcop.21540

Kastner, M., Sayal, R., Oliver, D., Straus, S. E., & Dolovich, L. (2017). Sustainability and scalability of a volunteer-based primary care intervention (Health TAPESTRY): A mixed-methods analysis. *BMC Health Services Research, 17*, Article 514. https://doi.org/10.1186/s12913-017-2468-9

Kingsland, M., Doherty, E., Anderson, A. E., Crooks, K., Tully, B., Tremain, D., Tsang, T. W., Attia, J., Wolfenden, L., Dunlop, A. J., Bennett, N., Hunter, M., Ward, S., Reeves, P., Symonds, I., Rissel, C., Azzopardi, C., Searles, A., Gillham, K., Elliott, E. J., & Wiggers, J. (2018). A practice change intervention to improve antenatal care addressing alcohol consumption by women during pregnancy: Research protocol for a randomised stepped-wedge cluster trial. *Implementation Science, 13*, Article 112. https://doi.org/10.1186/s13012-018-0806-x

Kingsland, M., Wolfenden, L., Tindall, J., Rowland, B., Sidey, M., McElduff, P., & Wiggers, J. H. (2015). Improving the implementation of responsible alcohol management practices by community sporting clubs: A randomised controlled trial. *Drug and Alcohol Review, 34*(4), 447–457. https://doi.org/10.1111/dar.12252

Kumpfer, K., Magalhães, C., & Xie, J. (2017). Cultural adaptation and implementation of family evidence-based interventions with diverse populations. *Prevention Science, 18*(6), 649–659. https://doi.org/10.1007/s11121-016-0719-3

Lau, R., Stevenson, F., Ong, B. N., Dziedzic, K., Treweek, S., Eldridge, S., Everitt, H., Kennedy, A., Qureshi, N., Rogers, A., Peacock, R., & Murray, E. (2015). Achieving change in primary care—Effectiveness of strategies for improving implementation of complex interventions: Systematic review of reviews. *BMJ Open, 5*(12), e009993. https://doi.org/10.1136/bmjopen-2015-009993

Lewis, C. C., Fischer, S., Weiner, B. J., Stanick, C., Kim, M., & Martinez, R. G. (2015). Outcomes for implementation science: An enhanced systematic review of instruments using evidence-based rating criteria. *Implementation Science, 10*, Article 155. https://doi.org/10.1186/s13012-015-0342-x

Llauradó, E., Aceves-Martins, M., Tarro, L., Papell-Garcia, I., Puiggròs, F., Prades-Tena, J., Kettner, H., Arola, L., Giralt, M., & Solà, R. (2018). The "Som la Pera" intervention: Sustainability capacity evaluation of a peer-led social-marketing intervention to encourage healthy lifestyles among adolescents. *Translational Behavioral Medicine, 8*(5), 739–744. https://doi.org/10.1093/tbm/ibx065

Luke, D. A., Calhoun, A., Robichaux, C. B., Elliott, M. B., & Moreland-Russell, S. (2014). The Program Sustainability Assessment Tool: A new instrument for public health programs. *Preventing Chronic Disease, 11*, 130184. https://doi.org/10.5888/pcd11.130184

Maher, L., Gustafson, D., & Evans, A. (2010). *Sustainability model and guide*. National Health Service Institute for Innovation and Improvement. http://www.institute.nhs.uk/index.php?option=com_joomcart&main_page=document_

Malone, S., Prewitt, K., Hackett, R., Lin, J. C., McKay, V., Walsh-Bailey, C., & Luke, D. (2021). The Clinical Sustainability Assessment Tool: Measuring organizational capacity to promote sustainability in healthcare. *Implementation Science Communications, 2*(77). https://doi.org/10.1186/s43058-021-00181-2

McFadyen, T., Wolfenden, L., Kingsland, M., Tindall, J., Sherker, S., Heaton, R., Gillham, K., Clinton-McHarg, T., Lecathelinais, C., Rowland, B., & Wiggers, J. (2019). Sustaining the implementation of alcohol management practices by community sports clubs: A randomised control trial. *BMC Public Health, 19*, Article 1660. https://doi.org/10.1186/s12889-019-7974-8

Mettert, K., Lewis, C., Dorsey, C., Halko, H., & Weiner, B. (2020). Measuring implementation outcomes: An updated systematic review of measures' psychometric properties. *Implementation Research and Practice, 1* (Jan–Dec 2020), 1–29. https://doi.org/10.1177/2633489520936644

Michie, S., Atkins, L., & West, R. (2014). *The behaviour change wheel: A guide to designing*. Silverback Publishing.

Michie, S., Richardson, M., Johnston, M., Abraham, C., Francis, J., Hardeman, W., Eccles, M. P., Cane, J., & Wood, C. E. (2013). The behavior change technique taxonomy (v1) of 93 hierarchically clustered techniques: Building an international consensus for the reporting of behavior change interventions. *Annals of Behavioral Medicine, 46*(1), 81–95. https://doi.org/10.1007/s12160-013-9486-6

Moore, J. E., Mascarenhas, A., Bain, J., & Straus, S. E. (2017). Developing a comprehensive definition of sustainability. *Implementation Science, 12*, Article 110. https://doi.org/10.1186/s13012-017-0637-1

Moullin, J. C., Sklar, M., Green, A., Dickson, K. S., Stadnick, N. A., Reeder, K., & Aarons, G. A. (2020). Advancing the pragmatic measurement of sustainment: A narrative review of measures. *Implementation Science Communications, 1*, Article 76. https://doi.org/10.1186/s43058-020-00068-8

Nathan, N., Hall, A., McCarthy, N. J., Sutherland, R., Wiggers, J., Bauman, A. E., Rissel, C., Naylor, P.-J., Cradock, A., Lane, C., Hope, K., Elton, B., Shoesmith, A., Oldmeadow, C., Reeves, P., Gillham, K., Duggan, B., Boyer, J., Lecathelinais, C., & Wolfenden, L. (2021). Multi-strategy intervention increases school implementation and maintenance of a mandatory physical activity policy: Outcomes of a cluster randomised controlled trial. *British Journal of Sports Medicine*, Advance online publication. https://doi.org/10.1136/bjsports-2020-103764

Nathan, N., Sutherland, R., Hope, K., McCarthy, N. J., Pettett, M., Elton, B., Jackson, R., Trost, S. G., Lecathelinais, C., Reilly, K., Wiggers, J. H., Hall, A., Gillham, K., Herrmann, V., & Wolfenden, L. (2020). Implementation of a school physical activity policy improves student physical activity levels: Outcomes of a cluster-randomized controlled trial. *Journal of Physical Activity and Health, 17*(10), 1–10. https://doi.org/10.1123/jpah.2019-0595

Nathan, N., Wiggers, J., Bauman, A., Rissel, C., Searles, A., Reeves, P., Oldmeadow, C., Naylor, P. J., Cradock, A., Sutherland, R., Gillham, K., & Duggan, B. (2019). A cluster randomised controlled trial of an intervention to increase the implementation of school physical activity policies and guidelines: Study protocol for the physically active children in education (PACE) study. *BMC Public Health, 19*, Article 170. https://doi.org/10.1186/s12889-019-6492-z

Nathan, N., Yoong, S. L., Sutherland, R., Reilly, K., Delaney, T., Janssen, L., Robertson, K., Reynolds, R., Chai, L. K., Lecathelinais, C., Wiggers, J., & Wolfenden, L. (2016). Effectiveness of a multicomponent intervention to enhance implementation of a healthy canteen policy in Australian primary schools: A randomised controlled trial. *International Journal of Behavioral Nutrition and Physical Activity, 13*, Article 106. https://doi.org/10.1186/s12966-016-0431-5

Palinkas, L. A., Chou, C.-P., Spear, S. E., Mendon, S. J., Villamar, J., & Brown, C. H. (2020). Measurement of sustainment of prevention programs and initiatives: The sustainment measurement system scale. *Implementation Science, 15*, Article 71. https://doi.org/10.1186/s13012-020-01030-x

Powell, B. J., Waltz, T. J., Chinman, M. J., Damschroder, L. J., Smith, J. L., Matthieu, M. M., Proctor, E. K., & Kirchner, J. E. (2015). A refined compilation of implementation strategies: Results from the Expert Recommendations for Implementing Change (ERIC) project. *Implementation Science, 10*, Article 21. https://doi.org/10.1186/s13012-015-0209-1

Proctor, E., Luke, D., Calhoun, A., McMillen, C., Brownson, R., McCrary, S., & Padek, M. (2015). Sustainability of evidence-based healthcare: Research agenda, methodological advances, and infrastructure support. *Implementation Science, 10*, Article 88. https://doi.org/10.1186/s13012-015-0274-5

Proctor, E., Silmere, H., Raghavan, R., Hovmand, P., Aarons, G., Bunger, A., Griffey, R., & Hensley, M. (2011). Outcomes for implementation research: Conceptual distinctions, measurement challenges, and research agenda. *Administration and Policy in Mental Health, 38*(2), 65–76. https://doi-org.ezproxy.cul.columbia.edu/10.1007/s10488-010-0319-7

Rabin, B. A., Glasgow, R. E., Kerner, J. F., Klump, M. P., & Brownson, R. C. (2010). Dissemination and implementation research on community-based cancer prevention: A systematic review. *American Journal of Preventive Medicine, 38*(4), 443–456. https://doi.org/10.1016/j.amepre.2009.12.035

Robertson-Wilson, J. E., Dargavel, M. D., Bryden, P. J., & Giles-Corti, B. (2012). Physical activity policies and legislation in schools: A systematic review. *American Journal of Preventive Medicine, 43*(6), 643–649. https://doi.org/10.1016/j.amepre.2012.08.022

Scheirer, M. A. (2005). Is sustainability possible? A review and commentary on empirical studies of program sustainability. *American Journal of Evaluation, 26*(3), 320–347. https://doi.org/10.1177/1098214005278752

Scheirer, M. A. (2013). Linking sustainability research to intervention types. *American Journal of Public Health, 103*(4), e73–80. https://doi.org/10.2105/ajph.2012.300976

Scheirer, M. A., & Dearing, J. W. (2011). An agenda for research on the sustainability of public health programs. *American Journal of Public Health, 101*(11), 2059–2067. https://doi.org/10.2105/AJPH.2011.300193

Scheirer, M. A., Santos, S. L., Tagai, E. K., Bowie, J., Slade, J., Carter, R., & Holt, C. L. (2017). Dimensions of sustainability for a health communication intervention in African American churches: A multi-methods study. *Implementation Science, 12*, Article 43. https://doi.org/10.1186/s13012-017-0576-x

Schell, S. F., Luke, D. A., Schooley, M. W., Elliott, M. B., Herbers, S. H., Mueller, N. B., & Bunger, A. C. (2013). Public health program capacity for sustainability: A new framework. *Implementation Science, 8*, Article 15. https://doi.org/10.1186/1748-5908-8-15

Scudder, A. T., Taber-Thomas, S. M., Schaffner, K., Pemberton, J. R., Hunter, L., & Herschell, A. D. (2017). A mixed-methods study of system-level sustainability of evidence-based practices in 12 large-scale implementation initiatives. *Health Research Policy and Systems, 15*, Article 102. https://doi.org/10.1186/s12961-017-0230-8

Shediac-Rizkallah, M. C., & Bone, L. R. (1998). Planning for the sustainability of community-based health programs: Conceptual frameworks and future directions for research, practice and policy. *Health Education Research, 13*(1), 87–108. https://doi.org/10.1093/her/13.1.87

Shelton, R. C., Chambers, D. A., & Glasgow, R. E. (2020). An extension of RE-AIM to enhance sustainability: Addressing dynamic context and promoting health equity over time [Perspective]. *Frontiers in Public Health, 8*, Article 134. https://doi.org/10.3389/fpubh.2020.00134

Shelton, R. C., Charles, T.-A., Dunston, S. K., Jandorf, L., & Erwin, D. O. (2017). Advancing understanding of the sustainability of lay health advisor (LHA) programs for African-American women in community settings. *Translational Behavioral Medicine, 7*(3), 415–426. https://doi.org/10.1007/s13142-017-0491-3

Shelton, R. C., Cooper, B. R., & Stirman, S. W. (2018). The sustainability of evidence-based interventions and practices in public health and health care. *Annual Review of Public Health, 39*(1), 55–76. https://doi.org/10.1146/annurev-publhealth-040617-014731

Shelton, R. C., Dunston, S. K., Leoce, N., Jandorf, L., Thompson, H. S., Crookes, D. M., & Erwin, D. O. (2016). Predictors of activity level and retention among African American lay health advisors (LHAs) from The National Witness Project: Implications for the implementation and sustainability of community-based LHA programs from a longitudinal study. *Implementation Science, 11*, Article 41. https://doi.org/10.1186/s13012-016-0403-9

Shelton, R. C., & Lee, M. (2019). Sustaining evidence-based interventions and policies: Recent innovations and future directions in implementation science. *American Journal of Public Health, 109*(S2), S132–S134. https://doi.org/10.2105/ajph.2018.304913

Shoesmith, A., Hall, A., Wolfenden, L., Shelton, R. C., Powell, B. J., Brown, H., McCrabb, S., Sutherland, R., Yoong, S. L., Lane, C., Booth, D., & Nathan, N. (2021). Barriers and facilitators influencing the sustainment of health behaviour interventions in schools and childcare services: A systematic review. *Implementation Science, 16*, Article 62. https://doi.org/10.1186/s13012-021-01134-y

Stoll, S., Janevic, M., Lara, M., Ramos-Valencia, G., Stephens, T. B., Persky, V., Uyeda, K., Ohadike, Y., & Malveaux, F. (2015). A mixed-method application of the Program Sustainability Assessment Tool to evaluate the sustainability of 4 pediatric asthma care coordination programs. *Preventing Chronic Disease, 12*, 150133. https://doi.org/10.5888/pcd12.150133

Strong, W. B., Malina, R. M., Blimkie, C. J., Daniels, S. R., Dishman, R. K., Gutin, B., Hergenroeder, A. C., Must, A., Nixon, P. A., Pivarnik, J. M., Rowland, T., Trost, S., & Trudeau, F. (2005). Evidence based physical activity for school-age youth. *Journal of Pediatrics, 146*(6), 732–737. https://doi.org/10.1016/j.jpeds.2005.01.055

Sutherland, R., Nathan, N., Brown, A., Yoong, S. L., Finch, M., Lecathelinais, C., Reynolds, R., Walton, A., Janssen, L., Desmet, C., Gillham, K., Herrmann, V., Hall, A., Wiggers, J., & Wolfenden, L. (2019). A randomized controlled trial to assess the potential efficacy, feasibility and acceptability of an m-health intervention targeting parents of school aged children to improve the nutritional quality of foods packed in the lunchbox 'SWAP IT'. *International Journal of Behavioral Nutrition and Physical Activity, 16*, Article 54. https://doi.org/10.1186/s12966-019-0812-7

Tabak, R. G., Duggan, K., Smith, C., Aisaka, K., Moreland-Russell, S., & Brownson, R. C. (2016). Assessing capacity for sustainability of effective programs and policies in local health departments. *Journal of Public Health Management and Practice, 22*(2), 129–137. https://doi.org/10.1097/PHH.0000000000000254

Tabak, R. G., Khoong, E. C., Chambers, D. A., & Brownson, R. C. (2012). Bridging research and practice: Models for dissemination and implementation research. *American Journal of Preventive Medicine, 43*(3), 337–350. https://doi.org/10.1016/j.amepre.2012.05.024

Vamos, S., Mumbi, M., Cook, R., Chitalu, N., Weiss, S. M., & Jones, D. L. (2014). Translation and sustainability of an HIV prevention intervention in Lusaka, Zambia. *Translational Behavioral Medicine, 4*(2), 141–148. https://doi.org/10.1007/s13142-013-0237-9

Vitale, R., Blaine, T., Zofkie, E., Moreland-Russell, S., Combs, T., Brownson, R. C., & Luke, D. A. (2018). Developing an evidence-based program sustainability training curriculum: A group randomized, multi-phase approach. *Implementation Science, 13*, Article 126. https://doi.org/10.1186/s13012-018-0819-5

Walkosz, B. J., Buller, D. B., Andersen, P. A., Scott, M. D., & Cutter, G. R. (2015). The sustainability of an occupational skin cancer prevention program. *Journal of Occupational and Environmental Medicine, 57*(11), 1207–1213. https://doi.org/10.1097/JOM.0000000000000544

Walugembe, D. R., Sibbald, S., Le Ber, M. J., & Kothari, A. (2019). Sustainability of public health interventions: Where are the gaps? *Health Research Policy and Systems, 17*, Article 8. https://doi.org/10.1186/s12961-018-0405-y

West, R., Michie, S., Atkins, L., Chadwick, P., & Lorencatto, F. (2019). *Achieving behaviour change: A guide for local government and partners*. Public Health England Publications. https://assets.publishing.service.gov.uk/government/uploads/system/uploads/attachment_data/file/875385/PHEBI_Achieving_Behaviour_Change_Local_Government.pdf

Wiltsey Stirman, S., Finley, E. P., Shields, N., Cook, J., Haine-Schlagel, R., Burgess, J. F., Jr., Dimeff, L., Koerner, K., Suvak, M., Gutner, C. A., Gagnon, D., Masina, T., Beristianos, M., Mallard, K., Ramirez, V., & Monson, C. (2017). Improving and sustaining delivery of CPT for PTSD in mental health systems: A cluster randomized trial. *Implementation Science, 12*, Article 32. https://doi.org/10.1186/s13012-017-0544-5

Wiltsey Stirman, S., Kimberly, J., Cook, N., Calloway, A., Castro, F., & Charns, M. (2012). The sustainability of new programs and innovations: A review of the empirical literature and recommendations for future research. *Implementation Science, 7*, Article 17. https://doi.org/10.1186/1748-5908-7-17

Wolfenden, L., Goldman, S., Stacey, F. G., Grady, A., Kingsland, M., Williams, C. M., Wiggers, J., Milat, A., Rissel, C., Bauman, A., Farrell, M. M., Légaré, F., Charif, A. B., Zomahoun, H. T. V., Hodder, R. K., Jones, J., Booth, D., Parmenter, B., Regan, T., & Yoong, S. L. (2018). Strategies to improve the implementation of workplace-based policies or practices targeting tobacco, alcohol, diet, physical activity and obesity. *Cochrane Database of Systematic Reviews*, (11), Article CD012439. https://doi.org/10.1002/14651858.CD012439.pub2

Wolfenden, L., Jones, J., Williams, C. M., Finch, M., Wyse, R. J., Kingsland, M., Tzelepis, F., Wiggers, J., Williams, A. J., Seward, K., Small, T., Welch, V., Booth, D., & Yoong, S. L. (2016). Strategies to improve the implementation of healthy eating, physical activity and obesity prevention policies, practices or programmes within childcare services. *Cochrane Database of Systematic Reviews*, (2), Article Cd011779. https://doi.org/10.1002/14651858.CD011779.pub2

Wolfenden, L., Nathan, N., Janssen, L. M., Wiggers, J., Reilly, K., Delaney, T., Williams, C. M., Bell, C., Wyse, R., Sutherland, R., Campbell, L., Lecathelinais, C., Oldmeadow, C., Freund, M., & Yoong, S. L. (2017). Multi-strategic intervention to enhance implementation of healthy canteen policy: A randomised controlled trial. *Implementation Science, 12*, Article 6. https://doi.org/10.1186/s13012-016-0537-9

Wolfenden, L., Nathan, N. K., Sutherland, R., Yoong, S. L., Hodder, R. K., Wyse, R. J., Delaney, T., Grady, A., Fielding, A., & Tzelepis, F. (2017). Strategies for enhancing the implementation of school-based policies or practices targeting risk factors for chronic disease. *Cochrane Database of Systematic Reviews*, (11), Article CD011677. https://doi.org/10.1002/14651858.CD011677.pub2

Yin, R. K. (1981). Life histories of innovations: How new practices become routinized. *Public Administration Review, 41*(1), 21–28. https://doi.org/10.2307/975720

13

De-Implementing Low-Value Practices in Healthcare and Public Health

Christian D. Helfrich, Barbara R. Majerczyk, and Elspeth Nolen

Learning Objectives

By the end of this chapter, readers will be able to:

- Define and provide examples of low-value practices and their cost
- Explain why low-value practices occur and persist
- Describe challenges and unintended consequences that make de-implementing low-value practices different than implementation
- Select from among de-implementation strategies and plan for adapting de-implementation strategies for a specific low-value practice

CASE STUDY 13.1 THE INHALER

Dr. B., a primary care provider in rural Washington State, was preparing for clinic by pulling up the electronic health records (EHRs) for patients she was scheduled to see that day and noticed a new note in one of the patient files. The EHR of Mr. L. had been flagged by a pulmonary team at the clinic's affiliated regional medical center. The note indicated that the pulmonary team was reviewing the charts of patients with chronic obstructive pulmonary disease (COPD) who were prescribed inhaled corticosteroids (ICS), which included Mr. L.'s. Mr. L. had been prescribed an ICS some time ago after an emergency department (ED) visit for breathing difficulty. Dr. B. recalled being uncomfortable when learning of the new prescription from the patient at a subsequent primary care appointment. Mr. L. was already on a combination inhaler of two long-acting agents that Dr. B. understood to be the current standard-of-care for COPD. But treatment guidelines for COPD had become significantly more complex in recent years. This complexity caused Dr. B. to be reluctant to second-guess the ED physician, who might have made the decision based on tests she did not have access to. However, what Dr. B. now read in the pulmonary team's note was that the innocuous inhaler posed a small but real health risk to Mr. L. The pulmonary team's note indicated that for every 62 patients on an ICS, within 1 year you could expect one of those patients to contract pneumonia who otherwise wouldn't. For a patient of Mr. L.'s age and history of breathing difficulties contracting pneumonia was a very serious risk.

The pulmonary team had made it simple to change the prescription for the ED-prescribed ICS, by including an unsigned order with the note. The order would go to the patient's pharmacy. It included instructions to separate the ICS from the long-acting agents, and to gradually eliminate the ICS. However, as the primary care provider, it was ultimately Dr. B.'s decision whether to sign the order or not. The pulmonary team's note vindicated her earlier doubts about the ICS, but Dr. B. still felt uncertain. Mr. L. was an anxious patient; he had been through several recent health scares and he was doing well right now. Dr. B. didn't want to cause her patient further anxiety, and momentarily considered not signing the order and leaving Mr. L.'s prescriptions alone. Ultimately, however, Dr. B. agreed with the pulmonary team's recommendation.

Later in the exam room with Mr. L., Dr. B. explained why she was recommending he no longer use the ICS. Mr. L. nodded in agreement, but Dr. B. sensed apprehension and asked if he had thoughts or questions about the change in inhalers. Mr. L. said he understood there were downsides to the medication, but that having it for an emergency felt like a security blanket. She asked what he meant by having it for an emergency? He talked about the trip to the ED when he couldn't breathe. He thought he was going to die. Dr. B. nodded and shared her worry that the ICS didn't prevent an episode like that; to the contrary, the ICS was going to be the cause of Mr. L. ending up in the ED with pneumonia. Dr. B. proposed a middle course, where Mr. L. would begin by gradually reducing ICS use over an agreed period, and then at their next appointment together they would discuss how it was going. If Mr. L. felt at that point like his breathing was getting worse with less use of the ICS, they could talk about doing something else. It didn't have to be an all-or-nothing choice. Mr. L. agreed to this plan, and at the end of the visit, Dr. B. electronically signed the order to change the prescription. Dr. B. reflected on the encounter with Mr. L. Primary care

(*continued*)

CASE STUDY 13.1 THE INHALER (*continued*)

physicians rarely had sufficient time for nuanced conversation with patients. It was clear that de-prescribing Mr. L.'s ICS would have caused the patient distress without that nuanced conversation to make sure he understood, and in turn that she had understood him and his concerns.

INTRODUCTION

This case study (13.1) is based on real physicians and real patients (Parikh et al., 2020; Stryczek et al., 2020) dealing with a real problem: ending use of an ineffective or harmful practice. **De-implementation** involves removing or reducing a routinely used treatment or practice that fails to deliver the expected benefits, and conversely actually increases risks of harm. This problem is not limited to ICSs, and it is not limited to medicine. In every field, whether public health, healthcare, or education, some practices that gain widespread use turn out to be ineffective or even counterproductive.

In some cases, practices are adopted based on the promise of early research that ultimately fails to deliver the expected results or that fails to anticipate harms. This usually happens when research findings are from highly controlled settings, from weak study designs, or when findings have not been replicated and evaluated adequately in real-world settings. In other cases, practices based on habit, tradition, or pseudoscience get passed along and are never examined against the available evidence or are never critically examined at all. As a result, we have a subset of public health and healthcare practices that we invest with limited resources for no benefit, and which often return a net harm. We broadly refer to these as **low-value practices and programs**, and we refer to systematic efforts to reduce low-value practices and programs as de-implementation.

The purpose of this chapter is to equip you with knowledge and tools to de-implement low-value practices. This chapter provides background on how to define low-value practices; highlights some of the reasons they occur and persist; discusses what makes de-implementing low-value practices particularly challenging; and reviews current knowledge about effective strategies to de-implement low-value practices. We also discuss potential unintended consequences from de-implementation and how we might avoid them. The chapter concludes with how to avoid compounding problems when de-implementing low-value practices.

DEFINING THE PROBLEM

Low-value practices are practices that either fail to provide any benefit, or where the risk of harm outweighs the expected benefit (Grimshaw et al., 2020; McKay et al., 2018). Low-value practices also occur when a practice does not align with the client's preferences (e.g., services that clients do not benefit from or do not want once they understand the benefits, risks, and cost [Berwick, 2019; Berwick & Hackbarth, 2012]). How common are low-value practices? It depends on the setting and the type of practice, but it appears to be a major problem in every country and healthcare system where the problem has been studied (Brownlee et al., 2017). In the U.S. healthcare system, where the most published research is available, studies have found a wide range of low-value practice prevalence. On the low-end, 10% to 16% of care represents unneeded or harmful care, and on the high end these low-value practices comprise 30% to 46% of care (Morgan et al., 2015; Niven et al., 2015; Scott, 2019). A 2019 study sought to estimate the total cost of low-value practices in the U.S. healthcare system, and concluded that the United States spends between $75.7 billion and $101.2 billion on low-value practices in healthcare (Shrank et al., 2019).

Undoubtedly these figures vary by country and healthcare or public health system. Yet we lack reliable figures in many settings, notably for non-healthcare settings, and for many low- and middle-income countries (LMICs). Nevertheless, there are two reasons to think that the burden of low-value practices and programs is likewise heavy for non-healthcare settings and for under-resourced healthcare settings often found in LMICs. First, there are well-documented examples of low-value practices and programs in these settings that have had profound costs while producing no benefits or documented harms. A notable example is the $1.4 billion dollars invested in abstinence-only sex education to reduce the spread of HIV in 22 sub-Saharan African countries that was found to have no effect on behavior or HIV risk (Lo et al., 2016). Second, as we'll discuss later in the chapter, many drivers of low-value care in healthcare appear to be equally applicable to public health programs and to non-U.S. healthcare settings. Additional research is needed to establish valid, reliable estimates of the extent of low-value practices and programs in a broader range of countries and settings, but in each instance where researchers have looked for low-value practices and programs, they have been found. Low-value practices and programs are widespread, pernicious, and costly.

DRIVERS OF LOW-VALUE CARE AND IMPLICATIONS FOR DE-IMPLEMENTATION

We can think of the drivers of low-value practices on two different levels: *Why do low-value practices exist in the first place? Why are those low-value practices still widely used even after we become aware of their harm and cost?* Understanding the answers to these questions can help us both reduce the likelihood that low-value practices gain a foothold in practice to begin with and help de-implementation teams better deal with the challenge of eliminating low-value practices when we inevitably discover them.

WHY DO LOW-VALUE PRACTICES EXIST?

Tradition-Based Practice

Practices and programs are often tradition-based, meaning they are taught as standard practice during training, or inherited when we join an organization or community (Hanrahan et al., 2015). Tradition-based practices are adopted uncritically without first posing the question: Does this work? Examples of tradition-based practices assumed to be effective include the use of episiotomies in obstetrics to prevent vaginal tearing during childbirth (Montini & Graham, 2015), and the D.A.R.E. (Drug Abuse Resistance Education) school-based program in the United States (West & O'Neal, 2004). Tradition-based practices and programs are often based on valid observations but inappropriate inferences. For example, in the case of episiotomies, obstetricians observed that vaginal tearing often occurred during childbirth (valid observation) but erroneously inferred that a pre-emptive incision (an episiotomy) was more desirable than allowing a tear to occur. As incisions heal less quickly than naturally occurring tears, this turned out to be untrue (Hartmann et al., 2005). In the case of D.A.R.E., the program was developed by police and teachers in Los Angeles based on their valid observation that the kids they interacted with faced peer pressure to use drugs. However, they incorrectly inferred that having police deliver anti-drug messages to kids in school would improve kids' self-esteem and therefore their abilities to resist invitations to try drugs and alcohol (Nordrum, 2014). Those working in specific professions, or working in a particular policy domain, may identify strongly with a tradition-based practice, and consequently feel attacked when these practices are questioned. We discuss the phenomenon of psychological reactance in more detail later in the chapter (see the section "Mitigating Unintended Consequences: Psychological Reactance").

While the evidence-based medicine movement has helped create a norm to establish evidence for biomedical practices, standards of evidence are generally much lower for public health practice, educational systems, health promotion and disease prevention, and for health and public-health policies and programs. For example, a recent literature review found that only 18% of healthcare delivery intervention studies (as opposed to biomedical intervention studies) used some form of randomization to better isolate the effects of the intervention and avoid drawing conclusions from spurious associations (Finkelstein & Taubman, 2015). This lower standard of evidence is also partly responsible for implementation of low-value care and the persistence of tradition-based practices in fields outside biomedicine.

Scientific Evolution

A hypothetical world where healthcare and public health programs were exclusively based on the best available evidence would still end up with low-value practices because science across fields constantly evolves. Consequently, what constitutes the best evidence today is different than what constituted the best evidence yesterday. This means that evidence-based practices that attain widespread use will sometimes turn out to be ineffective, inaccurate, or harmful. While some of the changes in evidence are modifications or elaborations of prior knowledge, in some cases knowledge is proven false. One example of this is the use of hormone replacement therapy (HRT) to reduce some of the uncomfortable symptoms of menopause. HRT turned out to have more risks than benefits, including increased risk of some of the same chronic diseases that HRT was originally thought to help prevent (Cagnacci & Venier, 2019).

In *The Half-life of Facts* (2013), Samuel Arbesman explores how our understanding of the objective facts of the world have evolved and will continue to evolve. Arbesman documents how in many fields knowledge evolves and decays at a predictable rate. We can't know for sure which "facts" will turn out to be incorrect, but it may be possible to predict what proportion of our knowledge will be overturned over time. An interesting example is Hall and colleagues' literature analysis (1997) of the half-life of accepted facts in surgery. The authors took a sample of studies from general surgery published in *Surgery, Gynaecology and Obstetrics* from 1935 to 1994 (260 studies total), summarized the findings from each study. A panel of seven surgeons then independently evaluated the veracity of the principal findings in each summary, judging each one as correct or incorrect according to current evidence. Based on their summaries, the authors calculated the half-life of facts in surgery at 47 years. This means that for an accepted set of facts in surgery, after a period of approximately 47 years, half of those facts were amended or overturned. To illustrate, among surgical practices once accepted as effective were many practices now known to be inappropriate, including prefrontal lobotomy to address patient anxiety, fear, or fear of impending death; lumbodorsal sympathectomy (i.e., cutting or blocking a nerve) for malignant hypertension; and surgery for gastric ulcer.

Poynard and colleagues (2002) conducted a similar analysis of research published from 1945 to 1999 on cirrhosis or hepatitis in adults and concluded that the half-life of facts in that literature was 45 years. It may be a coincidence that these two literature reviews both determined the half-life to be approximately 45 years, as the samples studied are far too limited to generalize from. Instead, these studies show that when there are vast literatures continuously producing new knowledge, some portion of the accumulated knowledge will cease to be true over time. Rates of change can be estimated, which may be useful in strategically planning to support clinicians updating their skills and knowledge over the course of a career.

There are three primary implications of scientific evolution for de-implementation. First, expect and plan for the underlying evidence base to evolve over time. Anticipate and plan for this eventuality through regular evaluation (see the section "Systems-Level De-implementation Strategies," and The Abdul Latif Jameel Poverty Action Lab, https://www.povertyactionlab.org/evidence-to-policy/scaling-back-evaluated-program). Systems can establish protocols for how to efficiently and systematically de-implement policies and programs once they have been evaluated and found to be ineffective or harmful. These protocols might include re-allocating budgeted funds, shifting personnel to new assignments, revising training programs, changing performance measures or goals, and planning for additional monitoring to ensure ineffective or harmful practices are in fact de-implemented. Second, evidence that has withstood the test of time ought to be viewed with greater confidence. This is not the same as accepting that something is appropriate simply because it's the way it has always been done. Rather, greater confidence should be placed in each practice or piece of knowledge the longer it has been subjected to scrutiny and has not yet been refuted (Ridley & Ganser, 2010).

Finally, we have less confidence in a completely new evidence-based practice, even when it is the result of very rigorous methods, and the measured effect is very strong (Ioannidis, 2005). Novel evidence-based practices have not yet survived repeated efforts to invalidate them, and the robustness of those findings across contexts is not yet known. This stands as a counterpoint to the impulse to speed innovations into practice, and to the popular concern about an average delay of 17 years to translate research into clinical practice (Balas & Boren, 2000). While delaying the dissemination and implementation of evidence-based care has serious implications, there can be an advantage to delayed adoption in terms of confidence in that the evidence base for the practice is robust.

Reproducibility and Pseudoscience

In addition to knowledge evolving as a function of science working correctly, there are serious threats to knowledge from the corruption of science. There are two distinct concerns: a crisis in the replication of findings on evidence-based practice in medicine and psychology (Resnick, 2016), and the promotion of pseudoscience (Bluestone, 2021; Caulfield, 2015; Oreskes, 2021).

The **replication crisis** is a failure to corroborate major findings in subsequent studies. This crisis first came to prominence in the field of psychology when a team of researchers attempted to replicate findings from 100 studies published in three of the top psychology journals (Open Science Collaboration, 2015). While 97% of the original studies reported a significant main finding, only 36% of the replications did, and the replication studies generally found approximately half the effect size (an indication of the strength of the associations being studied) of the original studies. While psychology remains the field where the replication crisis has been most examined and discussed, replication problems are emerging in nearly every field of science (Ritchie, 2019). Likely these crises are a function of bias in which findings get published and which do not, otherwise known as **publication bias**. Publication bias is often chalked up to journals' unwillingness to publish negative findings or replication studies. But authors also contribute to spurious findings through practices like *p*-hacking (i.e., defining outcomes different ways until you find a statistically significant result, as indicated by the *p*-value) and HARKing (hypothesizing after results are known). Additionally, scientists self-censor their research by declining to submit negative or null findings for publication.

One way to address the crisis of replication is simply more replication. Some research organizations are building replication into their missions and making the identification and elimination of failed practices an explicit part of their work. An example of this is the *International Initiative for Impact Evaluation* (3IE), which funds replication studies of public health and development programs, and reports on programs that fail to improve health outcomes and are recommended to close (3IE, 2021). In one instance, 3IE conducted and evaluated an intervention in Ghana to train women to build and use an improved clay cook stove design. The new stove design had been promoted as using less fuel and producing less pollution. 3IE evaluated the effect of the intervention on time spent collecting wood for fuel and respiratory-related health outcomes, but found the new stoves were no better than the traditional stoves. Because the new stoves were often constructed indoors instead of outdoors as traditional stoves often were, this could have unintentionally increased exposure to worse air quality (3IE, 2020). 3IE is now working to de-implement the new stoves.

Another challenge is the abundance of products and advice that present themselves as science-based while being pseudoscience. **Pseudoscience** adopts the language of science, but not the methods (Oreskes, 2021), and is used to persuade, often for the purpose of selling a product (Bluestone, 2021; Caulfield, 2015). A major barrier to eliminating pseudoscience is the effort it takes to refute it. While promoting a false health or policy claim requires little time or effort, the process of investigating, evaluating, and debunking such claims requires time and care (Williamson, 2016). It is impossible to prove a negative, so debunking a pseudoscientific claim often means documenting how an exhaustive search for evidence has turned up no evidence to support the original claim. As a result, many pseudoscientific claims go unchallenged. In healthcare and public health, we spend much more time evaluating and critiquing the products of scientific research than the pseudoscientific claims of product marketers.

WHY LOW-VALUE PRACTICES ARE USED

As Morgan and colleagues document, one of the challenges with low-value healthcare is that a range of factors condition us as individuals and as a society to be susceptible to it (see Table 13.1; Morgan et al., 2015). Morgan and colleagues draw two distinctions that are useful for thinking through the drivers of low-value practices in any setting: First, factors influencing those receiving the low-value practices (e.g., clients) versus factors influencing those delivering low-value practices (e.g., practitioners); second, factors internal (i.e., intrinsic) to the individuals (e.g., client and practitioner knowledge, beliefs, and tendencies), versus factors external (i.e., extrinsic) to the individuals (e.g., social, organizational, and political environments that client and practitioner inhabit).

Many intrinsic and extrinsic factors influence clients' and practitioners' use of low-value practices. Practitioners often lack knowledge (intrinsic factor) about the potential harms from overuse, such as downstream consequences of over testing, while at the same time over-estimating the potential benefits of the practice (Hoffmann & Del Mar, 2017). Clients feel discomfort with uncertainty about outcomes (intrinsic factor) that often arises when making changes to their care (Bokhof & Junius-Walker, 2016). Practitioners often rely on practice guidelines (extrinsic factor) to make decisions about care, but guidelines typically focus on recommending the practices clients should receive and focus less on

TABLE 13.1 Key Drivers of Low-Value Practices in Healthcare

	INTRINSIC	EXTRINSIC
Provider/healthcare system level	Lack of knowledge of harm from overuse Belief more care is better Discomfort with uncertainty Regret for errors of omission > commission Belief action better than inaction Use of therapeutics off label	Guidelines promoting overuse Medical culture Financial incentives for provider and hospital Process measures Inadequate time Positive publication bias Lack of training in shared decision-making Advocacy groups Medicalization of non-disease
Patient/public level	Discomfort with uncertainty Belief more care is better Lack of knowledge of harm from overuse	Media misrepresentation of research Financial—third party payment shielding from costs Culture of avoiding mortality Advocacy groups Medicalization of non-disease

Source: From Morgan, D. J., Brownlee, S., Leppin, A. L., Kressin, N., Dhruva, S. S., Levin, L., Landon, B. E., Zezza, M. A., Schmidt, H., Saini, V., & Elshaug, A. G. (2015). Setting a research agenda for medical overuse. *BMJ*, 351, h354. https://doi.org/10.1136/bmj.h4534

highlighting low-value practices that should be avoided (Morgan et al., 2015). For clients, the media often misrepresents research findings by promoting the implications of promising research while downplaying both the uncertainty about the highlighted research and any potential side effects (Bluestone, 2021). As discussed below under "Strategies to De-implement Low-Value Practices," distinguishing these different drivers of low-value practices may help identify promising strategies to eliminate them.

CASE STUDY 13.2: DE-IMPLEMENTING INHALED CORTICOSTEROIDS TO IMPROVE CARE AND SAFETY OF U.S. MILITARY VETERANS WITH COPD

COPD is one of the most frequent medical diagnoses among U.S. military veterans. People with COPD can have trouble breathing and are often put on medication to help alleviate these breathing problems. An ICS can help these patients if they have severe airflow limitation or frequent exacerbations. However, for patients who don't have airflow limitation or frequent exacerbations, ICSs do not provide any benefit beyond long-acting agents (LAMA/LABAs). At the same time, ICSs increase patients' risk of severe pneumonia. So why do providers keep patients on ICSs? Case Study 13.1 highlighted one challenge experienced by a primary care provider when de-implementing a low-value practice with an individual patient with COPD.

With rapidly changing guidelines for many chronic conditions, it can be challenging for primary care providers (PCPs) to stay current on standards of care for every

(*continued*)

CASE STUDY 13.2: DE-IMPLEMENTING INHALED CORTICOSTEROIDS TO IMPROVE CARE AND SAFETY OF U.S. MILITARY VETERANS WITH COPD *(continued)*

disease process and treatment. PCPs can refer patients to pulmonary specialists to ask for input about how the patient's care might be improved, but unless and until the patient has a problem, the PCP usually does not make a referral. In response to this barrier, the pulmonary specialty team in Case Study 13.1 decided to try to flip the way consultations were occurring and tested a de-implementation intervention where they proactively reviewed patient electronic health records (EHRs) to scan for patients with COPD with current prescriptions for ICSs. The de-implementation intervention included reviewing the charts of patients with COPD and determining if the patient should be on an ICS. If there was no indication for the medication, the pulmonary team made a recommendation (called an e-consult) to take the patient off the ICS. To make it as easy as possible for the PCP to de-implement the patient's low-value medication, the recommendation to discontinue or taper the ICSs was entered as a chart note accompanying a pharmacy order but was left unsigned. This meant that when the patient's PCP next opened the chart, they would see the note and the recommendation (see, e.g., Figure 13.1). This left the ultimate decision to de-implement ICSs to the PCP.

- What issues might emerge because of the proactive e-consult by the pulmonary team? Are there issues that could emerge among PCPs? What about among patients?
- As happened in Case Study 13.1, the pulmonary specialty team discovered that the inappropriate ICS prescriptions they identified were sometimes made by other providers and not by the patient's current PCP. How might that affect efforts to de-implement inappropriate ICS prescriptions?
- What issues might a health system want to consider before expanding implementation of a proactive e-consult program like this one?

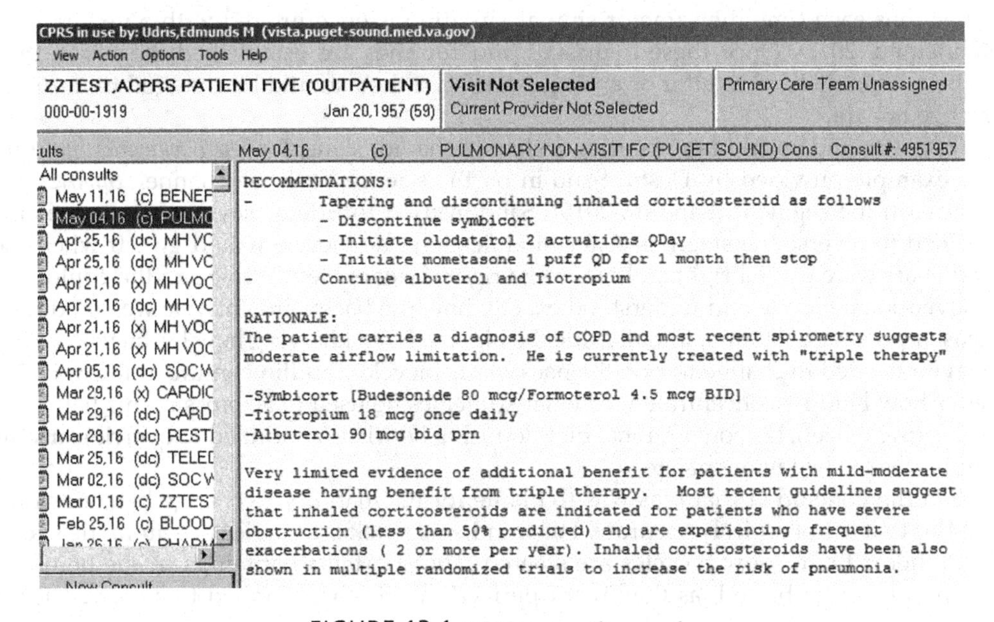

FIGURE 13.1 COPD e-consult example.

WHAT MAKES DE-IMPLEMENTATION DIFFERENT?

Is de-implementation meaningfully different from implementation? The frameworks that guide implementation look equally relevant to de-implementation (Grimshaw et al., 2020; Nilsen et al., 2020a), some implementation outcomes can be adapted for de-implementation (Prusaczyk et al., 2020), and some of the same strategies (e.g., audit and feedback) have been used for both implementation and de-implementation (Colla et al., 2017). In many respects, de-implementation is just the flipside of implementation (van Bodegom-Vos et al., 2017). However, there are at least three things that make de-implementing low-value practices fundamentally different from implementing evidence-based practices. The first is the challenge of changing behaviors and practices that are already routine; the second is the role of partisans and advocates for existing practices; and the third is an asymmetry in outcomes. These differences are important if de-implementation efforts are to be successful and to avoid creating new problems while de-implementing low-value practices. Let's discuss each in turn.

LOW-VALUE PRACTICES ARE ALREADY EMBEDDED IN HEURISTICS AND ROUTINES

Much of individual behavior and the collective behavior of teams and organizations is guided by heuristics and routines (Fiol & O'Connor, 2017a, 2017b; Kahneman, 2011). **Heuristics and routines** are decision rules and patterns of behavior that we enact in response to specific settings, events, or feelings, and which develop over time as we encounter the same or a similar problem. Examples in healthcare include when an individual clinician develops heuristics for how to help a patient who has recently begun experiencing severe shortness of breath climbing the stairs, or when a health promotion team develops a routine for conducting outreach and enrollment of employers in workplace wellness programs. These heuristics and routines are generally more reliable, effective, and efficient than consciously recreating an individualized set of decisions and actions each time the same or similar situation is encountered with a new patient (Kahneman, 2011). Once these heuristics and routines are established, however, they can be extremely hard to alter or extinguish even if they should be changed to improve practice or care.

To better understand how heuristics shape behavior, consider *The Backwards Brain Bicycle* example provided by Destin Sandlin on the science YouTube channel, *Smarter Every Day*. In the segment (Sandlin, 2015), Sandlin tried to ride a bicycle that a mechanic modified to reverse the steering. After modification, the bicycle would go left when the handlebars were turned right and would go right if steered left. While Sandlin could ride a conventional bicycle and understood exactly how the backwards bicycle was modified, it was impossible for him to initially ride the bicycle. Even knowing how his bicycle-riding behavior needed to change to ride the backwards bicycle, Sandlin continued to crash. No matter how hard he concentrated, or what strategies he used (e.g., crossing his hands on the steering wheel), his conventional bicycle-riding heuristic continued to override any attempts at rapid behavior change.

Sandlin concluded that bias was to blame for his inability to change behavior rapidly, but that is not entirely accurate. His mind was stuck on a series of automatic shortcuts: a heuristic for how bicycles are steered. The shortcuts contained in the heuristic are not inherently biased, as they work perfectly well when applied to a conventional

FIGURE 13.2 Scan to watch *The Backwards Brain Bicycle* on YouTube.

bicycle. What makes the conventional bicycle-riding heuristic maladaptive is the context. When the steering is reversed on the modified bicycle, the shortcuts involved in the conventional bicycle heuristic no longer work. Eventually, Sandlin was able to ride the bicycle by spending 8 months practicing, overriding the conventional-bicycle heuristic through careful concentration, effort, and practice. The process of unlearning an established heuristic was painful and at first any distraction caused him to crash, but through persistence Sandlin finally established a new heuristic for steering the backwards bicycle. Watch the video at https://youtu.be/MFzDaBzBlL0 or scan the QR code in Figure 13.2.

Low-value practices have sometimes been in use for years and are embedded both in habit and heuristics at an individual level (Ingvarsson et al., 2020), and embedded in policies, standards, and routines at a group or organizational level (Bourgault & Upvall, 2019; Hanrahan et al., 2015). A heuristic or routine that results in a low-value practice in one context (e.g., mammography guidelines that result in low-risk women receiving unnecessary invasive tests and erroneously believing they have cancer) might produce very positive outcomes in another (e.g., high-risk women having treatable cancers identified early; Woloshin & Schwartz, 2010). Even when what needs to happen to end a low-value practice or program is known, it can be difficult to not revert to the old practice or program without a great deal of attention, time, and effort. The time and effort necessary to suppress an old heuristic and routine while establishing a new one is a challenging part of what makes de-implementation distinct from implementation.

Key Points for Practice: Ways to Mitigate Effects of Heuristics and Routines During De-Implementation

It may be more effective to introduce a new, substitute practice or program instead of only trying to suppress or eliminate the old one (Helfrich et al., 2018; Patey et al., 2021). With this approach, the effort shifts to the adoption and implementation of the substitute practice or program, which is designed to displace the low-value practice or program. This replacement program or practice is sometimes termed an

(continued)

Key Points for Practice: Ways to Mitigate Effects of Heuristics and Routines During De-Implementation (*continued*)

incompatible substitute because continuing to use the low-value practice or program is incompatible with the adoption of the new practice. For example, a strategy referred to as "watchful waiting" is often proposed for people diagnosed with localized prostate cancer who have no symptoms, and who have low risk of dying from it (NCI, 2021). Prostate cancers typically grow slowly and if diagnosis is received at an advanced age, the patient is unlikely to die from it. Conversely, treating the cancer with a surgery called radical prostatectomy has a very high likelihood of causing major life-altering side effects such as permanent impotence and incontinence. The term *watchful waiting* was coined to communicate to patients that they and their providers can monitor symptoms and only proceed with treatment if there are signs the cancer is causing problems. As watchful waiting was adopted, use of radical prostatectomy declined. In this example watchful waiting serves as an incompatible substitute practice for a radical prostatectomy to treat low-risk prostate cancer (Mahal et al., 2019).

PARTISANS AND STAKEHOLDERS

Any established practice or program has partisans. **Partisans** are people or institutions that are invested literally or figuratively in the practice, whether financially, professionally, politically, or personally (Norton & Chambers, 2020). In some cases, the investment may be minor and amenable to persuasion. However, in many cases there are highly invested partisans and any efforts to de-implement the practice they have invested in can be met with a great deal of hostility. In addition to partisans who are invested in some way in the low-value practice, there are **stakeholders**, who affect or are affected by the low-value practice and might include clients, consumers, and community members (Prusaczyk et al., 2020). When we try to implement a new evidence-based practice, one of our challenges is recruiting stakeholders to champion and support the implementation effort (Greenhalgh et al., 2004). We identify and recruit stakeholders to make them aware of the existence of the evidence-based practice, its potential benefit and what needs to be done to make it available to patients (in the case of healthcare) or clients/the public (in the case of health promotion or public health practices). The inverse is the case in de-implementation. If a low-value practice continues to be delivered, there are one or more stakeholders.

Consequently, at the outset of a de-implementation effort you should ask: *Who could potentially be harmed by your de-implementation efforts? Who has invested in this practice and may resist its de-implementation?* For example, following controversies over the agency's clinical guidelines, in 1995 the U.S. *Agency for Health Care Policy and Research* (AHCPR, now the *Agency for Health Research and Quality*, AHRQ) was threatened with defunding by Congress (Deyo, 2008; Lo & Field, 2009). Interest groups comprised of practitioners and industry representatives were concerned that these clinical guidelines would lead to reductions in the services they provided and were perceived as a government infringement on private healthcare. These interest groups lobbied Congress to eliminate funding for AHCPR, which nearly succeeded, and the agency subsequently discontinued work on developing and disseminating evidence-based guidelines (Lo & Field, 2009).

Key Points for Practice: Ways to Counteract Efforts of Partisans

1. **Identify who bears the burden or cost of de-implementation:** Typically, a relatively small number of stakeholders (partisans) are invested in a low-value practice while a larger group bears the burden or cost. That cost may not be easily visible to other stakeholders or to the de-implementation team. See the example of avoidable deaths from anesthesiology in the section "Specific Strategies for De-Implementation: Systems and Organizations."
2. **Create a guiding coalition to balance competing interests:** There is often an interest mismatch between a small group of stakeholders who have an interest in supporting the low-value practice, and a much larger group of stakeholders (e.g., patients, payers) who have a comparatively weak interest or ability to oppose it. It is not unusual for proponents of the low-value practice to have greater leverage when advocating their interest to continue the low-value practice. This includes having the time, effort, knowledge, and resources available to do so, while those opposed to the low-value practice generally have diffused interests and widely varying responsibilities. This can be countered at least in part by creating a large coalition made up of representatives from parties with mutual interest in *reducing or eliminating low-value practices*. One example of this is the *Choosing Wisely* campaign in healthcare (Wolfson et al., 2014). *Choosing Wisely* is a coalition of consumer-rights advocates (Consumer Reports) and professional societies (e.g., American College of Cardiology) led by the American Board of Internal Medicine Foundation that engages with health systems and payers to act on overuse of low-value practices (Wolfson et al., 2014). This includes promoting the use of five questions in conversations between patients and clinicians: *Do I really need this test or procedure? What are the risks? Are there simpler, safer options? What happens if I don't do anything? How much does it cost?* (ABIM Foundation, 2018).
3. **Use their power against them:** Sometimes partisans try to resist change by discrediting those raising the alarm about a harmful practice. However, efforts to resist or discredit can increase the visibility of the work of those trying to de-implement the low-value practice. One example of this occurred in the mid-1990s, when a research team published findings questioning the effectiveness of new calcium channel blockers over older (and cheaper) medications for treating hypertension (Deyo, 2008). The researchers were attacked for their efforts by multiple partisans. One of the manufacturers of the new medications complained to the dean of the lead researcher's medical school about the researcher's scientific integrity. Another manufacturer encouraged partisan physicians to submit "Dear Doctor" letters to the editors at major scientific journals that criticized the researcher team's findings. The letters were authored by individual physicians who failed to disclose the involvement and influence of the manufacturer, and made it appear that the letter reflected consensus in the medical community against the researchers (MacCarthy, 1996). The research team even received a *Freedom of Information Act* request from one of the manufacturers. The effort by these partisans to discredit the research team's findings ultimately increased the visibility of their findings and encouraged other researchers to study the same issue. The original research team continued to maintain the integrity of their findings, which were subsequently corroborated multiple times (Deyo, 2008).

ASYMMETRY OF OUTCOMES FOR PRACTITIONERS

In most cases practitioners will experience successful de-implementation as "nothing." For example, a low-value medication is removed, and the patient does not get worse; a demonstrably ineffective health promotion program is eliminated, and clients' health behaviors do not regress; or erroneous recommendations on communicable-disease prevention in public health guidelines are removed, and the incidence of the disease does not increase. While there may be a statistical reduction in harm due to these de-implementation efforts, in contrast to something like cancer screening most often patients or clients do not notice a benefit. In part, this may be due to practitioners' reluctance to discuss the harms that could have been caused by something previously promoted as appropriate or high-value care.

The lack of discernible benefit from de-implementation creates an asymmetry of outcomes when paired with the knowledge that if a bad outcome does occur and is perceived to be due to de-implementation of low-value care, the practitioner will be held responsible. When it comes to de-implementation, practitioners can often see no immediate upside they'll feel good about or get credit for, and a possibility that they would be blamed for a bad outcome. Additionally, practitioners must weigh the potential for retaliation if partisans, clients, or the public believes the motives behind de-implementation are nefarious (see the section in "Mitigating Unintended Consequences: Psychological Reactance").

Even when not highly visible, there are many long-term benefits of de-implementing low-value practices and programs. In some cases (e.g., medications, healthcare procedures, invasive tests) the benefits include a reduction in measurable adverse events (e.g., stroke, infection, death). Resources previously spent on de-implemented practices can be freed up for pressing needs. In some cases (e.g., co-pays, travel time, unpaid time off, deductibles, program fees), de-implementation of low-value practices reduces drain on patient and client resources while increasing the quality of their care.

Nevertheless, many of these benefits will be invisible to the practitioners undertaking de-implementation. This means de-implementation teams need to be attentive to who does and does not see a direct benefit from de-implementation and not assume that all stakeholders view the risks and benefits of de-implementing low-value practices equally (see "Key Points for Practice: Ways to Counteract the Asymmetry of Outcomes").

Key Points for Practice: Ways to Counteract the Asymmetry of Outcomes

1. Counter support for the low-value practice by using real-world examples of the negative consequences: Ask patients or their loved-ones if they want to share their experiences with the negative consequences of the low-value practice (e.g., see Welch et al., 2011).
2. Create positive reinforcement for reducing low-value practices: Share information about the benefits of reducing the low-value practice, which can otherwise be invisible to the clinicians and agents who undertake the often-difficult process of de-implementation. Utilize the narratives shared by patients who have been taken off low-value care and some of the benefits they experience (e.g., reduced side effects, spending less time receiving or coordinating care, spending less money).
3. Support clinician decision-making: Endorse a colleague's decision to de-implement, particularly endorsements by a specialist (see Case Studies 13.1 and 13.2). Knowing

(continued)

Key Points for Practice: Ways to Counteract the Asymmetry of Outcomes (*continued*)

their peers support de-implementation can help practitioners feel they don't bear responsibility alone, and that their decision is well founded.
4. Create time-based check points: Examples of check points include setting dates when medications will be revisited or mandating a timeframe after which a service program is evaluated for revision. Time-based check points create an expectation at the outset that the care and services provided to patients, clients and the public will be periodically revisited and may change. These check points also help defeat inertia and increase the chance that a low-value practice will be de-implemented before significant harm occurs.

STRATEGIES TO DE-IMPLEMENT LOW-VALUE PRACTICES

The Big Picture

Before reviewing some specific de-implementation strategies, it is helpful to look at the big picture. Prior to actively de-implementing low-value practices, we need a thorough understanding of what led to and sustains the low-value practice or program. The principle known as *Chesterton's fence*, named for G. K. Chesterton, advises against undertaking reforms until you understand why a legacy policy or structure exists and what purposes it serves (Galef, 2021). Chesterton illustrated the principle by citing a hypothetical fence that someone encounters erected across a road they are traveling. The fence seems to impede traffic to no purpose, so the person is tempted to simply remove it. However, by precipitously removing the fence before understanding why it is there the person may cause unintentional harm.

Applied to de-implementation, we want to thoroughly understand the perspectives of all stakeholders involved in the low-value practice or policy. In doing so, stakeholders may help identify appropriate de-implementation strategies and avoid those strategies unsuited to the context. By soliciting broad stakeholder input de-implementation teams can take a step toward understanding (and possibly blunting) the partisans who are likely to oppose de-implementation. Conversely, deploying a de-implementation strategy without first understanding why the low-value practice is currently used is like prescribing a medication without confirming the illness being treated: It can cause harm. De-implementation strategies should be designed to address the drivers of the low-value practice. To do that, we ought to first spend some time investigating those drivers.

There are a range of tools and structured methods of observation that help to investigate the drivers of low-value practices. One method is using open-ended, grounded interviews with key stakeholders, paired with snowball sampling to identify additional stakeholder groups and individual stakeholders to interview. **Open-ended interviews** focus on one subject (the low-value practice) but are open to pursuing lines of inquiry based on what the interview participant sees as important. **Grounded interviews** use the participant's experience and understanding as the basis for the interview, using probes based on the participant's response and specific prompts to produce information rooted in their experience, (e.g., *Can you give me an example of…? Can you tell me about a time when…?*) or to better understand their meaning (e.g., *Can you tell me what you mean by…? Tell me more about…? Can you help me better understand…?*).

Visualizations can be useful. These include fishbone diagrams, process maps, and causal pathway diagrams (Lewis et al., 2018). These visualizations identify factors that contribute to a specific outcome (fishbone diagrams), the sequential or temporal flow of a given organizational process (process maps), or the decision points or conditions that led to an outcome (causal pathways). In some cases, visualizations of low-value practices can be shared with stakeholders as an intervention validity check. Presenting visualizations works best with stakeholders who are familiar with visualizations (e.g., patient advocates, community organizers, healthcare providers, and public health agents). Pareto charts, which display item frequencies (e.g., reasons low-value tests are ordered) with a cumulative proportion (e.g., percentage of low-value tests accounted for), can be a helpful visualization to use when determining where to intervene.

SPECIFIC DE-IMPLEMENTATION STRATEGIES

The de-implementation strategies reviewed in the following are split into three groups based on who the strategy targets: (a) clients receiving the low-value practice (e.g., patients, members of the public); (b) practitioners delivering low-value practices; and (c) the systems and organizations in which low-value practices are delivered. Each audience is briefly described, followed by an exemplar strategy and sources to identify additional strategies appropriate to that audience.

There are two caveats to sorting de-implementation strategies into these three groups. First, this is just one way of categorizing de-implementation strategies. Categorization is a convenient way to simplify a complex topic by grouping items that share traits. Second, de-implementation strategies employed with one audience must consider possible impact on other groups. While an intervention does not always target all three groups, it is important to consider what is happening with all three groups and what effects de-implementation strategies may have on each group.

Reviews of De-Implementation Strategies

To date at least five literature reviews have been published on strategies to promote de-implementation and/or factors influencing de-implementation of low-value care (Augustsson et al., 2021; Burton et al., 2021; Colla et al., 2017; Rietbergen et al., 2020; Sypes et al., 2020), including reviews specifically on studies of de-implementation strategies focused on patients (Sypes et al., 2020) and nurses (Rietbergen et al., 2020). This is a rapidly evolving literature, and readers should look for new scientific reviews to ensure they are operating with the most current knowledge on de-implementation strategies.

This is particularly important because the current body of research on de-implementation strategies lacks strength and is heterogeneous. The strategies most studied (i.e., clinician education, clinical decision support) score moderately for scientific quality, while the strategies with the highest quality research (i.e., risk sharing, patient education) have relatively fewer studies (Colla et al., 2017). Most of the findings reviewed in these four literature reviews come from cross-sectional comparisons, or uncontrolled pre-post comparisons that are highly susceptible to bias (Augustsson et al., 2021; Burton et al., 2021). The de-implementation literature also lacks replication studies.

Clients, Patients, and Members of the Public

Client-facing de-implementation strategies are actions directed at clients, often by practitioners, to discourage use of the low-value practice. These strategies seek to alter recipients' use of the low-value practice. Examples of client-facing de-implementation strategies include shared decision-making, client-directed education, and client cost-sharing (Colla et al., 2017; Sypes et al., 2020).

Shared decision-making in client-healthcare practitioner encounters is among the most effective client-facing strategies (Sypes et al., 2020). In shared decision-making the practitioner and client have a dialogue in which the practitioner explains different care options, including why they feel the identified low-value practice is inappropriate. Shared decision-making helps practitioners mitigate potential mistrust because the client has a chance to ask questions, share information, and explain their personal priorities. Shared decision-making is also applicable outside of healthcare to a wide range of contexts considering de-implementation of low-value practices.

Shared decision-making is time-consuming for practitioners, as it requires active engagement with clients in meaningful conversation. Depending on the options being considered, resources such as decision-support tools may be necessary (e.g., summarized information about care option advantages and disadvantages; Stiggelbout et al., 2015). Before deciding on shared decision-making, reflect on how such a resource-intensive strategy would be scaled up, and the effects on other audiences involved (e.g., if a practitioner was asked to engage in shared decision-making for several different low-value practices at the same time; see the section "Mitigating Unintended Consequences").

A less intensive strategy is a **trial period**, where the provider proposes a temporary suspension of the low-value practice (e.g., medication) or delaying the low-value practice (e.g., low-value test; Parikh et al., 2020). This strategy also occurs during a client–practitioner dialogue and entails active listening but focuses on the low-value practice instead of selecting from the array of potential alternatives. When using this strategy, the practitioner must follow through with revisiting the decision with the client later, otherwise they risk damaging patient trust.

Finally, **expectation management** occurs when practitioners set expectations that any decisions made will be revisited at an agreed upon point in time. Examples include: *In 1 year we'll revisit the diabetes medications you're prescribed to make sure they're still the best option;* or, *In 5 years we'll revisit whether annual mammograms are in your long-term interest.* Use of this strategy helps establish that practices can be thoughtfully changed and that the value of a treatment, test, or program to a client can change with time.

Practitioners

Practitioner-directed strategies influence how practitioners think about or act on a low-value practice, while generally preserving their decision-making prerogative. It may be helpful to think of two broad approaches to de-implementation strategies targeting practitioners: (a) de-implementation in which we try to change their patterns of thought through unlearning the low-value practice; and (b) de-implementation in which we try to change their behavior by introducing a substitute practice (Helfrich et al., 2018).

Unlearning is the systematic effort to recognize and change an established heuristic or routine. In the context of de-implementation, we speak of unlearning specifically as it applies to altering heuristics and/or routines that sustain low-value practices or programs (Helfrich et al., 2018). Unlearning strategies include practitioner education; report cards and benchmarking (e.g., providing information to practitioners on their performance relative to some standard); or audit and feedback (e.g., feedback to practitioners on specific examples of where their performance deviated from best practice or could be improved; Augustsson et al., 2021; Burton et al., 2021; Colla et al., 2017; Rietbergen et al., 2020). **Substitution** occurs when an alternative is introduced to replace or reduce use of a low-value practice. Most often, substitute practices are introduced among the individuals using the low-value practice or program, as opposed to individuals who do not directly engage with the low-value practice or program (Helfrich et al., 2018). Substitution approaches involve changes to the setting or process where practitioners choose low-value practices. Examples from healthcare include introducing new order sets for prescribing or testing (Burton et al., 2021); changing ordering defaults to favor an evidence-based medication or test in place of the low-value alternative (Scott et al., 2017); or performance incentives encouraging use of alternatives to low-value practices (Colla et al., 2017; Rietbergen et al., 2020).

Unlearning and substitution are not mutually exclusive. For example, in healthcare, clinical decision support tools often combine elements of both unlearning and substitution. Clinical decision support tools present structured information with branching recommendations based on client needs (Kawamoto et al., 2005), but often also provide brief summaries of evidence, clinician education, and clinician feedback (Augustsson et al., 2021; Burton et al., 2021; Colla et al., 2017). Unlearning and substitution strategies can also overlap with patient/client-facing strategies. For example, a practitioner-facing decision-support tool can be used to support shared decision-making.

Systems and Organizations

De-implementation strategies targeting a system or organization attempt to change policies or reconfigure services to eliminate or discourage low-value practices (Burton et al., 2021). Systems strategies include change to healthcare or public health policies; payment, funding, or reimbursement structures; and/or management, human resource, and information technology infrastructure.

Reducing low-value practices by raising awareness: Implementation scientists often say that it is not enough to just publish about the gaps in evidence-based practices if we want to close those gaps. While that is true, sometimes we underestimate the power of measuring and publicizing gaps in care. Often, stakeholders need to be aware of the problem before the problem can be addressed and raising awareness about the harms and frequency of a low-value practice or program can stimulate change. Brownlee and Korenstein (2021) cite the shocking reports on poor anesthesia practices in the 1980s that ultimately led to a host of changes from organizations around the world and major, sustained declines in deaths and harms. The reports signaling the problem were only the beginning. It took sustained, long-term efforts by the profession that involved changing anesthesia training, credentialing, and regulation, but the reporting on unnecessary deaths is what crystalized public anger that made large-scale change possible.

Change the care pathway: Care pathways are formal, documented steps in how to carry out care for a specific condition or process. Care pathways are interdependent and articulate decision points and resources needed to achieve a care goal. Care pathways help eliminate unintended variation in care and standardizing the overall care process can be effective in eliminating a low-value practice that occurs as part of the process. For example, Marchisio and colleagues describe how a hospital in Italy developed a care pathway for childbirth that was effective in reducing episiotomy by almost half, while improving maternal satisfaction with care (Marchisio et al., 2006). The care pathway was developed over many months with a multidisciplinary team of stakeholders including gynecologists, midwives, social workers, and administrators. The multidisciplinary team developed protocols for staff who would use the care pathway and conducted staff education on how to follow the care pathway. Staff documented their use of the pathway, including instances when they deviated from it and why. The multidisciplinary team performed daily audits of the pathway use and tracked and reported outcomes to promote accountability and transparency.

Leveraging information systems: Linked information systems, such as EHRs and client management systems, underpin much of modern care and service provision. Information systems can be used for system-level de-implementation through two broad approaches. The first makes expert input available at the point of decision-making where a low-value practice might otherwise occur or continue (see Case Study 13.1). The second is to create automated checks or stops that are triggered when a low-value practice is selected. An example of this second approach was developed at the Cleveland Clinic, where a hard-stop alert system identified when a laboratory test was ordered that had already been ordered that day (Procop et al., 2015). When a provider attempted to order a duplicate test, the alert system declined the request and provided the results from the already completed test. These alerts helped address the perceived need for the test while preventing waste and inconvenience to the patient. The development of system hard stops was only possible through collaboration with the providers who ordered tests, the pathologists and other laboratory specialists, the informatics team, and system leadership. This stakeholder-engaged approach ensured that new hard stops did not create more problems than they solve (Procop et al., 2019). In the rush of day-to-day work, much of what a clinician does is organized using heuristics and influenced by established organizational routines (see the section "Low-Value Practices Already Embedded in Heuristics and Routines"). This enables practitioners to continue reflexively opting for low-value practices in the absence of changes to the environment they operate in. This is one reason why hard stops were more effective in this case than a similar alert providing the same information but that did not preclude the order from being placed (Procop et al., 2015).

Prevention

It may be possible to prevent or slow the adoption of new low-value practices. Low-value practices based in pseudoscience may be targeted using strategies like those for countering disinformation. **Inoculation theory** posits that individuals can be pre-emptively sensitized to resist arguments intended to manipulate their attitudes, termed **counterattitudinal arguments**, by alerting individuals to the threat in advance (McGuire & Papageorgis, 1961). Inoculation theory has been used successfully in research interventions in a range of settings to counter a range of potentially negative beliefs (Compton & Pfau, 2005). Inoculation interventions target two mechanisms by explaining why the anticipated counterattitudinal argument is harmful and why it is wrong or incorrect.

In public health, approaches based on inoculation theory have been used to design successful health campaigns to sensitize adolescents to question and reject peer pressure to use tobacco and alcohol (Compton & Pfau, 2005). In healthcare, systems might send information to patients ahead of cold season alerting them to the inappropriate use of antibiotics to treat viral infections. While there is some evidence that improving general reasoning skills can protect against a harmful belief (Hameed et al., 2003), other research suggests that focusing on the factual refutation of a specific idea is more effective than trying to engage individuals in evaluating the logical reasoning underlying a harmful belief (Banas & Miller, 2013).

MITIGATING UNINTENDED CONSEQUENCES

When attempting to change established practices, it is important to avoid causing unintended consequences. This is particularly critical when de-implementing a low-value practice or program. As previously discussed, de-implementation of low-value practices is different from implementation because there are often stakeholders in the low-value practice (partisans) who are likely to oppose de-implementation efforts, and in some cases clients or patients favor low-value practices. A phenomenon discussed in the following termed **psychological reactance** can occur when people feel their freedom is being abridged. Psychological reactance is a risk during de-implementation, where the goal is curtailing a behavior or practice. It is also possible to inadvertently push people to use alternate lower-value practices that are not considered in the de-implementation intervention. Additionally, we want to be aware of the potential for unintended consequences when planning to scale-up an effective de-implementation strategy. Finally, any initiative or program should have a communication plan that includes informing stakeholders of the results. Communication with stakeholders at all phases of the intervention is especially critical to de-implementation efforts.

PSYCHOLOGICAL REACTANCE

Psychological reactance is negative thinking that occurs when an individual feels their freedom or rights are being threatened (Dillard & Shen, 2005). Psychological reactance has two distinct components: anger and counter-arguing (Dillard & Shen, 2005). **Anger** is hostility directed at the person or entity that the individual experiencing psychological reactance perceives as abridging their freedom. **Counter-arguing** is mistrust or disbelief in the person or entity perceived as abridging the individual's freedom, and in the message or idea that the individual perceives as threatening their freedom.

Psychological reactance can cause the **boomerang effect**, where individuals become more committed to the position, practice, or idea they feel is being threatened (Compton & Pfau, 2005). A recent example of psychological reactance and the boomerang effect is the energetic resistance to mask mandates for slowing the spread of COVID-19, most notably in the United States. The boomerang effect is a particular concern in the context of de-implementation because of the fear that poorly planned or poorly executed efforts at de-implementation could unintentionally increase use or commitment to the low-value practice; for example, in the early literature on audit-and-feedback interventions with clinicians, where a third of audit-and-feedback interventions were associated with an increase in the practice they were trying to curtail (Kluger & DeNisi, 1996).

While there is limited research assessing psychological reactance in the context of de-implementation of low-value practices, there is a history of backlashes in many countries against controlling access to healthcare for reasons of cost, typically referred to as rationing. For example, in 2019, the British National Health Service (NHS) sought to limit the use of 34 low-value tests and treatments, such as imaging for lower back pain. Unfortunately, the NHS failed to effectively communicate the reason for the changes to the public, and the British media reported the policy as motivated purely for reasons of cost and rationing care (Campbell, 2019). It can be tempting to dismiss the concerns of the public or to criticize the journalists for dangerously incorrect portrayals. However, directing blame at stakeholders is only likely to harden their positions. It could create mistrust that persists well after and well beyond a specific effort to reduce low-value care (Helfrich et al., 2018; Scott & McPhail, 2020).

Part of avoiding psychological reactance is employing the strategies related to inoculation theory described previously, in this case inoculating stakeholders in terms of what the purpose of the de-implementation strategy is. When a low-value practice or program is being ended or curtailed, the patients, clients, and practitioners will actively seek a rationale for the change, and in the absence of an explanation will imagine reasons for the change. Often, the assumed motives will be negative, such as saving money or political intrigues. When de-implementation of a low-value practice happens in a communication vacuum, that vacuum can quickly fill with inaccurate information (e.g., sensational media coverage). Even worse, an information vacuum can fill with misinformation, as when conspiracy theories began circulating that the reason health authorities were opposed to the use of ivermectin to treat COVID-19 was because ivermectin was an off-patent medication that was cheap and therefore not profitable to large drug manufacturers (Davey, 2021).

INADVERTENTLY INCREASING USE OF OTHER INEFFECTIVE PRACTICES WE ARE NOT TRACKING

Practitioners responsible for de-implementation efforts should consider how de-implementation might inadvertently encourage clients to seek other low-value services that are not being tracked. As discussed, psychological reactance and the boomerang effect can be triggered by de-implementation efforts. An additional consideration is how de-implementation efforts could drive clients and practitioners to inadvertently use another low-value practice to fill a perceived unmet need. One poignant example is the attempt to restrict the use of long-term prescription opioids among patients with chronic pain as the prescription opioid epidemic escalated, which may have resulted in patients seeking illicit drugs like heroin (Eisenstein, 2019). Another example is the well-documented ways that physicians circumvent policies to improve antimicrobial stewardship, including waiting until after hours to order restricted antibiotics because pre-authorization is only enforced during business hours in some systems, or listing an unconfirmed diagnosis to allow a non-formulary medication to be prescribed (Reed et al., 2013). The same can occur at the client level, as when patients circumvent antimicrobial stewardship policies by doctor-shopping until they find a doctor willing to prescribe them an antibiotic (Blaser et al., 2021).

One solution is to explore with stakeholders what needs the ineffective practice or program currently fills and to map out any options available to meet those needs once the ineffective practice or program is gone. It may be possible to anticipate the needs of stakeholders to better meet those needs at the same time the low-value practice is being eliminated, as with the example of a hard-stop intervention to reduce duplicate laboratory tests at the Cleveland Clinic discussed earlier. The de-implementation strategy used a technological solution (a hard stop alert to prevent the low-value test), but it was developed only after months of work with all the relevant stakeholders to ensure the solution was workable (Procop et al., 2015).

IT MATTERS HOW SCALE-UP AND SPREAD HAPPEN

Problems can arise in the future when scaling up and spreading de-implementation activities without engaging with stakeholders and thinking through the downstream and long-term implications of those activities. For example, shared decision-making may be highly effective in reducing a low-value practice, for example, to reduce MRIs for lower-back pain. In isolation, shared-decision-making related to lower-back pain treatment may be entirely feasible. But how might effectiveness change if shared decision-making is implemented simultaneously for multiple low-value practices in the same clinical setting? Some de-implementation strategies may be effective in isolation but create logistical problems when scaled-up and spread without considering broader implications. To avoid creating problems with scale-up and spread in healthcare, for example, ideally work is performed in a learning health system. This means institutional and programmatic structures need to be created to identify and tackle low-value practices within the context of the services and mission of the overall organization or institution, and within the overall delivery system. Establishing these new structures should not be left up to individuals or small teams but should be handled collectively and at the system level.

CLOSE THE LOOP AND EARN TRUST

When we make a change to reduce or eliminate a low-value practice or program, we need to inform stakeholders what impact these efforts had. This includes if things did not work as planned, as when de-implementation efforts fail to reduce the low-value practice or cause an unanticipated problem. As detailed earlier in the chapter, there are almost always partisans in favor of the low-value practice or program. When de-implementation teams do not communicate with stakeholders, a narrative vacuum can fill with a broad range of information, including misinformation. Actively communicating with stakeholders, including partisans, can build a sense of momentum and buy-in if de-implementation efforts are successful. If efforts do not work as expected and de-implementation teams communicate openly with stakeholders about challenges faced, they can strengthen credibility and limit the opportunity for false narratives (e.g., conspiracy theories).

SUMMARY

This chapter defined low-value practices and programs and described the distinct sources and drivers of low-value practices. There are three unique challenges to de-implementing low-value practice: embeddedness in habits and routines, the existence of partisans, and an asymmetry of outcomes for practitioners involved. De-implementation strategies can be directed to three audiences: patients or clients, practitioners, and systems or organizations. Systems thinking can be applied with all three audiences. Systems thinking can help to mitigate unintended consequences, including how to limit psychological reactance, how to avoid unintentionally increasing use of the low-value practice or program, and how to build credibility and trust with stakeholders.

KEY POINTS FOR PRACTICE

1. Mitigate the effects of heuristics and routines during de-implementation: Identify incompatible substitutes or alternatives to the low-value practice.
2. Counteract the efforts of partisans by revealing who bears the burden of the low-value practice, creating a guiding coalition to lead de-implementation, and, when partisans seek to discredit your work, use the opportunity to increase visibility of the low-value practice and its harms.
3. Counteract the asymmetry of outcomes experienced by practitioners and agents by providing stories and examples of the negative consequences of the low-value practice; create positive reinforcement by sharing information about how de-implementation efforts have helped patients or clients; have colleagues endorse or express support for actions to de-implement low-value practices; and create time-based check points when decisions about low-value practices can be revisited.

COMMON PITFALLS IN PRACTICE

1. Fail to consider how low-value practices are embedded in heuristics and routines that may be extremely difficult to change even if stakeholders want to change and even if they know exactly what needs to change.

2. Chesterton's Fence: Begin actively de-implementing a low-value practice before first understanding why it exists and what purpose it serves or served.
3. Focus de-implementation activities on one group or level (patients/clients, practitioners/agents, organizations/systems) without considering the role other groups or levels play, and how de-implementation strategies affect stakeholders in other groups or levels.
4. Inadvertently provoke psychological reactance among practitioners and agents, or among clients and patients; potentially cause a boomerang effect where individuals become more committed to the low-value practice because de-implementation efforts make them feel threatened.

DISCUSSION QUESTIONS

1. What is a low-value practice? How do we know that a low-value practice does not provide a benefit?
2. Why do we have low-value practices?
3. Why do low-value practices persist even after we have strong evidence that they produce more harms than benefits?
4. What challenges make de-implementing low-value practices different from implementing new evidence-based practices?
5. What unintended consequences can arise when we de-implement low-value practices and how can we reduce the threat of unintended consequences?
6. What steps might we take in selecting a de-implementation strategy? What factors might we consider in choosing to intervene at the client or patient level; at the practitioner or agent level; and the organization or system level?

KNOWLEDGE CHECK: DE-IMPLEMENTING DETRIMENTAL FEEDING PRACTICES

In some cultures, adults routinely hurry children through meals, coerce children to try foods, or require that they finish eating all the food they have been served. However, hurrying or coercing children to eat when they are not hungry can lead children to ultimately reject healthy foods, to lower their willingness to try new foods, and can inhibit their ability to manage impulses (Swindle et al., 2020).

Childcare is a setting that exerts substantial influence on children's diets, where early childhood educators (ECEs) influence the dietary practices of children in their care. However, the role of ECEs in influencing children's diet is typically unrecognized, and ECEs generally receive limited training about child feeding and nutrition. Unintentionally, ECEs can perpetuate detrimental feeding practices (e.g., coercing or rushing children to finish all their food).

U.S. based researchers worked with ECEs along with other stakeholders to implement evidence-based nutrition practices while de-implementing harmful practices (Swindle et al., 2020), using the WISE program (*Together, We Inspire Smart Eating*). The researchers encouraged ECEs to use WISE components at meals and to build them into classroom instruction. These included role-modeling nutrition and using a puppet to engage with children to promote fruits and vegetables. The researchers sought to use a participatory approach by engaging with school directors, ECEs, and parents of school children on how this should be done. The goal of the stakeholder engagement process was to understand local knowledge and to tailor the WISE strategies to the schools.

Questions to Consider:

- What resistance might be seen when the researchers discuss detrimental feeding practices with stakeholders?
- Are there additional stakeholders the team could or should involve?
- In what ways is the WISE approach an example of de-implementation through unlearning?
- In what ways is the WISE approach an example of de-implementation through substitution?
- If the WISE program is successful in improving children's nutrition in participating classrooms, are there ways to determine if WISE has influenced ECEs' practices through unlearning versus substitution?
- Are there any unintended consequences that could emerge from efforts to de-implement detrimental feeding practices in the participating classrooms? If so, are there things the researchers can do to reduce the risk of unintended consequences?

ACKNOWLEDGMENTS

Research used for case studies funded by the VA Quality Enhancement Research Initiative (QUE 15–271), David H Au, MD, MS, Christian D. Helfrich, MPH, PhD, and Christine Hartmann, PhD.

We are grateful to Diana E. Naranjo, MPH, PHD, for drafting the case study, "De-implementation of Detrimental Feeding Practices" and a Spotlight segment on the World Health Organization statement on abuse and disrespect in facility-based childbirth across the globe.

REFERENCES

ABIM Foundation. (2018). Choosing wisely: A special report on the first five years. *Choosing Wisely*. Retrieved August 11, 2021, from https://www.choosingwisely.org/wp-content/uploads/2017/10/Choosing-Wisely-at-Five.pdf

Arbesman, S. (2013). *The half-life of facts: Why everything we know has an expiration date*. Penguin.

Augustsson, H., Ingvarsson, S., Nilsen, P., von Thiele Schwarz, U., Muli, I., Dervish, J., & Hasson, H. (2021). Determinants for the use and de-implementation of low-value care in health care: A scoping review. *Implementation Science Communications*, *2*(1), 1–17. https://doi.org/10.1186/s43058-021-00110-3

Balas, E. A., & Boren, S. A. (2000). Managing clinical knowledge for health care improvement. *Yearbook of Medical Informatics*, *9*(01), 65–70. https://pubmed.ncbi.nlm.nih.gov/27699347/

Banas, J. A., & Miller, G. (2013). Inducing resistance to conspiracy theory propaganda: Testing inoculation and metainoculation strategies. *Human Communication Research*, *39*(2), 184–207. https://doi.org/10.1111/hcre.12000

Berwick, D. M. (2019). Elusive waste: The Fermi paradox in US health care. *JAMA*, *322*(15), 1458–1459. https://doi.org/10.1001/jama.2019.14610

Berwick, D. M., & Hackbarth, A. D. (2012). Eliminating waste in US health care. *JAMA*, *307*(14), 1513–1516. https://doi.org/10.1001/jama.2012.362

Blaser, M. J., Melby, M. K., Lock, M., & Nichter, M. (2021). Accounting for variation in and overuse of antibiotics among humans. *BioEssays*, *43*(2), 2000163. https://doi.org/10.1002/bies.202000163

Bluestone, G. (2021). *Hype: How scammers, grifters, and con artists are taking over the internet—and why we're following*. Harlequin.

Bokhof, B., & Junius-Walker, U. (2016). Reducing polypharmacy from the perspectives of general practitioners and older patients: A synthesis of qualitative studies. *Drugs & Aging*, *33*(4), 249–266. https://doi.org/10.1007/s40266-016-0354-5

Bourgault, A. M., & Upvall, M. J. (2019). De-implementation of tradition-based practices in critical care: A qualitative study. *International Journal of Nursing Practice*, *25*(2), e12723. https://doi.org/10.1111/ijn.12723

Brownlee, S., Chalkidou, K., Doust, J., Elshaug, A. G., Glasziou, P., Heath, I., Nagpal, S., Saini, V., Srivastava, D., Chalmers, K., & Korenstein, D. (2017). Evidence for overuse of medical services around the world. *The Lancet*, *390*(10090), 156–168. https://doi.org/10.1016/S0140-6736(16)32585-5

Brownlee, S. M., & Korenstein, D. (2021). Better understanding the downsides of low value healthcare could reduce harm. *BMJ*, *372*. https://doi.org/10.1136/bmj.n117

Burton, C., Williams, L., Bucknall, T., Fisher, D., Hall, B., Harris, G., Jones, P., Makin, M., Mcbride, A., Meacock, R., Parkinson, J., Rycroft-Malone, J., & Waring, J. (2021). Theory and practical guidance for effective de-implementation of practices across health and care services: A realist synthesis. *Health Services and Delivery Research*, *9*(2). https://doi.org/10.3310/hsdr09020

Cagnacci, A., & Venier, M. (2019). The controversial history of hormone replacement therapy. *Medicina*, *55*(9), 602. https://doi.org/10.3390/medicina55090602

Campbell, D. (2019). Revealed: NHS plans to ration 34 everyday tests and treatments. *The Guardian*. Fri 29 Nov 2019 13.09 EST. Retrieved March 30, 2021, from https://www.theguardian.com/society/2019/nov/29/revealed-nhs-plans-to-ration-34-unnecessary-tests-and-treatments

Caulfield, T. (2015). *Is Gwyneth Paltrow wrong about everything?* Viking Press. ISBN-10: 067006758X

Colla, C. H., Mainor, A. J., Hargreaves, C., Sequist, T., & Morden, N. (2017). Interventions aimed at reducing use of low-value health services: A systematic review. *Medical Care Research and Review*, *74*(5), 507–550. https://doi.org/10.1177/1077558716656970

Compton, J. A., & Pfau, M. (2005). Inoculation theory of resistance to influence at maturity: Recent progress in theory development and application and suggestions for future research. *Annals of the International Communication Association*, *29*(1), 97–146. https://doi.org/10.1080/23808985.2005.11679045

Davey, M. (2021). Fraudulent ivermectin studies open up new battleground between science and misinformation. *The Guardian*, News: Health. Retrieved September 24, 2021, from https://www.theguardian.com/australia-news/2021/sep/25/fraudulent-ivermectin-studies-open-up-new-battleground-between-science-and-misinformation

Deyo, R. (2008). "Hope or hype: The conflict between science and profit in health care." Hilde and Bill Birnbaum Endowed Lecture. *Kaiser Permanente Washington Health Research Institute*. Retrieved 8/3/2021, from https://www.kpwashingtonresearch.org/news-and-events/events/birnbaum-lecture-2016/past-birnbaum-lectures

Dillard, J. P., & Shen, L. (2005). On the nature of reactance and its role in persuasive health communication. *Communication Monographs*, *72*(2), 144–168. https://doi.org/10.1080/03637750500111815

Eisenstein, M. (2019). Treading the tightrope of opioid restrictions: US efforts to control opioid prescriptions are having unintended effects on people with chronic pain. *Nature*, Outlook. Retrieved September 11, from https://www.nature.com/articles/d41586-019-02687-1

Finkelstein, A., & Taubman, S. (2015, February). *Using randomized evaluations to improve the efficiency of US healthcare delivery*. J-PAL North America. https://www.povertyactionlab.org/sites/default/files/Using%20Randomized%20Evaluations%20to%20Improve%20the%20Efficiency%20of%20US%20Healthcare%20Delivery_0.pdf

Fiol, M., & O'Connor, E. (2017a). Unlearning established organizational routines—Part I. *The Learning Organization*, *24*(1), 13–29. https://doi.org/10.1108/TLO-09-2016-0056

Fiol, M., & O'Connor, E. J. (2017b). Unlearning established organizational routines—Part II. *The Learning Organization*, *24*(2), 82–92. https://doi.org/10.1108/TLO-09-2016-0063

Galef, J. (2021). *The scout mindset: Why some people see things clearly and others don't*. Penguin.

Greenhalgh, T., Robert, G., Macfarlane, F., Bate, P., & Kyriakidou, O. (2004). Diffusion of innovations in service organizations: Systematic review and recommendations. *The Milbank Quarterly*, *82*(4), 581–629. https://doi.org/10.1111/j.0887-378X.2004.00325.x

Grimshaw, J. M., Patey, A. M., Kirkham, K. R., Hall, A., Dowling, S. K., Rodondi, N., Ellen, M., Kool, T., van Dulmen, S. A., Kerr, E. A., Linklater, S., Levinson, W., & Bhatia, R. S. (2020). De-implementing wisely: Developing the evidence base to reduce low-value care. *BMJ Quality & Safety*, *29*(5), 409–417. https://doi.org/10.1136/bmjqs-2019-010060

Hall, J. C., & Platell, C. (1997). Half-life of truth in surgical literature. *The Lancet*, *350*(9093), 1752. https://doi.org/10.1016/S0140-6736(05)63577-5

Hameed, S., Robinson, G. M., & Moulton, J. (2003, December). Bashing Pseudoscience in Academia. In *American Astronomical Society Bulletin*, *35*, 1237.

Hanrahan, K., Wagner, M., Matthews, G., Stewart, S., Dawson, C., Greiner, J., Pottinger, J., Vernon-Levett, P., Herold, D., Hottel, R., & Cullen, L. (2015). Sacred cow gone to pasture: A systematic evaluation and integration of evidence-based practice. *Worldviews on Evidence-Based Nursing*, *12*(1), 3–11. https://doi.org/10.1111/wvn.12072

Hartmann, K., Viswanathan, M., Palmieri, R., Gartlehner, G., Thorp, J., & Lohr, K.N. (2005). Outcomes of routine episiotomy: A systematic review. *JAMA*, *293*(17), 2141–2148. https://doi.org/10.1001/jama.293.17.2141

Helfrich, C. D., Rose, A. J., Hartmann, C. W., van Bodegom-Vos, L., Graham, I. D., Wood, S. J., Majerczyk, Chester B. R., Good, B., Pogach, L. M., Ball, S. L., Au, D. H., & Aron, D. C. (2018). How the dual process model of human cognition can inform efforts to de-implement ineffective and harmful clinical practices: A preliminary model of unlearning and substitution. *Journal of Evaluation in Clinical Practice, 24*(1), 198–205. https://doi.org/10.1111/jep.12855

Hoffmann, T. C., & Del Mar, C. (2017). Clinicians' expectations of the benefits and harms of treatments, screening, and tests: A systematic review. *JAMA Internal Medicine, 177*(3), 407–419. https://doi.org/10.1001/jamainternmed.2016.8254

Ingvarsson, S., Augustsson, H., Hasson, H., Nilsen, P., von Thiele Schwarz, U., & von Knorring, M. (2020). Why do they do it? A grounded theory study of the use of low-value care among primary health care physicians. *Implementation Science, 15*(1), 1–10. https://doi.org/10.1186/s13012-020-01052-5

International Initiative for Impact Evaluation. (2020). *Informing a cook stoves programme in Ghana* [online summary], Evidence Impact Summaries. 3IE.

Intervention Initiative for Impact Evaluation. (2021). Unable to replicate. Retrieved October 20, from https://www.3ieimpact.org/our-expertise/replication/unable-to-replicate

Ioannidis, J. P. (2005). Why most published research findings are false. *PLoS Medicine, 2*(8), e124. https://doi.org/10.1371/journal.pmed.0020124

Kahneman, D. (2011). *Thinking fast and slow*. Farrar, Straus and Giroux. ISBN: 9780141033570.

Kawamoto, K., Houlihan, C. A., Balas, E. A., & Lobach, D. F. (2005). Improving clinical practice using clinical decision support systems: A systematic review of trials to identify features critical to success. *BMJ, 330*(7494), 765. https://doi.org/10.1136/bmj.38398.500764.8F

Kluger, A. N., & DeNisi, A. (1996). The effects of feedback interventions on performance: A historical review, a meta-analysis, and a preliminary feedback intervention theory. *Psychological Bulletin, 119*(2), 254–284. https://doi.org/10.1037/0033-2909.119.2.254

Lewis, C. C., Klasnja, P., Powell, B.J., Lyon, A.R., Tuzzio, L., Jones, S., Walsh-Bailey, C., & Weiner, B. (2018). From classification to causality: Advancing understanding of mechanisms of change in implementation science. *Frontiers in Public Health, 6*, 136. https://doi.org/10.3389/fpubh.2018.00136

Lo, B., & Field, M. J. (2009). *Conflict of interest in medical research, education, and practice*. National Academies Press. ISBN 9780309145442.

Lo, N. C., Lowe, A., & Bendavid, E. (2016). Abstinence funding was not associated with reductions in HIV risk behavior in Sub-Saharan Africa. *Health Affairs, 35*(5), 856–863. https://doi.org/10.1377/hlthaff.2015.0828

MacCarthy, E. P. (1996). Dear doctor... regarding calcium channel blockers. *JAMA, 275*(7), 518. https://doi.org/10.1001/jama.1996.03530310023020

Mahal, B. A., Butler, S., Franco, I., Spratt, D. E., Rebbeck, T. R., D'Amico, A. V., & Nguyen, P. L. (2019). Use of active surveillance or watchful waiting for low-risk prostate cancer and management trends across risk groups in the United States, 2010–2015. *JAMA, 321*(7), 704–706. https://doi.org/10.1001/jama.2018.19941

Marchisio, S., Ferraccioli, K., Barbieri, A., Porcelli, A., & Panella, M. (2006). Care pathways in obstetrics: The effectiveness in reducing the incidence of episiotomy in childbirth. *Journal of Nursing Management, 14*(7), 538–543. https://doi.org/10.1111/j.1365-2934.2006.00704.x

McKay, V. R., Morshed, A. B, Brownson, R. C., Proctor, E. K., & Prusaczyk, B. (2018). Letting go: Conceptualizing intervention de-implementation in public health and social service settings. *American Journal of Community Psychology, 62*(2 Jan), 189–202. https://doi.org/10.1002/ajcp.12258.

Montini, T., & Graham, I. D. (2015). "Entrenched practices and other biases": Unpacking the historical, economic, professional, and social resistance to de-implementation. *Implementation Science, 10*, 24. https://doi.org/10.1186/s13012-015-0211-7

Morgan, D. J., Brownlee, S., Leppin, A. L., Kressin, N., Dhruva, S. S., Levin, L., Landon, B. E., Zezza, M. A., Schmidt, H., Saini, V., & Elshaug, A. G. (2015). Setting a research agenda for medical overuse. *BMJ, 351*, h354. https://doi.org/10.1136/bmj.h4534

National Cancer Institute. (2021). *Prostate cancer treatment (PDQ®)–Patient version*. Updated October 15, 2021. https://www.cancer.gov/types/prostate/patient/prostate-treatment-pdq

Nilsen, P., Ingvarsson, S., Hasson, H., von Thiele Schwarz, U., & Augustsson, H. (2020). Theories, models, and frameworks for de-implementation of low-value care: A scoping review of the literature. *Implementation Research and Practice, 1*. https://doi.org/10.1177/2633489520953762

Niven, D. J., Mrklas, K. J., Holodinsky, J. K., Straus, S. E., Hemmelgarn, B. R., Jeffs, L. P., & Stelfox, H. T. (2015). Towards understanding the de-adoption of low-value clinical practices: A scoping review. *BMC Medicine*, 13(1), 255. https://doi.org/10.1186/s12916-015-0488-z

Nordrum, A. (2014). The new D.A.R.E. program—This one works: The "keepin' it REAL" substance-abuse curriculum focuses on elementary and middle-school students' decisions, not drugs. *Scientific American*. Retrieved September 10, 2014, from https://www.scientificamerican.com/article/the-new-d-a-r-e-program-this-one-works/

Norton, W. E., & Chambers, D. A. (2020). Unpacking the complexities of de-implementing inappropriate health interventions. *Implementation Science, 15*(1), 1–7. https://doi.org/10.1186/s13012-019-0960-9

Open Science Collaboration. (2015). Estimating the reproducibility of psychological science. *Science, 349*(6251), aac4716. https://doi.org/10.1126/science.aac4716

Oreskes, N. (2021). *Why trust science?* Princeton University Press.

McGuire, W. J., & Papageorgis, D. (1961). The relative efficacy of various types of prior belief-defense in producing immunity against persuasion. *The Journal of Abnormal and Social Psychology, 62*(2), 327. https://doi.org/10.1037/h0042026

Parikh, T. J., Stryczek, K. C., Gillespie, C., Sayre, G. G., Feemster, L., Udris, E., Majerczyk, B., Rinne, S. T., Wiener, R. S., Au, D. H., & Helfrich, C. D. (2020). Provider anticipation and experience of patient reaction when deprescribing guideline discordant inhaled corticosteroids. *PLoS One, 15*(9), e0238511. https://doi.org/10.1371/journal.pone.0238511

Patey, A. M., Grimshaw, J. M., & Francis, J. J. (2021). Changing behaviour, 'more or less': Do implementation and de-implementation interventions include different behaviour change techniques? *Implementation Science, 16*(1), 1–17. https://doi.org/10.1186/s13012-021-01089-0

Poynard, T., Munteanu, M., Ratziu, V., Benhamou, Y., Martino, V. D., Taieb, J., & Opolon, P. (2002). Truth survival in clinical research: An evidence-based requiem? *Annals of Internal Medicine, 136*(12), 888–895. https://doi.org/10.7326/0003-4819-136-12-200206180-00010

Procop, G. W., Keating, C., Stagno, P., Kottke-Marchant, K., Partin, M., Tuttle, R., & Wyllie, R. (2015). Reducing duplicate testing: A comparison of two clinical decision support tools. *American Journal of Clinical Pathology, 143*(5), 623–626. https://doi.org/10.1309/AJCPJOJ3HKEBD3TU

Procop, G. W., Weathers, A. L., & Reddy, A. J. (2019). Operational aspects of a clinical decision support program. *Clinics in Laboratory Medicine, 39*(2), 215–229. https://doi.org/10.1016/j.cll.2019.01.002

Prusaczyk, B., Swindle, T., & Curran, G. (2020). Defining and conceptualizing outcomes for de-implementation: Key distinctions from implementation outcomes. *Implementation Science Communications, 1*, 1–10. https://doi.org/10.1186/s43058-020-00035-3

Reed, E.E., Stevenson, K. B., West, J. E., Bauer, K. A., & Goff, D. A. (2013). Impact of formulary restriction with prior authorization by an antimicrobial stewardship program. *Virulence, 4*(2), 158–162. https://doi.org/10.4161/viru.21657

Resnick, B. (2016). What psychology's crisis means for the future of science. Retrieved September 26, 2021, from https://www.vox.com/2016/3/14/11219446/psychology-replication-crisis. Updated Mar 25, 2016.

Ridley, M., & Ganser, L. J. (2010). *The rational optimist.* HarperAudio.

Ritchie, S. (2019). *Science fictions: Exposing fraud, bias, negligence and hype in science.* Henry Holt.

Rietbergen, T., Spoon, D., Brunsveld-Reinders, A. H., Schoones, J. W., Huis, A., Heinen, M., Persoon, A., van Dijk, M., Vermeulen, H., Ista, E., & van Bodegom-Vos, L. (2020). Effects of de-implementation strategies aimed at reducing low-value nursing procedures: A systematic review and meta-analysis. *Implementation Science, 15*, 1–18. https://doi.org/10.1186/s13012-020-00995-z

Sandlin, D. (2015, April 24). *The backwards brain bicycle - Smarter every day 133* [Video]. YouTube. https://www.youtube.com/watch?v=MFzDaBzBlL0

Scott, I. A. (2019). Audit-based measures of overuse of medical care in Australian hospital practice. *Internal Medicine Journal, 49*(7), 893–904. https://doi.org/10.1111/imj.14346

Scott, I. A., & McPhail, S. M. (2020). Sociocognitive approach to behaviour change for reducing low-value care. *Australian Health Review, 45*(2), 173–177. https://doi.org/10.1071/AH20209

Scott, I. A., Soon, J., Elshaug, A. G., & Lindner, R., (2017). Countering cognitive biases in minimising low value care. *Medical Journal of Australia, 206*(9), 407–411. https://doi.org/10.5694/mja16.00999

Shrank, W. H., Rogstad, T. L., & Parekh, N. (2019). Waste in the US health care system: Estimated costs and potential for savings. *JAMA, 322*(15), 1501–1509. https://doi.org/10.1001/jama.2019.13978

Stiggelbout, A. M., Pieterse, A. H., & De Haes, J. C. (2015). Shared decision making: Concepts, evidence, and practice. *Patient Education and Counseling, 98*(10), 1172–1179. https://doi.org/10.1016/j.pec.2015.06.022

Stryczek, K., Lea, C., Gillespie, C., Sayre, G., Wanner, S., Rinne, S. T., Wiener, R. S., Feemster, L., Udris, E., Au, D. H., & Helfrich, C. D. (2020). De-implementing inhaled corticosteroids to improve care and safety in COPD treatment: Primary care providers' perspectives. *Journal of General Internal Medicine, 35*(1), 51–56. https://doi.org/10.1007/s11606-019-05193-2

Swindle, T., Rutledge, J. M., Johnson, S. L., Selig, J. P., & Curran, G. M. (2020). De-implementation of detrimental feeding practices: A pilot protocol. *Pilot and Feasibility Studies, 6*(1), 1–10. https://doi.org/10.1186/s40814-020-00720-z

Sypes, E. E., de Grood, C., Whalen-Browne, L., Clement, F. M., Parsons Leigh, J., Niven, D. J., & Stelfox, H. T. (2020). Engaging patients in de-implementation interventions to reduce low-value clinical care: A systematic review and meta-analysis. *BMC Medicine, 18*, 1–15. https://doi.org/10.1186/s12916-020-01567-0

van Bodegom-Vos, L., Davidoff, F., & Marang-van de Mheen, P. J. (2017). Implementation and de-implementation: Two sides of the same coin? *BMJ Quality & Safety, 26*(6), 495–501. https://doi.org/10.1136/bmjqs-2016-005473

Welch, H. G., Schwartz, L., & Woloshin, S. (2011). *Overdiagnosed: Making people sick in the pursuit of health.* Beacon Press.

West, S. L., & O'Neal, K. K. (2004). Project DARE outcome effectiveness revisited. *American Journal of Public Health, 94*(6), 1027–1029. https://doi.org/10.2105/ajph.94.6.1027

Williamson, P. (2016). Take the time and effort to correct misinformation. *Nature, 540*(7632), 171. https://doi.org/10.1038/540171a

Wolfson, D., Santa, J., & Slass, L. (2014). Engaging physicians and consumers in conversations about treatment overuse and waste: A short history of the choosing wisely campaign. *Academic Medicine, 89*(7), 990–995. https://doi.org/10.1097/ACM.0000000000000270

Woloshin, S., & Schwartz, L. M. (2010). The benefits and harms of mammography screening: Understanding the trade-offs. *JAMA, 303*(2), 164–165. https://doi.org/10.1001/jama.2009.2007

14

Implementation Science in Policy

Heather L. Bullock, Michael G. Wilson, and John N. Lavis

Learning Objectives

By the end of this chapter, readers will be able to:

- Articulate the phases in the policy cycle
- Identify when and how research evidence can influence policy
- Apply frameworks to conduct a policy analysis in support of implementation planning
- Distinguish among the different types of process, products, infrastructure, and capacities needed to support evidence-informed policy processes

CASE STUDY 14.1 SUSTAINING EFFECTIVE EVIDENCE-BASED INNOVATIONS AND IMPLEMENTING PUBLIC POLICIES—A TALE OF TWO POLICY-RELATED IMPLEMENTATION CHALLENGES

An organization has gathered together stakeholders, decided what evidence-based intervention (EBI) it will implement, done an assessment of organizational context, identified an implementation team, and developed a sound implementation plan replete with measures to help the organization learn and improve. Now the organization is ready to get going. . . . or is it? This case study introduces two implementers, Mathilde and Jorge, in two different countries, facing different but related implementation challenges.

In response to distressing suicide rates for youth in their remote Indigenous community in Nunatsiavut in northern Labrador, Mathilde and her team have co-designed a land-based program together with community youth to support positive mental well-being and foster connections with other community members and with the land. They used start-up funds from their local public health unit to plan and launch the program. After 2 years, they have found encouraging results: Youth participation in the program is high and suicide rates for youth have plummeted; however, the money to staff and run the program is running low. They need a stable ongoing source of funding to keep the program alive over the long-term but do not know where to turn.

Mathilde's experience is a relatively common one. Many successful EBIs that are built from the ground-up or are adapted from other settings or jurisdictions are not able to be sustained over time. Other times, a successful EBI is not scaled-up or scaled-out wide enough for there to be population-level impacts. The need to continually seek out short-term funding to sustain programs and services that work can be a distraction to the EBI team that takes away focus and momentum from the program and its successful implementation. Thus, it is important to plan for sustainability and scaling as early as possible in an implementation process. If an EBI team has not considered the "outer setting" for implementation (Damschroder et al., 2009)—generally understood as factors that start outside of the organizational context but excerpt influence within it, such as public policies or organized interests—the EBI team may find it challenging to sustain or scale an EBI.

But starting from the perspective of a local EBI implementation effort ("bottom-up") is only one pathway for implementation. The drive for implementation can also start from the "top-down," beginning instead with policy makers who are often seeking to develop and implement policies that reduce death and improve the health and well-being of citizens. In this case, the policy (or policies) is the EBI that must be implemented effectively.

Jorge works for his state government in its Ministry of Health. Recently his government has learned from a research group at the state university that the smoking and vaping rates have recently increased at an alarming rate for young people in his state, after a prolonged period of low and stable smoking rates for this population group. He and his team have been tasked with recommending actions that his government can implement to reduce smoking/vaping rates in young people. He learns about an approach taken by another state that had some success. The approach includes: (a) raising taxes on tobacco and vape products; (b) restricting the number and location of places that are permitted to sell these products, including a minimum

(*continued*)

CASE STUDY 14.1 SUSTAINING EFFECTIVE EVIDENCE-BASED INNOVATIONS AND IMPLEMENTING PUBLIC POLICIES—A TALE OF TWO POLICY-RELATED IMPLEMENTATION CHALLENGES (*continued*)

distance away from schools; and (c) investing in an evidence-based tobacco cessation mobile phone application targeted to young people. He decides to present an adapted version of it as one of three options for the minister to consider. The minister endorses this policy option and the associated budget. Now Jorge has to figure out how to implement this strategy effectively to get the outcomes they are expecting. How can he do this?

Jorge faces a different challenge than Mathilde, but each has its own complexity. Most policy makers have a strong understanding of what makes "good" policy and what policy instruments they have available to them. Yet they tend to know less about effective implementation, and the science behind it. It is clear that Jorge could benefit from a better understanding of implementation science and Mathilde could benefit from a better understanding of public policy. However, despite the many advancements in implementation science, there have been relatively few attempts to draw from the scholarship on the public policy and political science literature and vice versa (Bullock et al., 2021; Nilsen et al., 2013).

INTRODUCTION

The goal of this chapter is to introduce the world of implementation from a policy perspective. The chapter starts by unpacking what is meant (and not meant) by policy and its implementation, sharing a heuristic (a mental shortcut) that is often used in public policy to identify the phases through which ideas become policy, with a focus on the policy implementation phase. Next, the chapter briefly discusses the instruments used to make policy. The chapter then shifts to exploring how research evidence can shape policy, including its implementation, and introduces a framework that can help conduct policy analyses to support better implementation. The chapter concludes with an overview of the approaches that can be taken to support evidence-informed policymaking and provides some current examples of such initiatives.

The focus of this chapter is on public policy broadly defined, such as legislation, technical guidance, strategies, and other funding initiatives by governments or agencies of government at the supra-national, national, regional (e.g., province/state), or local (e.g., municipal) level. The chapter does not focus on organizational policy or policymaking in the context of professional associations, although much of this content may still be applicable. Through this lens, the chapter begins by developing a richer understanding of the policy process so the reader can understand how implementation fits within it.

THE POLICY PROCESS

Public health, other health or social system actors, and those supporting implementation efforts in community, clinical, or academic networks will likely encounter public policy during their careers. Yet many education and training programs for these professionals offer little content on how to work with policy makers or shed light on their (often quite different) contexts. This is especially perplexing given that the evidence shows that enabling effective implementation and understanding the role of "outer context" variables (Damschroder et al., 2009) are both dependent on implementers having a sound understanding of the policy process to work with, and perhaps even influence, policy-related implementation decisions over time. So, we begin by building a collective understanding with definitions: What is public policy exactly?

There is no widely accepted definition of public policy (see Colebatch, 1998; Howlett & Ramesh, 2003; Smith & Larimer, 2009); however, put simply, **public policy** is "anything a government chooses to do or not to do" (Dye, 1972, as cited in Birkland, 2005). The choices a government makes are relatively easy to discern, as they entail a statement or action produced or led by a public authority. These statements or actions tend to: (a) focus on a goal that defines one or more problems affecting the population they govern (or one or more groups within it), as well as a response to that problem in terms of objectives, actions, and actors; or (b) limit or increase the presence of certain phenomena within the population (National Collaborating Centre for Healthy Public Policy, 2021). The things the government chooses not to do are more difficult to observe or quantify. Making a choice to not do something suggests the government has complete visibility on all the issues within a population at a given point in time as well as all of the possible actions that could be taken to address the problem. This is simply not possible. However, governments do indeed choose not to act on certain issues or by selecting some policy levers or approaches over others when responding to an issue. Both governmental actions and inactions, and the reasons for them, can signal policy intentions. These signals often indicate when EBIs and their associated implementation efforts will be more likely to result in greater support from policy makers at the outset, as well as when implementers might expect that adequate time would be invested in the EBI or resources allocated to sustain the EBI over time. This concept will be explored further later in the chapter, where frameworks will be presented that help analyze the policy environment(s) relevant to implementation efforts.

With this general definition of public policy in mind, it is helpful to understand how public policy gets made and where implementation fits within this process. It is important to understand that policymaking is indeed a process, not an event (Lomas, 2007). Policymaking, like implementation, is a complex, multi-faceted process that unfolds over time. A common way to understand the policymaking process is to break it down into identifiable stages; collectively these stages are often referred to as "the policy cycle" or the "stages heuristic." Different countries and different policy scholars have developed slight modifications to the policy cycle and the number of stages (e.g., see Anderson, 2011; Cairney, 2020; Howlett & Ramesh, 2003). For the purposes of this chapter, the policy cycle will be broken down into six stages, as seen in Figure 14.1. As the focus of this chapter is on policy implementation, following this general introduction to the policy cycle the chapter will elaborate further on the policy implementation stage and present an overview of the scholarship behind it.

Stage 1: Agenda Setting

Before the making of policy can take place, a policy problem must come to the attention of policy makers. In other words, an issue needs to be on the government's agenda to become subject to public policy. There are two broad types of agendas. The first is the governmental (or public) agenda, which is the longer list of subjects or issues getting the attention of policy makers. The second type is the decision agenda, the smaller list of subjects on the

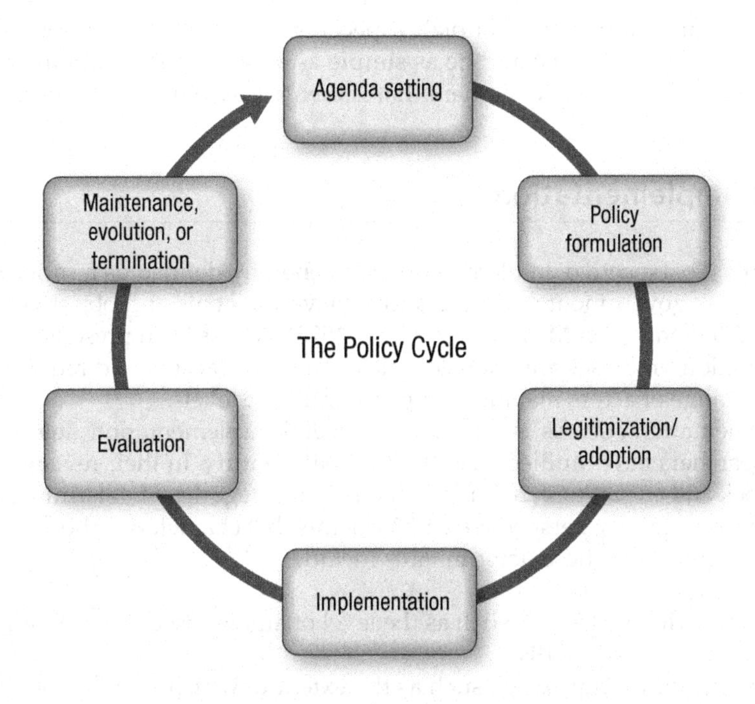

FIGURE 14.1 The policy cycle.

governmental agenda that are up for active decision. Ideas compete for government attention. When looking to garner implementation support from government, it is important to understand if there is awareness of the problem the EBI is attempting to address and if they are looking to make decisions about it. Knowing whether or not the issue or problem is on the governmental or decision agenda is key.

Stage 2: Policy Formulation

Once a problem is on a government's agenda, those working in the government (often public administrators) will develop policy options that the government can take to address the problem. These options are usually comprised of multiple policy instruments (such as making changes to the governance, financial or delivery arrangements within a policy area) and implementation guidance. Public administrators can get their ideas from a range of sources, such as successful initiatives from elsewhere (policy learning), interest groups who bring forward (or advocate for) specific solutions, research evidence, influential individuals or experts, or their perception of what the public values and would deem acceptable.

Stage 3: Legitimization/Adoption

Once a particular policy option has been selected, it often (but not always) needs to undergo some type of legitimization or adoption process. At its most formal, this can be a governmental vote on a new piece of legislation, but often decision-making authority is delegated (in the health field, decisions are often delegated to Ministries of Health or

Departments of Health, for example), especially in complex, high-resourced democratic systems, so adoption could be as simple as a senior public administrator giving approval on a final strategy document that is then released to stakeholders.

Stage 4: Implementation

From a policy perspective, implementation is generally defined as a series of activities undertaken by government and others to achieve the goals and objectives articulated in policy statements (Van Meter & Van Horn, 1975). As has been presented in this book, implementation processes are often complex and multi-faceted and require the participation of a range of actors making changes at multiple levels.

Implementation success is affected by several implementation determinants that policy researchers have studied over the past half century. In their review of the literature, Bullock and colleagues (2021) identified eight categories of determinants of implementation from a policy perspective and 35 factors that characterize those determinants. The main categories of these determinants include:

1. **Characteristics of the EBI**, such as the level of ambiguity of the EBI or its relative advantage over other EBIs.
2. **Policy formulation process**, such as the extent to which stakeholders have an opportunity to provide input and feedback in the process of formulating the policy.
3. **Vertical public administration and thickness of hierarchy**, such as the number and complexity of institutions, departments, and agencies involved in decision-making as well as the number and of socio-political levels (i.e., national, province/state, municipal) needed for implementation.
4. **Networks/inter-organizational relationships**, such as types of pre-existing networks and the degree of coordination among the actors involved.
5. **Implementing agency responses**, such as attitudes of implementers toward the EBI and the resources available to organizations to support implementation.
6. **Attitudes and responses of those affected by the EBI**, such as the diversity of target group behavior.
7. **Timing and sequencing**, such as the timing and pace of cycles, such as political, policy, and funding cycles.
8. **External environment or overall policy context**, such as the prevailing ideas and societal norms, and how far the EBI is from them, or external events (such as a pandemic) that may facilitate, or create barriers to, implementation.

Stage 5: Evaluation

Once implemented, policies must be evaluated to determine whether they have achieved their objectives. It is important to note that there is usually some accordance with the other outcomes articulated in implementation, such as individual, service/organizational, and implementation outcomes (Proctor et al., 2011), but there may be additional policy- or system-level outcomes important to policy makers that should also be measured. Examples of this category of outcomes include policy outputs (e.g., enforcement variables, change of perspective of street-level staff), policy outcomes (e.g., unemployment levels, life-expectancy of population, crime levels) or indices of policy system change (e.g., administrative re-organization, privatization; Bullock et al., 2021). Evaluation can be done by government actors, consultants, or civil society (Howlett & Ramesh, 2003).

Stage 6: Maintenance, Evolution, or Termination

The final stage involves what happens after policy makers receive the evaluation feedback. Depending on the feedback, the current policy climate, competing priorities, and other considerations, policy makers have the option to maintain the current policy initiative, make changes or tweaks to it to optimize it, or to choose to stop investing in the policy (termination).

The policy cycle is a helpful heuristic for policy actors, including implementers, to understand where the current policy "energy" is focused on a particular issue. For example presenting policy makers with an EBI as a policy solution to a problem that is not currently on their agenda is unlikely to be effective. However, it is commonly acknowledged that the policy cycle is a large oversimplification of what is a complex, and much less linear, policy process (Cairney, 2020; Howlett & Ramesh, 2003). In practice, stages are not discrete and there is blurring and interdependence across the stages. Take, for example, policy development and policy implementation. The way policy is developed (including the level of engagement with civil society and interest groups or how much implementation guidance or funds for implementation are included in the policy package) has a strong bearing on how it is implemented. As colleagues at the Centre for Effective Services (CES) state: "There is no good way to implement bad policy. Poor policy design is a common reason for poor implementation. Likewise, a well-designed policy can be poorly implemented" (CES, 2021; Gold, 2014). This is especially important when considering equity and disparities for groups within the population. When public administrators and their advisors fail to use health equity impact assessments to carefully and consciously consider the potential negative impacts of policies for certain groups within the policy development process, implementers may be faced with implementing policy that may actually worsen pre-existing disparities. Additionally, a poor or uneven implementation effort that is not tailored appropriately to particular groups may result in an implementation failure to the very groups that could benefit most from the policy being implemented.

A Short History on Policy Implementation

The *policy implementation* stage of the policy cycle receives considerably less attention than the *problem definition* and *policy formulation* stages in many academic circles, yet implementation is the lynchpin that makes policy decisions meaningful and realizable to citizens and leads to population-level health impact. How have policy scholars tackled policy implementation to date and what have they learned? This short journey through the policy implementation literature will highlight some of the thinking and advances that have shaped the state of the current field policy implementation. It makes "pit stops" at some of the more pivotal models and influential thinking but is not an exhaustive description of the policy implementation scholarship landscape.

What Is Policy Implementation?

Policy implementation can be defined as those actions taken by people that are directed at the achievement of objectives set forth in the policy decision (Van Meter & Van Horn, 1975).

It is what develops between an intention of the government to do something and its ultimate impact following action (O'Toole, 2000). Most works on this subject cite Pressman and Wildavsky's (1973) book, *Implementation. How Great Expectations in Washington Are Dashed in Oakland*, as the first study to systematically explore policy implementation. Pressman and Wildavsky argued that successful implementation relied upon good linkages between levels of government and organizations at the local level. An absence or breakdown of these linkages results in an implementation deficit. Their book gained traction in the policy community, although a careful inspection of the history and contributions to the policy implementation literature by Satetren in 2005 demonstrated that doctoral students had been publishing theses on the subject for many years prior to that. So more accurately, Pressman and Wildavsky should be cited as the most widely available early work related to policy implementation.

Evolution of Policy Implementation Theories

Policy implementation models are now generally described as spanning three "generations." First-generation models were mainly focused on exploring the concept of policy implementation and developing case examples of implementation processes, usually related to single authoritative decisions in single locations or multiple sites (Goggin et al., 1990). These studies were described using a top-down approach, where factors explaining the implementation gap were identified from the perspective of central government policy makers, such as unclear or flawed policy, insufficient resources, unfavorable socio-economic conditions, and so forth (Schofield, 2001). An example of the first-generation models is the previously mentioned study by Pressman and Wildavsky (1973). This generation of models was effective at elucidating implementation failures, dubbed "misery research," which resulted in many theorists moving away from the field and on to more promising enterprises.

The second generation of models emerged in the late 1970s and early 1980s and is distinguished by a move away from success or failure perspectives toward the analysis of variables that explicate the implementation process (Schofield, 2001). This generation is characterized by both top-down and bottom-up models. In top-down models, the central actors in implementation are those who design policy. The focus is on factors for which they have influence at a central level (Matland, 1995). Perhaps the most well-known of these models was developed by Sabatier and Mazmanian in the early 1980s (Mazmanian & Sabatier, 1983; Sabatier & Mazmanian, 1980). Their model includes a set of three factors important for implementation success: tractability of the problem (e.g., how clearly defined the problem is and how simple it is to address it), ability of the policy to structure implementation, and non-statutory variables affecting implementation (e.g., support from stakeholder groups or socio-economic conditions). These factors can be analyzed to explain implementation and ultimately tie policy to outcomes.

In general, top-down models face three sets of criticisms, as outlined in Matland (1995). They take statutory language as their starting point, which means they fail to consider actions from earlier in the policymaking process or history of the area that may be important for implementation success. Top-down models also conceive of implementation as a mainly administrative process, ignoring or trying to eliminate the political aspects of the process. Finally, they fail to account for the role of front-line staff who are responsible for putting the policy into action, instead focusing on policy designers.

Bottom-up theorists argued that a more realistic understanding of implementation is gained by viewing implementation from the perspective of the target population and the service deliverers (Matland, 1995). They focus more on the contextual and field variables at the "bottom" of the policy implementation process (Nilsen et al., 2013). Benny Hjern and several colleagues have done extensive empirical work using this approach (see Hjern, 1982). According to Schofield (2001), there are three core elements of the bottom-up approach: the focus on the actions of local implementers rather than the central government (also called "street level bureaucrats" by Lipsky [1980]); the emphasis on the nature of the social problem (what the policy is intended to address) rather than the goals of the policy itself; and the aim to describe networks of implementation, identifying the diverse range of people and organizations that are responsible for implementing policy. This third element was an important methodological contribution to the field of implementation analysis (Schofield, 2001). The bottom-up approach is inductive in nature and tends to be more descriptive than prescriptive, which means it results in few explicit policy recommendations (Matland, 1995).

Criticisms of the bottom-up approach are generally twofold. First is a normative argument based on the notion that in a democracy, policy control should be exercised by actors whose power derives from their accountability to sovereign voters. Local service deliverers do not hold this power (Matland, 1995; Schofield, 2001). Second, these models tend to overemphasize the autonomy of local actors, failing to take into consideration the role of the central actors and the importance of the centrally determined policy in defining the range of actions local actors can take (Matland, 1995; Schofield, 2001).

While the top-down and bottom-up approaches were helpful in elucidating certain aspects of the policy implementation process, they were not satisfactory in providing a holistic view of the process. The top-down models over-emphasized the role of government actors and their influence in making implementation happen as well as the legislation and the related processes. In contrast, the bottom-up models placed too much emphasis on the local implementer's ability to achieve large-scale policy outcomes. Convergence was deemed necessary for the field to develop (Nilsen et al., 2013) leading to the third generation of policy implementation research (Goggin et al., 1990). This generation sought to either reconcile the two approaches by synthesizing the "macro" world of policy makers with the "micro" world of individual implementers into new models and frameworks, or to develop the conceptualization of learning and negotiation within different policy environments. These models aimed to look at implementation holistically, integrating both top-down and bottom-up perspectives. They also attempted to develop theories and frameworks that would lend themselves to being tested with empirical research, to encourage policy implementation researchers to use more rigorous research methodologies, longitudinal study designs, and comparative multiple case studies with more explanatory power than single case descriptions (Nilsen et al., 2013).

Some notable examples include the Ambiguity-Conflict Model (Matland, 1995) and the Communication Model of Inter-Governmental Policy Implementation (Goggin et al., 1990). Matland's model is an example of a third-generation policy implementation model. His model posits that the level of ambiguity of the policy package (e.g., how vague or specific the policy package is as interpreted by stakeholders), and the amount of conflict among stakeholders with respect to the policy package (e.g., to what extent is there agreement among stakeholders that the policy is the "right" thing to do) help to characterize the implementation process and also to explain its outcomes. Using this thinking, and putting these variables in a 2×2 table where each variable is measured as either "high" or "low," there are four possible types of implementation processes: (a) administrative implementation when there is low policy ambiguity and low policy conflict (e.g., eradication of a deadly disease); (b) political implementation when there is low ambiguity but high levels of conflict (e.g., investing in public transit); (c) experimental implementation when there is high ambiguity but low conflict (e.g., Head Start programs for pre-school age children);

and (d) symbolic implementation when both ambiguity and conflict are high and policies only have a referential goal and differing perspectives on how to translate the abstract goal into instrumental actions (e.g., establishing youth wellness hubs). Matland's model creates a testable hypothesis for empirical implementation researchers, allowing them to interrogate whether the type of implementation process could be predicted by ambiguity and conflict alone. It also allows researchers to examine whether their results hold across different policy areas (e.g., child services or justice).

A Short Gap

There was a pause in the development of the policy implementation literature in the 1990s, mainly attributed to major shifts in state–society relationships in many industrialized countries. This decade saw shifts away from unilateral and hierarchical governance arrangements toward more horizontal accountabilities and reciprocal approaches whereby government bodies and agencies endeavored to work together across silos with shared accountabilities (Saetren, 2005). This retreat from government intervention was replaced by an increased focus on market-based policy instruments such as developing taxes on processes or products to account for the external costs of production or consumption. Perhaps the best example of this approach is taxing companies for the pollution they cause. Policy scholars became interested in governance and policy networks to address these new institutional and inter-organizational relationships, moving away from the language of policy implementation as originally conceived (O'Toole, 2000; Saetren, 2005).

Policy Implementation Literature Today

Twenty-first century scholars have continued to address implementation by expanding the range of disciplinary approaches it utilizes to include public management and organizational theories (Schofield & Sausman, 2004). Some of these models are not focused on implementation as a discrete stage of the policy cycle, but are inclusive of it, such as Sabatier's Advocacy Coalition Framework (Sabatier & Jenkins-Smith, 1993). Implementation research continues to grow but much of it is found outside the traditional fields, as several calls for revival and renewal have noted (Barrett, 2004; Saetren, 2005; Schofield, 2001). This has the potential to result in the development of novel theories of policy implementation and new analytic approaches (for an example of advocating for cross-fertilization between fields, see Nilsen et al., 2013). In general, the literature faces a valid criticism that most models originate in the United Sates or to a lesser extent, Western Europe, limiting our understanding of the generalizability and applicability of these theories in low- and middle-income country settings. Furthermore, with advancements in fields such as implementation science as well as dissemination and knowledge translation (KT) science, perspectives on policy implementation are slowly broadening and scholarship is becoming more interdisciplinary. While each field has much to offer, the fields all approach implementation through different lenses and with different goals in mind (Table 14.1).

One example of an interdisciplinary effort at theory building comes from Bullock and colleagues (2021), who conducted a systematic review of the policy implementation models theories and frameworks from these three fields and used the findings interpretively to build a process model and a policy determinants framework.

The integration of these fields is viewed as an important future direction of implementation science and this sub-field of "policy implementation science" is seen as critical

TABLE 14.1 The Lens Through Which Implementation Is Viewed and the Goal of Implementation by Field of Research

FIELD	LENS	GOAL OF IMPLEMENTATION
Public management	Policy	Realizing policy decisions
Knowledge translation/ dissemination	Research evidence	Improving the use of research evidence in policy and practice
Implementation science	Practice	Creating improvements in the delivery of services and interventions

to reducing health and social disparities across populations. As Emmons and Chambers (2021) point out, policies are made every day, and these policies interact with local contexts, with differential effects across different groups in a population. Using rigorous methods to study the implementation of policies will support our understanding of how to reduce inequities across the population and support better population health.

To sum up, the policy cycle is just one way of describing the policy process. It may be overly simplistic, but it is useful, nonetheless. Situating the problem an implementation effort or an EBI is trying to address in the context of policy, understanding whether it is on the government's agenda, how to present it as a viable policy option during the formulation stage, offering evidence-informed implementation support, and data for evaluative purposes can be valuable to any type of change effort. In fact, many of the tools for policy analysis connect in some way to one or more of the stages, including those introduced later in this chapter. Furthermore, understanding how policy makers approach implementation, and the related scholarship arising from the public management field is crucial to proactively identify and address issues that may arise because of these competing paradigms and the way each party is framing implementation. Additionally, the advancement of more integrated policy implementation science will support a stronger understanding of how to implement not just effectively, but equitably. With this understanding of the policy process in mind, the chapter next explores policy makers' toolboxes to learn more about the tools they have at their disposal.

POLICY INSTRUMENTS

The tools in policy makers' toolboxes are often called "policy instruments" or "policy levers." They are the myriad of techniques that governments have at their disposal to implement public policy objectives. Policy levers can be classified in many ways (Howlett, 2004), but can be grouped according to whether they are legal and regulatory instruments, economic instruments, voluntary instruments, or information and education instruments (Treasury Board of Canada Secretariat, 2007). Legal and regulatory instruments include acts and regulations, self-regulation regimes (e.g., health professions), and performance-based regulations. Economic instruments include taxes and fees, public expenditure and loans, public ownership, insurance schemes, and contracts among others, and is by far the most common type of instrument in the implementation literature and usually described as "funding." Voluntary instruments can include things like standards and guidelines and both formalized partnerships and support for less formalized networks. Finally, information and education instruments are usually targeted to citizens in general or specific groups and can be an important instrument when a behavior change of the public or the workforce is needed. There is usually a mix of levers in any policy package. Depending on the level of specificity, the policy package can also include some implementation guidance such as a description of the overall implementation strategy architecture, the major streams of activity, timing of events and milestones, and roles and responsibilities.

USING EVIDENCE TO INFORM THE POLICY PROCESS

Many people with scientific training assume that governments have access to and use research evidence to inform their decisions as a matter of course. The reality is that while some governments and some policy areas within a particular government are better at this than others, most policy makers would tell you that their use of evidence is not optimized. So why is this?

Some of the reasons why research evidence (including pre-packaged evidence, such as evidence-based practices and EBIs) is not always part of the process include (Oliver et al., 2014):

1. Research evidence must compete with other sources of information as well as the values and previously stated policy directions of elected officials and political parties.
2. Research evidence is not valued as an information input.
3. Research evidence is not relevant.
4. Research evidence is not easy for decision-makers to use, meaning:
   a. Research is not communicated effectively.
   b. Research is not available when policy makers need it and in a form that they can use.
   c. Policy makers lack mechanisms to prompt them to use research in decision-making.
   d. Policy makers lack forums where health-system challenges can be discussed with key stakeholders who are informed about the best available research evidence.

Approaches to Informing the Policy Process With Research Evidence

Even given these challenges, there are many ways that research can inform the policy process. Following are a few of the more common ways, as well as some of the types of research that are particularly helpful at informing certain stages.

Informing the Policy Agenda

This method involves bringing attention to an issue, framing a problem and/or getting it on the "decision" agenda for action. An example of this can be found in the earlier case study of Jorge the policy analyst and the tobacco cessation policy. In this case study, a research group informed Jorge that smoking and vaping rates were increasing at an alarming rate for young people. In this case the research group was monitoring a social problem through survey methods, identified a change in an indicator (smoking/vaping rates), and was able to share this information with a policy partner (Jorge) who was able to get it on the Ministry's decision agenda. Using research to bring attention to inequities and disparities among the population is an important aspect of this. Epidemiological, observational, and some types of qualitative research are particularly informative at this stage.

Informing Policy Options

Informing policy options involves identifying choices about how to address an issue. Often researchers and implementers simply start with an EBI that they "know works" (see Case Study 14.1). However, that EBI is likely just one of several policy options a government could take. There are likely other groups lobbying the government for different solutions, such as means restrictions, other types of effective EBIs, or better postvention approaches that are also evidence-based. Positioning an EBI as the preferred option for policy makers requires a sound understanding of the political and policy climate as well as having information that will address and not only demonstrate that it is feasible, implementable, cost-effective, and will get the outcomes they are looking for (preferable quickly), but also that it aligns with the government's mandate, will be acceptable to the public, among many other considerations. Health and social systems and services research, economic analyses, and qualitative research that speaks to the experience of the EBI are helpful at this stage.

Informing Implementation

In order to inform implementation, one must identify effective implementation strategies, manage challenges, and monitor the implementation process. This is the area where implementation science plays a particularly important role. As mentioned, implementation guidance is sometimes (although not always) part of a policy package. Whether part of an initial policy or used after as the government begins to plan the policy roll-out, guidance about the optimal, most cost-effective way to get their policy intentions realized across services and systems is important knowledge for policy partners. Comparative costing of various implementation strategies or approaches (not just costing related to the EBI itself) is an important input for policy makers so that they understand the value and trade-offs between strategies in terms of time and money.

Providing Policy Feedback

Evaluating the effectiveness of the policy/intervention against the policy and system goals as well as the effectiveness of the implementation of it is another way for research to inform policy. This is a critical step for policy learning and improvement and one to which research can certainly contribute. Systems and services research, implementation outcomes research, policy analyses, as well as evaluation research are key contributions here.

USING A FRAMEWORK TO CONDUCT POLICY ANALYSIS

Policy analysis is a systematic way of scanning the policy landscape and looking for factors that can explain why (or why not) a particular policy decision was made, or to identify features that could be important to consider during the implementation process that could either act as facilitators or barriers to it. If we think back to Jorge in Case Study 14.1, he may wish to conduct a policy analysis prior to bringing forward the policy options related to tobacco cessation for youth. His policy analysis might be focused on the political landscape to determine what interests or interest groups might be opposed to his policy proposal (such as the tobacco companies, tobacco farmers, or youth themselves) and how to mitigate their opposition. This information may inform which policy option he recommends and/or may influence the overall design and implementation plan for the policy option. Alternatively, for Mathilde and the land-based program she and her team are trying to sustain, a policy analysis could help them to identify how to position their EBI for long-term adoption and scaling. For example, instead of just seeking funding for the service, a careful consideration of the policy landscape may reveal that land-based programs are not currently defined as mental health services and, thus, are not eligible for funding (at least from the health system). This knowledge may influence who from the public administration Mathilde will seek to work with (e.g., working with the provincial policy unit responsible for maintaining the roster of publicly funded community mental health services rather than the mental health services unit that focuses on contracting with services). These are just two examples of the many ways policy analyses can support better implementation planning and execution. In the following, we focus on one of the many frameworks available to conduct policy analyses that can inform implementation.

Policy Analysis Framework: 3I+E

When attempting to understand the political and policy landscape surrounding an implementation effort, it is helpful to draw on the **3I+E framework**, which identifies the *Institutions, Interests, Ideas* and *External factors* that might influence implementation or act as a facilitator or barrier to it (Lavis, 2013). While originally developed to identify the factors that influence policy choices, it has proven to be equally salient to policy implementation, particularly in the planning or exploration phases. Here each of the framework elements are briefly described as well as presented in Table 14.2 that includes specific prompts to use when conducting an analysis.

Institutions

Often defined as "the rules of the game," **institutions** include things like government structures that are currently in place that are connected with an EBI and where decisions related to the EBI or its implementation get made. It is important to think about all of the structures that might be influential within a particular level of a system (e.g., the institutional structures within the province/state level such as government ministries, agencies of government, professional associations, unions, service-delivering organizations, patient, client or family groups, non-governmental organizations) as well as vertically across policy levels (such as "up" to the national level or "down" to the municipal level).

TABLE 14.2 3I+E Policy Analysis

INSTITUTIONS	INTERESTS	IDEAS	EXTERNAL FACTORS
Government structures Policy legacies Policy networks	Interest groups (e.g., unions, professional associations, patient groups, community groups) Individual interests	Research evidence Peoples' values (including cultural norms)	Events or other factors that are outside of the policy area of interest (election, pandemic, weather event, etc.)

Past policies ("policy legacies") are a second type of institutional influence that may make current implementation efforts easier or more difficult (Pierson, 1993). Policy legacies are created by past decisions that have generated the structures and rules that are presently in operation. These structures and rules that are already in place can create some inertia in the system and can constrain decisions. The way health insurance is organized and delivered is a good example of this. It is much easier to try and improve the system of health insurance that already exists rather than to overhaul it by changing a mostly private system to a mostly public one or vice versa. Evidence-informed innovations that align with existing institutional structures or policies often have an easier time being successfully implemented. This is a particularly important point when it comes to considering EBIs that address disparities. If there is a system of institutional structures and decisions that have favored some groups over others, it may be inherently easier to continue to build new policies onto those existing decisions, thus leading to a potential of increasing disparities over time.

The third type of institutional influence is policy networks. Policy networks reflect the formal and informal relationships between governmental and other actors related to a particular policy area. These relationships are not static and are continually negotiated among network members. The structure of these relationships on a given policy issue at a particular moment in time and the amount of conflict among actors can influence the success of an implementation effort. Understanding what structures and past policy decisions will constrain or enable the implementation of an EBI can help plan implementation better by identifying where system inertia might be pushing against the implementation effort.

Interests

Interests are defined as the individuals or groups of people who are interested in a particular policy issue. While theoretically everyone in the public has an interest in public policy decisions, people tend to engage personally or professionally only in some policy areas and only on some decisions. Identifying interest groups, such as patient groups, professional associations, unions, and others that can influence (positively or negatively) the will and the ability to implement the intervention are key. It can also include other interests, such as elected officials, civil servants, trusted members of civil society (including researchers or professionals), or community members who may be influential as individuals in the ability to effectively implement an EBI. Individuals and interest groups can often be identified through the media (they may issue statements, press releases, or tweets, when certain policy decisions are made, or may be quoted by news outlets) or by using self-knowledge of the policy area. Developing skills in stakeholder identification and analysis are key to doing this well. Identifying those individuals and groups who will support or oppose an implementation effort can influence the process by shaping the EBI itself or the implementation approach. Early engagement of stakeholders in the implementation process can help build consensus and remove barriers to implementation as it proceeds.

Ideas

Ideas are the thoughts and norms that are circulating related to an EBI at any given time. This includes the research evidence, technical knowledge, and evaluation findings related to an EBI that exists, in addition to consideration of whether people know about the research and whether they believe it. It also includes current societal values and norms that need to be taken into consideration and that may affect implementation. Some policy areas are more visible to the public and can be more affected by values. For example, in substance use policy, prevailing values and norms may drive different responses to addiction, such as abstinence-based treatments, harm-reduction approaches, or legal responses (e.g., criminalization or decriminalization). If the EBI is a significant departure from the current way of doing things and/or if it does not align with the prevailing values of the mass public, it may be more difficult to gain support for its implementation. If the EBI is tailored to a sub-population group and it does not align with the values and norms of the broader public or the values and norms of the political leaders in power, it may be more challenging to get or sustain support for the implementation activities. So how does one understand societal values and norms when planning implementation? There is a range of techniques to identify prevailing values and norms. One approach might be to look to credible polling organizations to see if they have done any recent polling related to the policy area of an EBI. Media outlets are also a source for understanding the overall public mood and current values. Protests and social movements can indicate a shift in public mood or that policy decisions are being made that do not align with the prevailing values and norms. Researchers (political scientists in particular) often have a very good handle on the values, norms, and beliefs in specific jurisdictions and for certain policy areas. A phone or video chat with a knowledgeable expert is a useful source of feedback. Finally, the policy platforms of the political parties, especially those parties that garner large popular support, may give a sense of the norms and values of the elected officials in the jurisdiction(s) in which implementation is situated.

External Factors

External factors are things that fall outside of the area of implementation focus but can influence the success or failure of implementation efforts. Some visible examples include pandemics, stock market crashes, elections, environmental disasters, or wars. Often not much can be done about this, and they are difficult or impossible to predict in advance, but it is still important to understand the larger context in which an implementation effort is occurring and can help to interpret implementation outcomes (or the lack thereof) appropriately.

APPROACHES TO SUPPORTING EVIDENCE-INFORMED POLICY PROCESSES

While understanding and analyzing the policy process may be helpful in unpacking the complexity in the outer context of implementation, it is not necessarily instructive about how exactly the process itself can be influenced. This section introduces how policymaking processes can be supported to be evidence-based in both high- and low- or middle-income countries. This is done by considering four different elements of support:

1. The role of individuals and groups in influencing the policy process
2. The infrastructure (the organizations, programs, or networks) to support this function
3. The processes and products being generated
4. The capacities (skills and expertise) required

This section concludes by sharing some examples of entities that have experience supporting policy processes to be evidence-informed.

How Can Individuals or Groups Influence the Policy Process, Including Implementation?

Let's start with a look at what the evidence says about what is effective at influencing the policy process to become more evidence informed. Fortunately, there is some research examining the factors associated with the use of research evidence in policymaking that can guide us. In fact, there are now several reviews of the literature that include hundreds of observational studies (e.g., Liverani et al., 2013; Lawrence et al., 2019; Mitton, Adair, McKenzie, et al., 2007; Murthy, Sheppard, Clark, et al., 2012; Perrier et al., 2011). Despite the growing number of reviews, all authors point to the limitations of the existing literature, including its lack of precision, and the (over)reliance on case descriptions rather than effectiveness studies or comparative analyses or other more rigorous designs. Even with these shortcomings, these reviews suggest that several factors are important in promoting evidence-informed policymaking, including (but not limited to):

1. Timing/timeliness—Being very strategic about when the evidence is shared and how it is shared and tailoring it in response to the stage of policymaking. Turn-around times for policy makers can be very fast (sometimes only a matter of hours) and windows of opportunity for influence may not remain open for very long.
2. Accordance between the beliefs, values, and strategies of policy makers with the available research evidence—Positioning the evidence to demonstrate its alignment with current policies and strategies or with the values and beliefs of citizens.
3. Trust—Developing trusting relationships with policy makers over time by being an "honest broker" and speaking with some impartiality about the benefits and risks of a particular policy choice or EBI.

Individuals, such as influential researchers, clinicians or other system leaders that accomplish policy influence independently are often called "policy entrepreneurs." This term was first used by John Kingdon (1984) to describe individuals who were influential in the policy agenda-setting process. Kingdon describes these individuals as people who are very familiar with the policy environment and who can effectively "couple" a particular societal problem within a particular political context with a particular policy solution (e.g., an EBI) to make change happen. They usually come into the policy environment with a policy solution in mind and are skilled at getting traction for it. Depending on the context, sometimes these individuals are visible to an observer, but other times they work quietly in the background. Individuals who wish to influence the adoption or implementation of an EBI can consider if they have the ability, skills, and network to become a policy entrepreneur themselves. Of course, the label does not come through official channels but rather through a proven track record of working effectively with the policy process and the individuals within it. An alternative approach might be to scan the policy environment to see if there is a policy entrepreneur who might take on the work of encouraging adoption, implementation, or scaling of an EBI. Individuals may wish to think carefully about whether they might attempt to become a policy entrepreneur or whether there may be someone else who believes in their intervention and has built strong and trusting relationships with government, who may wish to work with them to bring more visibility to the EBI. Either approach may increase changes at influencing the policy process as an individual.

Beyond policy entrepreneurs, many governments are now using more inclusive approaches to policymaking that involve the engagement of system stakeholders in the policy process, sometimes referred to as a "new public governance" (Osborne, 2006, 2010; Torfing & Triantafillou, 2013). New public governance thinking includes the concept of co-production, whereby state and non-state actors collectively produce or inform public service delivery (Howelett et al., 2017; Pestoff, 2006). The overarching hypothesis is that the development and implementation of public policy is improved by cooperation, negotiation, and the active participation of relevant stakeholders who contribute knowledge, ideas, and resources. Of course, the type of involvement of stakeholders, the extent of involvement, and the stage of the policymaking process will vary by jurisdiction and by policy area; however, it is increasingly clear that many more opportunities are being created for active participation in policy processes, including at the implementation stage.

So far, this chapter has focused on the role that individuals can play to influence the policymaking process to be more evidence informed; however, it is becoming more common for organizations, programs, or networks to play this support function. Whether support happens through individuals or groups, many of the same lessons apply. The authors' own observation is that trusting relationships are built between people and not organizational entities. While it is possible and often even necessary for organizations, programs, or networks to be involved in supporting evidence-informed policy processes, the individual people really matter. The main advantages of using an organization, program, or network for this function are that it provides for increased capacity (both by increasing the output volume and improving response time), encourages a more diverse range ideas and approaches than one individual alone can generate, and increases sustainability. There are a variety of opportunities for organizations, programs, and networks to support evidence-informed policymaking. In the next section, the chapter delves more deeply into the infrastructure and how different jurisdictions are organizing these support functions.

What Infrastructure Is Needed to Support This Function?

There are many different types of organizations, programs, and networks that support evidence-informed policymaking. They are distinguished according to the phase of the policymaking process (e.g., agenda setting, policy development, or policy implementation); what area of the system they intend to support (e.g., clinical programs, services or products that target individuals; public health programs or services that target groups and populations; or the health system as a whole, including its governance, financial and service delivery arrangements); and their location in the system (e.g., academic institution, service-delivering organization or non-governmental organization; Bullock & Lavis, 2019; Lavis et al., 2012; Partridge et al., 2020). These system support initiatives are labeled variably in the literature as intermediaries, technical assistance centers, KT platforms, centers of excellence, or backbone organizations, to name a few; for example, clinical practice guideline initiatives that focus on supporting clinicians to deliver care that is evidence-based and often located in either academic settings or attached to an academic health sciences center. In the past two decades, many of these guideline groups have collaborated to create a global network of guideline developers known as the Guidelines International Network (GIN) that works to create common standards across different country settings (Ollenschläger et al., 2004). Another example is the mental health system policy intermediaries described by Bullock and Lavis (2019) from several different countries. In their study, they defined intermediaries as organizations or programs that have an explicit and recognized role to support the implementation of government mental health policy goals and employ specific methods of implementation support. These two examples, as well as the following case study, underpin the wide array of entities that exist to support the use of evidence in systems.

CASE STUDY 14.2 McMASTER HEALTH FORUM, ONTARIO, CANADA (www.mcmasterforum.org)

The McMaster Health Forum's goal is to generate action on pressing health- and social-system issues, based on the best available research evidence and systematically elicited citizen values and stakeholder insights. They aim to strengthen health systems—locally, nationally, and internationally—and get the right programs, services, and drugs to the people who need them. In operation now for over a decade, they work to:

1. Make evidence available when policy makers and stakeholders need it and in a form that they can use (facilitating pull) by:
   - Maintaining a one-stop shop for pre-appraised global evidence, and including links to local evidence (www.healthsystemsevidence.org and www.socialsystemsevidence.org)
   - Preparing rapid syntheses in 3, 10, and 30 business days for policy makers, stakeholders, and writers of election platforms
   - Building capacity to find and use research evidence efficiently through workshops for decision-makers
2. Communicate evidence effectively (packaging and push) by:
   - Preparing evidence/citizen briefs on high-priority topics and with the input of those who will need to act on the briefs
3. Convene stakeholder dialogues and citizen panels where policy challenges can be discussed with key stakeholders who are informed about the best available research evidence (exchange)

The McMaster Health Forum has also played a key role during the COVID-19 pandemic. In Ontario it has developed new relationships and networks (such as participating in the province's Evidence Synthesis Network; www.esnetwork.ca), expanded on existing ones, and created tailored products and tools (such as rapid evidence profiles—summarizing the evidence in as little as 3 hours) in response to the emergent needs of decision-makers. Internationally, it co-developed, and provides secretariat support to, a large international collaboration the COVID-19 Evidence Network to Support Decision-making (COVID-END; www.covid-end.org). COVID-END is a time-limited network that brings together more than 50 of the world's leading evidence-synthesis, technology-assessment, and guideline-development groups around the world. It covers the full spectrum of the pandemic response, from public-health measures and clinical management to health-system arrangements and economic and social responses. It also covers the full spectrum of contexts where the pandemic response is playing out, including low-, middle- and high-income countries.

Housed at McMaster University in Hamilton, Ontario, it is staffed by a core team of research, operations, and communications experts, and is supported by students at the graduate and undergraduate levels, as well as a number of adjunct faculty and fellows. Depending on the initiative, it partners with other research institutes across the world, such as Monash University for Social Systems Evidence, and the Ottawa Hospital Research Institute for COVID-END.

It is important to note that if when the goal is to implement or scale an EBI, there may be an organization, program, or network in the system that is focused on supporting policymaking and may have tools, resources, relationships, expertise, and capacity to support EBI implementation efforts. Using existing system capacity where possible, instead of trying to create it from scratch for each new EBI implementation, is a more efficient use of system resources and may accelerate implementation as well as increasing the likelihood of implementation success. This seems to be especially important in settings where evidence resources are scarce, such as low- and middle-income countries, but all jurisdictions and policy areas would benefit from this approach.

What Are the Processes and Products Available to Support Evidence-Informed Policymaking?

Encouraging the use of research evidence in the policymaking process requires processes and outputs (or products) that are tailored to policy makers and system leaders and their context. One mistake that researchers and public health practitioners can make is to assume that what they find most useful, or what is useful for a clinical audience, will resonate equally with policy makers. The lack of a tailor-made approach is part of the reason why there is an evidence-to-policy gap. Fortunately, there are several processes and products that have been developed by research groups across the world that have been found to be effective. It is helpful to think of the activities and outputs according to what they are trying to accomplish with policy makers or the "domain" of **Knowledge Translation (KT)**. Common KT goals include:

- Building demand for evidence
- Prioritization of evidence and co-production of evidence and/or evidence-informed policy
- Packaging evidence for a policy audience, "push" strategies (from the evidence producers to the policy makers) and support to implementation
- Facilitating "pull" (encouraging the use of evidence by making it easy for policy makers to access and use evidence)
- Exchange (interactive approaches to building partnerships and creating a common understanding of needs and constraints)

These domains have been adapted from the Cochrane Collaboration KT Framework building on the work of other KT scholars (Cochrane Collaboration, 2017; Ellen et al., 2011; Lavis et al., 2006). Using these domains, Partridge and colleagues (2020) reviewed descriptions and evaluations of KT platforms that support evidence-informed policymaking in low- and middle-income countries. They sorted the most common processes and activities they identified in the studies by these domains of KT. They found that evidence briefs (packaging, push, and support to implementation domain) and deliberative dialogues (exchange domain) were well-studied and viewed as helpful. Put simply, an evidence brief is a type of document that provides a summary of the research evidence about what is known about a problem, possible ways to address the problem, and considerations for implementation (Alvarez et al., 2019). They are often used in conjunction with other activities, such as deliberative dialogues, that bring policy makers, researchers, and other stakeholders together to discuss these issues with the goal of informing policy. The review also found that rapid evidence services (facilitating pull domain) and capacity-building workshops (focusing specifically on evidence use—also a facilitating pull domain) were less studied but also viewed as helpful. These findings from low- and middle-income countries echo the approaches being taken in jurisdictions in high-income countries, and what has reportedly been found useful to policy makers (Boyko et al., 2014; Wilson et al., 2012).

CASE STUDY 14.3 K2P CENTER, BEIRUT, LEBANON (www.aub.edu.lb/k2p)

The Knowledge to Policy (K2P) Center aims to serve as a leading hub in the Arab world for strengthening public policy and practice and improving health and social outcomes using a collective problem-solving approach. Their goal is to bridge the gap between evidence, policy, and politics. They do this by:

1. Building KT capacity of research networks, civil society, researchers, policy makers and the media, including capacity of health policymaking institutions (facilitating pull)
2. Informing the production, packaging, and sharing of evidence from public health research in an objective manner and based on current and emerging policy priorities (packaging and push—research supply side)
3. Using the best available evidence to inform policy making in an objective and timely manner (facilitating pull and exchange—policy demand side)
4. Developing and testing models of KT that are culturally appropriate, relevant, and effective for the region (innovating and tailoring for context)

Some of their products and activities include:

- Policy briefs—Analysis of the context, problem, policy options, and implementation barriers for a particular policy-relevant issue
- Briefing notes—Quick and effective advice to policy makers and stakeholders about a pressing public issue by bringing together global research evidence and local evidence
- Rapid responses—Respond to urgent requests from policy makers and stakeholders by delivering optimally packaged, relevant, and high-quality evidence for decision-making
- Evidence summaries—Use of global research evidence to provide insight on public health priority topics that are ambiguous or uncertain
- Media bites—Short, media-friendly summaries to communicate evidence to the media and support evidence-based health reporting
- Policy dialogues—Events that convene policy makers and stakeholders to capture contextual information, tacit knowledge, views, and experiences including potential options to address high-priority issues
- Citizen consultations—Events that convene citizens from different Lebanese areas and backgrounds to capture contextual information, tacit knowledge, views, values, and experiences on potential options to address high-priority issues and their implementation considerations

Located at the American University of Beirut, the K2P Center is a WHO Collaborating Center for Evidence Informed Policy and Practice and has been selected as a lead mentor institute for developing sustainable institutional capacity for evidence-informed decision-making in health in low- and middle-income countries.

What Capacities (Skills and Expertise) Are Required?

Effectively supporting evidence-informed policymaking (including implementation) is dependent on highly skilled individuals. In a multi-sector review of research on these positions, Neal et al., (2021) identified a range of skills necessary to successful undertake the processes and develop the products identified previously. Some skills were important regardless of the process or product while others were specific to certain strategies. The cross-functional skills they identified include communicating clearly, expertise in research and policy, and knowledge of change processes. They also identified 16 function-specific skills that range from scanning the horizon, translating, and tailoring and packaging evidence for dissemination, to mediating differences, understanding roles and power, being responsive to stakeholder needs, and navigating social networks to find alignment. While there are some certificate-type training programs that do exist that support the development of some of these skills, there is currently no internationally recognized, post-graduate (i.e., masters level) training program available. Thus, individuals recruited to these roles are drawn from diverse settings, often with different types of formal education. Because of the high number of skills and level of expertise these individuals possess, recruitment and retention have been identified as a challenge, especially in low-resource settings (Partridge et al., 2020).

SUMMARY

This chapter introduced implementation from the perspective of public policy and through the eyes of policy makers. The chapter began by unpacking what is meant by policy and its implementation, sharing a heuristic that is often used to identify the phases through which ideas become policy. This was followed by a brief discussion about the instruments used to make policy, and a whirlwind tour of policy implementation models, theories, and frameworks. It then explored how research evidence can shape policy, including its implementation, and introduced a framework that can help you conduct policy analyses to support better implementation. The chapter concluded with an overview of the approaches that can be taken to support evidence-informed policymaking.

KEY POINTS FOR PRACTICE

1. Policies can be both the evidence-based innovation that is being implemented or a facilitator or barrier to implementation success.
2. When implementing, it is important to look outside of the organizational context for policy or system factors that could affect the success of implementation efforts over the long term.
3. Policies, and the effective implementation of them, can increase or reduce disparities in a population. It is important to assess the potential impacts of a policy and its implementation on equity, both intended and unintended, prior to and during, implementation.
4. There are whole "generations" of policy implementation models, theories, and frameworks from which to draw! Find one that resonates with the implementation effort and use it to help guide implementation.
5. The policy process can be influenced by locating an issue within the policy cycle, conducting an analysis of political factors that impact the EBI using the 3I+E framework, and/or seeking out individuals or organizations that are skilled at supporting an evidence-informed policy process.

COMMON PITFALLS IN PRACTICE

1. The late-comer: Ignoring outer context/public policy factors until late in the implementation process.
2. Over-simplifying: Assuming that good evidence will automatically inform the policy process (or that policy maker knowledge about "what works" is "enough").
3. Ignorance is not bliss: Not understanding the factors that drive the policy process, the pace of policymaking (timing/sequencing), the influence of politics, or how to effectively position the EBI for implementation or scaling within that context.
4. The hero complex: Overlooking existing capacity in systems (such as organizations, programs, or networks viewed as KT or implementation intermediaries) that have expertise in supporting evidence-informed policymaking and can facilitate implementation or scaling efforts.

DISCUSSION QUESTIONS

1. What public policies have influenced your life so far? Can you describe the policy level (local, state/province, national, international)? Were the effects on your life positive, negative, or neutral in your view? Why or why not?
2. Identify a public policy or a policy area that is having differential effects on certain groups in the population.
   a. What disparities are being created, exacerbated, or sustained and for whom?
   b. In your assessment, does the policy area you identified have a "good" policy but it is not implemented well or is the policy itself creating the disparities?
   c. In your assessment, what are the reasons why the policy still exists? What are the institutional, interest, and ideational factors that are contributing to its sustainment?
   d. What would need to happen to improve the policy or replace it with a new one?
3. How should a policy implementation process be designed? What elements are critical to ensuring an implementation process that reflects an equity, diversity, and inclusion lens?
4. What policy lever(s) do you think can enable EBI implementation the most? What lever(s) is the biggest barrier to implementation? Can you see any patterns regarding what policy lever(s) seem to be favored by your current government? Can they be distinguished from past governments, by political party, or by policy area?
5. How does policy implementation differ in low- and middle-income countries (as compared to high-income countries)? Are there additional barriers? If so, how can they be minimized or overcome?

REFERENCES

Alvarez, E., Lavis, J. N., Brouwers, M., Clavijo, G. C., Sewankambo, N., Solari, L., & Schwartz, L. (2019). Developing evidence briefs for policy: A qualitative case study comparing the process of using a guidance-contextualization workbook in Peru and Uganda. *Health Research Policy and Systems, 17*(1), 1–11. https://doi.org/10.1186/s12961-019-0488-0

Anderson, J. E. (2011). *Public policy making* (7th ed.). Wadsworth, Cengage Learnings.

Barrett, S. M. (2004). Implementation studies: Time for a revival? Personal reflections on 20 years of implementation studies, *Public Administration, 82*(2), 249–262. https://doi.org/10.1111/j.0033-3298.2004.00393.x

Birkland, T. (2005) *An introduction to the policy process: Theories, concepts and models of public policy making* (2nd ed.). ME Sharpe.

Boyko, J. A., Lavis, J. N., & Dobbins, M. (2014). Deliberative dialogues as a strategy for system-level knowledge translation and exchange. *Healthcare Policy, 9*(4), 122. https://doi.org/10.12927/hcpol.2014.23808

Bullock, H. L. & Lavis, J. N. (2019). Understanding the supports needed for policy implementation: A comparative analysis of the placement of intermediaries across three mental health systems. *Health Research Policy & Systems, 17*, 82. https://doi.org/10.1186/s12961-019-0479-1

Bullock, H. L., Lavis, J. N., Wilson, M. G., Mulvale, G., & Miatello, A. (2021). Understanding the implementation of evidence-informed policies and practices from a policy perspective: A critical interpretive synthesis. *Implementation Science, 16*(1), 1–24. https://doi.org/10.1186/s13012-021-01082-7

Cairney, P. (2020). *Understanding public policies: Theories and issues* (2nd ed.). Red Globe Press (Palgrave Macmillan).

Cochrane Collaboration. (2017). *Cochrane knowledge translation framework*. Retrieved September 1, 2021 from https://community.cochrane.org/sites/default/files/uploads/Cochrane%20Knowledge%20Translation%20Framework%281%29.pdf

Colebatch, H. (1998). *Policy*. Open University Press.

Damschroder, L. J., Aron, D. C., Keith, R. E., Kirsh, S. R., Alexander, J. A., & Lowery, J. C. (2009). Fostering implementation of health services research findings into practice: A consolidated framework for advancing implementation science. *Implementation Science, 4*(1), 1–15. https://doi.org/10.1186/1748-5908-4-50

Ellen, M. E., Lavis, J. N., Ouimet, M., Grimshaw, J., & Bédard, P. O. (2011). Determining research knowledge infrastructure for healthcare systems: A qualitative study. *Implementation Science, 6*(1), 1–5. https://doi.org.10.1186/1748-5908-6-60

Emmons, K. M., & Chambers, D. A. (2021). Policy implementation science: An unexplored strategy to address social determinants of health. *Ethnicity & Disease, 31*(1), 133–138. https://doi.org/10.18865/ed.31.1.133

Goggin, M. L., Bowman, A. O. M., Lester, J. P., & O'Toole, L. J. Jr. (1990). *Implementation theory and practice: Toward a third generation*. Foreman/Little Brown.

Gold, J. (2014). *International delivery: Centres of government and the drive for better policy implementation*. Mowat Centre for Policy Innovation.

Hjern, B. (1982). Implementation research – The link gone missing. *Journal of Public Policy, 2*(3), 301–308. https://doi.org/10.1017/S0143814X00001975

Howlett, M. (2004). Beyond good and evil in policy implementation: Instrument mixes, implementation styles, and second generation theories of policy instrument choice. *Policy and Society, 23*(2), 1–17. https://doi.org/10.1016/S1449-4035(04)70030-2

Howlett, M. & Ramesh, M. (2003). *Studying public policy: Policy cycles and policy subsystems*. Oxford University Press Canada.

Howlett, M., Kekez, A., & Poocharoen, O. O. (2017). Understanding co-production as a policy tool: Integrating new public governance and comparative policy theory. *Journal of Comparative Policy Analysis: Research and Practice, 19*(5), 487–501. https://doi.org/10.1080/13876988.2017.1287445

Kingdon, J. W. (1984). *Agendas, Alternatives, and Public Policies*. Little, Brown & Co.

Lavis J. N. (2013). Studying health-care reforms. In: H. Lazar, J. N. Lavis, P. Forest, J. Church, (Eds.), *Paradigm freeze: Why it is so hard to reform health care in Canada*. McGill-Queen's University Press.

Lavis, J. N., Lomas, J., Hamid, M., & Sewankambo, N. K. (2006). Assessing country-level efforts to link research to action. *Bulletin of the World health Organization, 84*, 620–628. https://doi.org/10.2471/blt.06.030312

Lavis, J. N., Røttingen, J. A., Bosch-Capblanch, X., Atun, R., El-Jardali, F., Gilson, L., Lewin, S., Oliver, S., Ongolo-Zogo, P., & Haines, A. (2012). Guidance for evidence-informed policies about health systems: Linking guidance development to policy development. *PLoS Medicine, 9*(3), e1001186. https://doi.org/10.1371/journal.pmed.1001186

Lawrence, L. M., Bishop, A., & Curran, J. (2019). Integrated knowledge translation with public health policy makers: A scoping review. *Healthcare Policy, 14*(3), 55–77. https://doi.org/10.12927/hcpol.2019.25792

Lipsky, M. (1980). *Street-level bureaucracy: Dilemmas of the individual in public services*. Russell Sage Foundation.

Liverani, M., Hawkins, B., & Parkhurst, J. O. (2013). Political and institutional influences on the use of evidence in public health policy. A systematic review. *PLoS One, 8*(10), e77404. https://doi.org/10.1371/journal.pone.0077404

Lomas J. (2007). The in-between world of knowledge brokering. *BMJ (Clinical Research Ed.), 334*(7585), 129–132. https://doi.org/10.1136/bmj.39038.593380.AE

Matland, R. (1995). Synthesizing the implementation literature: The ambiguity-conflict model of policy implementation. *Journal of Public Administration Research and Theory, 5*(2), 145 174. https://doi.org/10.1093/oxfordjournals.jpart.a037242

Mazmanian, D.A., & Sabatier, P.A. (1983). *Implementation and public policy*. Scott, Foresman.

Mitton, C., Adair, C. E., McKenzie, E., Patten, S. B., & Waye Perry, B. (2007). Knowledge transfer and exchange: review and synthesis of the literature. *The Milbank Quarterly, 85*(4), 729–768. https://doi.org/10.1111/j.1468-0009.2007.00506.x

Murthy, L., Shepperd, S., Clarke, M. J., Garner, S. E., Lavis, J. N., Perrier, L., Roberts, N. W., & Straus, S. E. (2012). Interventions to improve the use of systematic reviews in decision-making by health system managers, policy makers and clinicians. *The Cochrane Database of Systematic Reviews*. https://doi.org/10.1002/14651858.CD009401.pub2

National Collaborating Centre for Healthy Public Policy. (2021, April 21). *Defining public policy*. http://www.ncchpp.ca/62/what-we-do.ccnpps

Neal, J. W., Posner, S., & Brutzman, B. (2021, September 2). Understanding brokers, intermediaries, and boundary spanners: A multi-sectoral review of strategies, skills, and outcomes. https://doi.org/10.31234/osf.io/bn7ya

Nilsen, P., Ståhl, C., Roback, K., & Cairney, P. (2013). Never the twain shall meet? – A comparison of implementation science and policy implementation research. *Implementation Science, 8*, 63. https://doi.org/10.1186/1748-5908-8-63

Ollenschläger, G., Marshall, C., Qureshi, S., Rosenbrand, K., Burgers, J., Mäkelä, M., & Slutsky, J. (2004). Improving the quality of health care: Using international collaboration to inform guideline programmes by founding the Guidelines International Network (GIN). *BMJ Quality & Safety, 13*(6), 455–460. https://doi.org/10.1136/qhc.13.6.455

Oliver, K., Innvar, S., Lorenc, T., Woodman, J., & Thomas, J. (2014). A systematic review of barriers to and facilitators of the use of evidence by policy makers. *BMC Health Services Research, 14*(1), 1–12. https://doi.org/10.1186/1472-6963-14-2

Osborne, S. P. (2006). The New Public Governance? *Public Management Review, 8*(3), 377–387. https://doi.org/10.1080/14719030600853022

Osborne, S. P. (2010). *The New Public Governance: Emerging Perspectives on the Theory and Practice of Public Governance*. Routledge.

O'Toole, L. J. Jr. (2000). Research on policy implementation: Assessment and prospects. *Journal of Public Administration Research and Theory, 10*(2), 263–288. https://doi.org/10.1093/oxfordjournals.jpart.a024270

Partridge, A., Mansilla, C., Randhawa, H., Lavis, J. N., El-Jardali, F., & Sewankambo, N. K. (2020). Lessons learned from descriptions and evaluations of knowledge translation platforms supporting evidence-informed policy-making in low- and middle-income countries: a systematic review. *Health Research Policy and Systems, 18*(1), 127. https://doi.org/10.1186/s12961-020-00626-5

Perrier, L., Mrklas, K., Lavis, J. N. & Straus, S. E. (2011). Interventions encouraging the use of systematic reviews by health policy makers and managers: A systematic review. *Implementation Science, 6*, 43. https://doi.org/10.1186/1748-5908-6-43.

Pestoff, V. (2006). Citizens and co-production of welfare services. *Public Management Review, 8*(4), 503–519. https://doi.org/10.1080/14719030601022882

Pierson, P. (1993). When effect becomes cause: Policy feedback and political change. *World Politics, 45*(4), 595–628. https://doi.org/10.2307/2950710

Pressman, J. L. & Wildavsky, A. B. (1973). *Implementation. How great expectations in Washington are dashed in Oakland*. University of California Press.

Proctor, E., Silmere, H., Raghavan, R., Hovmand, P., Aarons, G., Bunger, A., Griffey, R. & Hensley, M. (2011). Outcomes for implementation research: conceptual distinctions, measurement challenges, and research agenda. *Administration and Policy in Mental Health and Mental Health Services Research, 38*(2), 65–76. https://doi.org/10.1007/s10488-010-0319-7.

Sabatier, P., & Mazmanian, D. (1980). The implementation of public policy: A framework of analysis. *Policy Studies Journal, 8*(4), 538–560. https://doi.org/10.1111/j.1541-0072.1980.tb01266.x

Sabatier, P. A., & Jenkins-Smith, H. C. (1993). The advocacy coalition framework, assessment, revisions, and implications for scholars and practitioners. In P. A. Sabatier, & H. C. Jenkins-Smith (Eds.), *Policy change and learning: An advocacy coalition approach*. Westview Press.

Saetren, H. (2005). Facts and myths about research on public policy implementation: Out-of-fashion, allegedly dead, but still very much alive and relevant. *Policy Studies Journal, 33*(4), 559–582. https://doi.org/10.1111/j.1541-0072.2005.00133.x

Schofield, J. (2001). Time for a revival? Public policy implementation: A review of the literature and an agenda for future research. *International Journal of Management Reviews, 3*(3), 245–263. http://dx.doi.org/10.1111/1468-2370.00066

Schofield, J., & Sausman, C. (2004). Symposium on implementing public policy: Learning from theory and practice: Introduction. *Public Administration, 82*(2), 235–248. http://dx.doi.org/10.1111/j.0033-3298.2004.00392.x

Smith, K., & Larimer, C. (2009). *The public policy theory primer*. Westview Press.

Torfing, J., & Triantafillou, P. (2013). What's in a name? Grasping new public governance as a political-administrative system. *International Review of Public Administration, 18*(2), 9–25. https://doi.org/10.1080/12294659.2013.10805250

Treasury Board of Canada Secretariat. (2007). *Assessing, selecting, and implementing instruments for government action*. Governement of Canada.

Van Meter, D., & Van Horn, C. (1975). The policy implementation process: A conceptual framework. *Administration and Society, 6*, 445–488. https://doi.org/10.1177/009539977500600404

Wilson, M., Lavis, J., & Grimshaw, J. (2012). Supporting the use of research evidence in the Canadian health sector. *Healthcare Quarterly, 15*, 58–62. http://dx.doi.org/10.12927/hcq.2013.23148

GLOSSARY

3I+E framework: Identifies the institutions, interests, ideas and external factors that might influence implementation or act as a facilitator or barrier to it.

7 Ps Framework: A framework offering a clear and simple taxonomy for identifying stakeholders involved within comparative effectiveness research. This framework can be readily applied to implementation efforts. The seven groups of stakeholders include patients and the public, providers, purchasers, payers, policy makers, product makers, and principal investigators

Active implementation: The process by which stakeholders provide feedback when interpreting implementation outcomes to inform ongoing implementation.

Actor: The person or entity at the center of any dissemination effort (e.g., a professional organization, a government agency, a passionate researcher, or a concerned citizen) making deliberate decisions and taking purposeful actions to communicate information about an EBI to target audiences.

Adaptation: The modification of messages for different types of people within a target population to align the message with the characteristics of the recipient. Messages can be adapted in terms of their content, the sources from which they are sent, and the modes through which they are delivered.

Adoption: A measure of the number, proportion, and representativeness of settings and providers who initiate the implementation or delivery of an intervention. Measures of adoption parallel those used to measure reach, but with a focus on settings and/or providers.

Anger: Hostility directed at the person or entity that the individual experiencing psychological reactance perceives as abridging their freedom.

Audit and feedback: A commonly used intervention to provide data about clinical processes (e.g., consistency of measuring and documenting blood pressure) and patient outcomes (e.g., rates of uncontrolled blood pressure and cardiovascular disease) to healthcare professionals.

Barriers and facilitators: The various factors in implementation science influencing implementation, referring to those things that make it harder or easier to get something implemented.

Boomerang effect: The condition by which individuals become more committed to a position, practice, or idea they feel is being threatened. A recent example of psychological reactance and the boomerang effect is the energetic resistance to mask mandates for slowing the spread of COVID-19, most notably in the United States.

Changeability: The ease or difficulty of changing a factor. This criterion is particularly relevant in identifying barriers and facilitators to be addressed through implementation strategies.

Characteristics of individuals: Characteristics influencing implementation such as knowledge, attitudes, and beliefs about the intervention, self-efficacy, or an individual's stage of change and identification with the organization.

Characteristics of the intervention: Characteristics relating to perceptions of the innovation by implementers (e.g., adaptability, complexity, cost, relative advantage, or evidence strength and quality). Perceptions of evidence strength and quality of the innovation may influence willingness to implement or deliver the innovation to patients.

Checklist Assess Organizational Readiness (CARI) for Evidence-Based Implementation: Applicable to the assessment of the domains of system, organization, staff capacities, functional considerations, organizational culture, senior leadership, and the implementation plan. The use of the CARI tool can enable the implementation team to systematically identify areas of concern and workshop potential solutions (e.g., gaining the support of managerial sponsorship).

Client-facing de-implementation strategies: Actions directed at clients, often by practitioners, to discourage use of the low-value practice. These strategies seek to alter recipients' use of the low-value practice. Examples of client-facing de-implementation strategies include shared decision-making, client-directed education, and client cost-sharing.

Context: Factors such as the culture and history of the implementing organization, characteristics of the individuals involved in the implementation effort, leadership, or local policies and regulations, which can affect the success or failure of implementation. Different disciplines use different lenses through which to conceptualize context.

Continuous quality improvement (CQI, or quality improvement [QI]): An implementation strategy used at a local level to test iterative small changes to determine which ones improve targeted process or implementation outcomes. CQI may use qualitative or quantitative data to evaluate the small changes, often testing adaptations of the small changes in iterative cycles.

Core functions: The "active ingredients" of a treatment that make it effective. Sometimes referred to as core components, core processes, or core elements.

Core processes: A set of helpful actions or tools that can provide a systematic way to answer questions raised while exploring potential barriers and facilitators to implementation. Using core processes can make it less likely that important factors will be missed and can help prioritize which ones should be addressed.

Counter-arguing: A mistrust or disbelief in the person or entity perceived as abridging the individual's freedom, and in the message or idea that the individual perceives as threatening their freedom.

Deep adaptations: Adaptations that integrate culture-specific conceptualizations of the target problem (e.g., explanatory models of illness), social norms (e.g., gender roles, family composition), and cultural beliefs (e.g., stigma related to mental illness) into the EBI to enhance cultural sensitivity and facilitate desired outcomes.

De-implementation: A process that involves removing or reducing a routinely used treatment or practice that fails to deliver the expected benefits, and conversely actually increases risks of harm.

Demographic separation approaches to audience segmentation: Approaches that involve dividing an audience into segments based on demographic characteristics. Segmenting demographics could include characteristics such as race/ethnicity, gender, and age, as well as professional role (e.g., frontline clinician or administrative manager), type of organization (e.g., government versus nongovernment), or political ideology, as well as differences in knowledge, attitudes, intentions, and behaviors related to an EBI.

Determinant models: Models that aid in understanding or describing the factors (barriers and facilitators) influencing implementation.

Difference-in-difference (DID): A type of nonrandomized design that extends the simple pre–post design to strengthen internal validity. It is used when there is only one or a few observations before and after implementation, such as when surveys are conducted every year or less frequently. The most common DID design measures changes in key evaluation outcomes before and after implementation in both an implementation group and a comparison group.

Discontinuation and de-adoption: The failure to sustain the EBI or cessation of the EBI over time.

Dissemination: The strategic communication of information about EBIs to audiences who affect the population health impact of these interventions. The communication is strategic because the content of messages, the sources from which they are distributed, and the channels through which they are delivered are intentionally selected to influence specific knowledge, attitudes, intentions, and ultimately behaviors related to the EBI among target audiences.

Dissemination strategies: Strategies that target knowledge, attitudes, and intentions to adopt an EBI and implementation strategies that target the execution of behaviors related to an EBI.

Dynamic Sustainability Framework (DSF): A framework for rethinking the relationships among fidelity, adaptation, effectiveness, and sustainability. The DSF recognizes that it is not realistic to think about sustainability as a static end goal and reframes sustainability amid the dynamic, complex, real-world contexts in which intervention delivery and impact occur over time.

Ecological models: Models that focus on the interdependence of environmental levels and individuals.

Effectiveness: The impact an intervention has when delivered in real-world conditions. Because they are conducted in real-world conditions, studies of intervention effectiveness may yield findings with greater potential for implementation in real-world practice.

Efficacy: The impact an intervention has when tested under controlled conditions that limit the influence that factors other than the intervention may have on outcomes.

Empirical clustering approaches to audience segmentation: Statistical techniques used to identify relationships among multiple variables within a target population. Survey data are typically used to conduct empirical clustering audience segmentation analyses, but administrative data on the practice patterns of a dissemination audience could also be used for such analyses.

Engaged participation: An arrangement in which stakeholders have shared decision-making authority and collaboratively manage the implementation effort. Implementation projects adopting a model of engaged participation with stakeholders often involve concerted efforts for collaboration between the stakeholders and implementers where both groups are actively involved in designing and implementing the project.

Engagement: An iterative process of actively soliciting the knowledge, experience, judgment, and values of individuals selected to represent a broad range of direct interest in a particular issue, for the dual purposes of creating a shared understanding and making relevant, transparent, and effective decisions.

EPIS framework of implementation: A framework providing a conceptual model that maps the implementation process across four distinct phases of implementation: exploration, preparation, implementation, and sustainment. Engaging stakeholders across each phase of implementation can lead to more meaningful and sustained implementation.

Evaluation models: Models that provide guidance about implementation outcomes.

Evidence pyramid: A means of determining the quality of evidence. The evidence pyramid underscores that not all evidence is of the same strength; weaker evidence (e.g., expert opinions, case reports) are placed at the bottom of the pyramid while higher quality evidence (e.g., meta analyses, systematic reviews) placed at the top.

Evidence-based interventions (EBIs): Include programs, practices, principles, procedures, policies, and the use of new products. Evaluation of EBIs might include testing the clinical efficacy of a new vaccine in a controlled setting or evaluating the real-world effectiveness of a clinical procedure.

Expectation management: An arrangement by which practitioners set expectations that any decisions made will be revisited at an agreed upon point in time.

Exploration: A phase of implementation that includes identifying a practice gap or conducting a needs assessment to identify a potential implementation need.

External factors: Factors that fall outside the area of implementation focus but can influence the success or failure of implementation efforts. Some visible examples include pandemics, stock market crashes, elections, environmental disasters, or wars.

Feedback-tailored messages: Communications that provide recipients with information about themselves as it relates to the EBI and their knowledge, attitudes, intentions, or behaviors.

Fidelity: The extent to which an EBI is delivered or executed as designed (e.g., with fidelity). Measure of fidelity may include (a) adherence to intervention or implementation protocols, (b) dose or amount of the intervention delivered, and (c) quality of intervention delivery. Evidence on intervention fidelity may be found in the materials included with a packaged intervention or in reports of intervention studies.

Framing: The selective emphasis of certain aspects of an EBI to influence specific knowledge, attitudes, intentions, and behaviors among a target audience. Framing is similar to the tailoring strategy of adaptation but broader because information can be deliberately framed regardless of whether audience segmentation and message tailoring are conducted.

Grounded interviews: Interviews that use the participant's experience and understanding as the basis for the interview, using probes based on the participant's response and specific prompts to produce information rooted in their experience.

Health Equity Implementation (HEI) framework: Incorporates both an implementation science framework and a healthcare disparities framework and can be useful for ensuring the consideration of health-equity related barriers and facilitators to implementation. A key feature of the HEI framework is its attention to multilevel healthcare disparities factors that influence implementation, and it considers factors negatively impacting vulnerable populations caused by social and historical sidelining.

Heuristics and routines: Decision rules and patterns of behavior enacted in response to specific settings, events, or feelings, which develop over time as the same or similar problems are encountered.

Ideas: The thoughts and norms circulating that relate to an EBI at any given time. These includes the research evidence, technical knowledge, and evaluation findings related to an EBI, in addition to consideration of whether people know about the research and whether they believe it.

Implementation: Purposeful actions taken to put an EBI into practice or into use. Implementation can be viewed as a stage or phase of activity that is preceded by the decision to make use of an EBI (often referred to as adoption) and followed by continued use of an EBI (sometimes referred to as sustainment).

Implementation determinant: Factors determining whether and/or how well an innovation gets implemented. Whether these factors are referred to as barriers and facilitators or determinants, they can be encompassed by the global term *context*.

Implementation mapping (IM): A multi-step process that includes (a) identifying determinants that need to be addressed with a strategy and what change is needed, (b) describing potential mechanisms of change and which implementation strategies could be used, and (c) prioritizing strategies based on team/organizational input or pilot data as well as feasibility. Tools within IM that are particularly helpful include a logic model to illustrate causal relationships (which and how various factors affect outcomes), and a table to organize information from various sources and help in prioritization.

Implementation research: Defined by the U.S. National Institutes of Health as "the scientific study of the use of strategies to adopt and integrate EBIs into clinical and community settings to improve individual outcomes and benefit population health."

Implementation Research Logic Model (IRLM): A model that builds on the traditional logic model by more explicitly linking implementation determinants to strategies, calling out the mechanisms through which they will work and identifying which outcomes (implementation and/or clinical and systems) are targeted.

Implementation science: A multidisciplinary field designed to generate evidence to explain and predict translation of research results and EBIs into practice settings to improve public health and to yield effective methods uncovered through this process.

Implementation strategies: The methods or techniques used by a program or clinical team to support the adoption, integration, and sustainability of an EBI in practice. A team may need to include more than one strategy to successfully address multiple determinants.

Implementation team: The group responsible for identifying and assessing the know-do gap and who are responsible for the day-to-day accountability, implementation, and scale-up of the evidence-based practices identified. The implementation team is typically composed of a small group of individuals who have dedicated time to support the process of implementing evidence-based practices in response to the know-do gap.

Inner setting: A grouping of constructs including structural characteristics, networks and communications, culture, implementation climate, and readiness for implementation. The many aspects of the inner setting reflect the complex array of influences within clinical settings.

Inoculation theory: The theory that individuals can be pre-emptively sensitized to resist arguments intended to manipulate their attitudes (termed counterattitudinal arguments) by alerting individuals to the threat in advance. Inoculation theory has been used successfully in research interventions in a range of settings to counter a range of potentially negative beliefs.

Institutionalization or routinization: The maintenance of organizational practices, procedures, and policies started during implementation or integration into existing organizational routines, policies, or budgets within an institution.

Institutions: Entities (e.g., government structures) currently in place that are connected with an EBI and where decisions related to the EBI or its implementation get made.

Integrated knowledge translation: The process of involving stakeholders (such as decision-makers, clinicians and practitioners, policymakers, patients, and members of the public) throughout the lifecycle of an implementation project.

Integrated Sustainability Framework: An empirically informed framework that identifies multi-level factors that have been commonly associated with sustainability across different settings, contexts, and populations. It can be used as a starting place for identifying and refining understanding of factors that are important to consider within a certain setting.

Interests: The individuals or groups of people who are interested in a particular policy issue. While theoretically everyone in the public has an interest in public policy decisions, people tend to engage personally or professionally only in some policy areas and only on some decisions.

Interrupted time series (ITS): Nonrandomized designs often used in implementation evaluations, which can be used to evaluate policy implementation. ITS considers the same group (people, regions, or other groups) at numerous time points before and after a strategy is introduced.

Intersectionality: Rooted in Black feminist thought and the advocacy work of Black feminists in the 1980s, this concept underscores that an individual's experience is shaped by a combination of individual factors (e.g., gender, age, ability, race/ethnicity, social capital, religion) occurring within connected systems, cultures, and structures of power.

Judging importance: The determination of how likely it is that a particular factor is causally related to implementation.

Know-do gaps: Gaps between what we know that works and what we do in practice, which have in some cases contributed to racial/ethnic, socio-economic, and other disparities in health outcomes.

Knowledge brokers: Individuals whose responsibilities relate to the spread of information about EBIs. Knowledge brokers facilitate, translate, and diffuse knowledge by developing positive relationships between knowledge producers (e.g., researchers) and knowledge users (e.g., clinicians, policymakers) to encourage the use of EBIs.

Knowledge to action cycle: The iterative process of generating and synthesizing evidence to create evidence-based recommendations and then adapting, implementing, and evaluating that evidence to fit the implementation context, stakeholder needs, and implementation challenges. Notably, the first step in the Knowledge to Action implementation cycle is to connect knowledge syntheses (know) to the practice (do) gap.

Knowledge translation (KT): The science and practice of disseminating and implementing evidence into practice. The first step to implementing knowledge is to determine what the evidence says versus what is actually done in practice. This gap between evidence and practice is sometimes referred to as the "know-do" gap.

Logic model: A planning and evaluation tool frequently used to understand what is needed (inputs), what actions should be happening (activities), and how they link to targeted outcomes and longer term impact. Logic models have been used to help design implementation of projects, communicate the planned steps and goals, ensure required resources are available, and determine the methods for measuring progress from start to completion.

Long-term implementation: The continued delivery of an EBI (e.g., the extent to which all components of a program continue to be delivered over time).

Maintenance: The extent to which the implementation and effectiveness of an intervention are sustained or have the potential to be sustained over time.

Monitoring, Evaluation, and Learning (MEL) plan: A tool that improves overall project performance by helping implementation teams identify where they will need to measure the process of implementation, including what is working or being done and what is not.

Non-participation: The informing of stakeholders, rather than engaging them, in the planning or decision-making of implementation efforts.

Normalization process theory (NPT): Explains the social process by which new treatments are implemented, embedded, and fully integrated to ensure that new treatments are routinely used within clinical settings to improve patient outcomes. NPT focuses specifically on what people do within organizations.

Open-ended interviews: Interviews focusing on one subject but open to pursuing lines of inquiry based on what the interview participant sees as important.

Opinion leaders: Individuals who have a substantial interpersonal influence on others in their social network. They are often referred to as "change agents" in the literature. Opinion leaders can help successfully introduce new ideas, depict old ideas in newly positive light, and change the behavior of peers within their social networks.

Packaged intervention: Defined broadly to include any intervention that is disseminated in a format that provides information about the intervention together with additional guidance, protocols, and/or materials to support intervention delivery and implementation.

Partisans: People or institutions invested literally or figuratively in the practice, whether financially, professionally, politically, or personally. In some cases, the investment may be minor and amenable to persuasion, but often there are highly invested partisans and any efforts to de-implement the practice they have invested in can be met with hostility.

Peripheral elements: Elements not essential for an EBI to be effective.

Personalization: The integration of recognizable aspects of message recipients (e.g., their name, professional title, organization) into messages.

Preparation: The process of selecting an EBI to implement, identifying the implementation setting, identifying implementers, identifying consumers, selecting outcomes of interest, and providing input on the implementation plan.

Process: The procedure for implementation, containing four constructs: planning, executing the plan, engaging key individuals, and reflecting and evaluating progress.

Process models: The steps, stages, or phases that characterize the process of translating research into practice generally or implementing EBIs specifically.

Pseudoscience: The adoption of the language of science without the methods, used to persuade, often for the purpose of selling a product.

Psychological reactance: Negative thinking that occurs when an individual feels their freedom or rights are being threatened. Psychological reactance has two distinct components: anger and counter-arguing.

Public policy: Anything a government chooses to do or not to do.

Publication bias: The bias informing publications' decisions on which findings get published and which do not.

Purchasers: Entities responsible for underwriting healthcare costs, such as employers and other agencies in charge of sponsoring healthcare costs.

Quality improvement or implementation science: The framework or model guiding the process of measuring the know-do gap.

Quality indicator: A process or healthcare outcome measure that provides a clear description on the measure of interest and how data should be collected and reported for this measure of interest. The description should include the ideal timing and frequency of data collection (how often, and when the measure of interest should be assessed), population of interest (among whom is the measure of interest being evaluated), method of analysis (how is the measure of interest assessed), and the format of results (how is the measure of interest presented and used).

Randomized controlled trials (RCT): A method by which researchers recruit participants or settings and then randomly assign them to groups that either receive an intervention or not and then determine which group(s) had the best outcomes. RCTs are the gold standard for determining an intervention's efficacy because randomization increases the likelihood that the intervention caused the differences in outcomes rather than other systematic differences between those who did or did not receive the intervention.

Readiness: The tangible and immediate indicators or organizational commitment to a decision to implement, including sub-constructs of leadership engagement, available resources, and access to knowledge and information.

RE-AIM: A framework in implementation science that can be used to assess an EBI's potential for implementation in practice. The intervention must **R**each the intended population, be **E**ffective at improving targeted outcomes, and be **A**dopted, **I**mplemented, and **M**aintained over time.

Regression discontinuity (RD): A nonrandomized design that can be used to evaluate public health programs is the regression discontinuity (RD) design. The RD design can be applied when there is a natural "cutoff score," such as socio-economic status of a community or size of a hospital, that dictates if the group has access to an intervention, program, or implementation strategy.

Replication crisis: A failure to corroborate major findings in subsequent studies. This crisis first came to prominence in the field of psychology when a team of researchers attempted to replicate findings from 100 studies published in three of the top psychology journals.

Shared decision-making: The process by which a practitioner and client have a dialogue in which the practitioner explains different care options (e.g., why they feel the identified low-value practice is inappropriate). Shared decision-making helps practitioners mitigate potential mistrust because the client has a chance to ask questions, share information, and explain their personal priorities.

Social Ecological Model (SEM): A framework that can help illuminate the multiple levels of contextual factors that can influence implementation. Developed by psychologists over 50 years ago and applied commonly in the field of health promotion, the SEM describes the interaction between individual, organizational, community, and societal factors.

Stakeholder analysis: The evaluation of stakeholders from the perspective of an organization, or to determine their relevance to a project or policy. Questions are asked about a stakeholder's position, influence, interest, and networks and how each of those relate to the implementation effort. A stakeholder analysis is an iterative and ongoing process that can be conducted prior to and during the implementation process.

Stakeholders: Commonly, individuals who help inform contextual assessment of constructs and may include individuals at many levels of the organization (clinicians, administrators, and leaders) or community setting, along with potential beneficiaries (e.g., patients) of a newly implemented program. Stakeholders are simply all individuals who influence or are influenced by implementation of a new program.

Substitution: The introduction of an alternative to replace or reduce use of a low-value practice. Most often, substitute practices are introduced among the individuals using the low-value practice or program, as opposed to individuals who do not directly engage with the low-value practice or program.

Surface adaptations: Adaptations made in response to observable social and behavioral characteristics of the population. These may include language translations or customizing metaphors to increase alignment with the target population's culture.

Sustainability: The continuing delivery of a program, clinical intervention, and/or implementation strategy and/or the maintenance of an individual behavior change for a defined period of time. The program or individual behavior may adapt while continuing to produce benefits for systems or individuals.

Sustainment: A process by which stakeholders disseminate implementation findings to larger audiences to garner support for implementation and long-term buy-in from consumers. The goal of most implementation initiatives is to transfer implementation oversight and responsibility to the community.

Symbolic participation: A process by which stakeholders are invited to participate in discussions about implementation plans and have a voice in the decision-making process. Activities involved in symbolic participation include coordination (stakeholders provide feedback that informs implementation decisions but are not involved in designing and carrying out implementation efforts) and cooperation (stakeholders provide help with implementation efforts instead of just providing advice).

Systematic review of the literature: The use of systematic and explicit methods to identify, select, and appraise reports of research studies and then extract and synthesize their findings with the goal of answering a specific research question. Systematic reviews of the literature are disseminated in peer-reviewed journals and on the websites of governmental and nongovernmental organizations.

Tailoring: The manipulation of dissemination materials and messages so that they are aligned with the personal attributes of individual message recipients. A large body of evidence from the fields of health communication and marketing indicate that tailored dissemination materials and messages are more effective than "one-size-fits-all" messages.

Transcreation Framework: A framework promoting evidence building with interventions that are initially tested in community settings and with populations who experience health disparities instead of traditional efficacy trials conducted under constrained circumstances with predominantly White populations.

Treatment adaptation: A process of thoughtful and deliberate alteration to the design or delivery of an intervention, with the goal of improving its fit or effectiveness in a given context. Ideally, this is done in a data-driven and stakeholder-engaged manner. Treatment adaptations typically aim to preserve the core functions of a treatment.

Treatment fidelity: The level at which treatment delivery is consistent with the original EBI protocol or as it was intended by its developers. Treatment fidelity is conceptualized as encompassing the delivery of key elements of a treatment protocol (i.e., adherence) and the skill (i.e., competence) with which the components are delivered.

Treatment modification: A concept encompassing any changes made to interventions, whether deliberately and proactively (adaptation) or in reaction to unanticipated challenges that arise in a given session or context.

Trial period: A period in which a provider proposes a temporary suspension of the low-value practice (e.g., medication) or delaying the low-value practice (e.g., low-value test). This strategy also occurs during a client–practitioner dialogue and entails active listening but focuses on the low-value practice instead of selecting from the array of potential alternatives.

Unlearning: The systematic effort to recognize and change an established heuristic or routine. In the context of de-implementation, we speak of unlearning specifically as it applies to altering heuristics and/or routines that sustain low-value practices or programs.

INDEX

Printed in the United States
by Baker & Taylor Publisher Services

Printed in the United States
by Baker & Taylor Publisher Services